Updates in Surgery

SOCIETÀ ITALIANA DI CHIRURGIA • FONDATA A ROMA NEL 1882 •

Angelo Di Giorgio • Enrico Pinto
Editors

Treatment of Peritoneal Surface Malignancies

State of the Art and Perspectives

In collaboration with
Paolo Sammartino
Franco Roviello

Foreword by
Giorgio De Toma

Springer

Editors
Angelo Di Giorgio
Department of Surgery "Pietro Valdoni"
Sapienza University of Rome
Rome, Italy

Enrico Pinto
Department of Medical, Surgical,
and Neurological Sciences
University of Siena
Siena, Italy

In collaboration with
Paolo Sammartino and Franco Roviello

The publication and the distribution of this volume have been supported by the Italian Society of Surgery

ISSN 2280-9848
ISBN 978-88-470-5882-8 ISBN 978-88-470-5711-1 (eBook)

DOI 10.1007/978-88-470-5711-1

Springer Milan Dordrecht Heidelberg London New York

Cover design: eStudio Calamar S.L.
Typesetting: Graphostudio, Milan, Italy

Springer-Verlag Italia S.r.l. – Via Decembrio 28 – I-20137 Milan
Springer is a part of Springer Science+Business Media (www.springer.com)

Foreword

On the basis of the latest epidemiological data, peritoneal surface malignancies (PSM) represent a pathology characterized by a high annual incidence, between those of stomach and colorectal cancer.
The integration of cytoreduction surgery (CRS) and hyperthermic intraperitoneal chemotherapy (HIPEC), variously combined with other adjuvant and neoadjuvant chemotherapeutic regimens, is an example of the increasingly complex care strategy for PSM.

There is a strong rationale behind combining CRS with HIPEC to create a procedure based on the evolutionary history of PSM, once considered to be caused only by locally advanced malignancies of the abdominal cavity free of distant metastases. Over the past 20 years, the consistency of results of this integrated procedure has led to it now being considered the treatment of choice for carcinomatosis from pseudomyxoma peritonei, mesothelioma and, recently, the colon, with low peritoneal spread. Furthermore, the trend in using this procedure is increasingly being applied to treat gastric and ovarian carcinomatosis and rarer forms of peritoneal diseases, such as peritoneal metastases from breast and pancreatic cancer and sarcomatosis.

Experience to date using this treatment modality has identified the most significant prognostic parameters and the most important risk factors associated with the procedure. This monograph is thus based on contributions from some of the major Italian centers devoted to treating PSM. It provides the most significant updates on diagnosis, treatment, and outcomes obtained so far. The text thoroughly summarizes the state of the art on CRS plus HIPEC and identifies future development perspectives on related research.

Rome, September 2014

Giorgio De Toma
President, Italian Society of Surgery

Preface

A variety of tumors originating from intra- or extra-abdominal viscera and, more rarely, from the peritoneal membrane, spread or metastasize to the visceral and parietal peritoneum. The term peritoneal surface malignancy (PSM) encompasses all these forms and thus identifies a heterogeneous family of primary or metastatic tumors with epithelial or mesenchymal origin. The inclusion of various forms of primary and secondary PSM under a unique definition is justified by the substantial uniformity of their clinical evolution within the abdominal and pelvic cavity, leading to production of tumor implants and ascites until fatal obstruction occurs. Prognosis is poor, and palliative therapy has long represented the only treatment option. In the natural history of PSM, evolution can be slow and metastatic development late, so that many forms represent ideal targets for aggressive locoregional therapies.

In the 1980s, Paul Sugarbaker theorized – following countless pharmacokinetic and pharmacodynamic studies – about advantages of the association between maximal surgical cytoreduction [peritonectomy (PRT)], aimed at removing all visible implants, and hyperthermic intraperitoneal chemotherapy (HIPEC), aimed at treating microscopic or millimetric residues. Since the 1990s, this concept has gradually gained acceptance and currently is the intervention of choice for pseudomyxoma peritonei and mesothelioma, but it is also diffusely used to treat carcinomatosis from colorectal, gastric, and ovarian cancer and peritoneal sarcomatosis. For the most common forms of PSM treated with PRT plus HIPEC, experiences available to date consistently show overall results better than or highly competitive with traditional treatment modalities. PSM forms that until two decades ago were considered untreatable surgically and for which progression was fatal within months of diagnosis, today, after appropriate patient selection, are routinely treated with PRT plus HIPEC, resulting in improved patient quality of life and long-term survival rates. The combined procedure achieves acceptable postoperative morbidity and mortality rates in relation to its complexity and duration (median 10 h) similar to those of major abdominal and pelvic surgery.

However, the procedure has limited application considering the high overall incidence of various forms of PSM and is not exempt from criticism. The limited diffusion of PRT plus HIPEC treatment is related to the long learning curve; availability of relevant human, technical, and economic resources; and skepticism toward its effectiveness, particularly in reference to HIPEC, which is considered potentially risky during the postoperative course. Furthermore, the main criticisms concern the lack of prospective randomized phase III studies to define clearly the role of HIPEC, given that the validity of maximum cytoreduction is accepted worldwide. Indeed, to date, overall results of prospective trials for HIPEC are scarce and heavily criticized for the general treatment approach, lack of homogeneity of surgical techniques, and wide dispersion of enrolled cases. Therefore, results regarding overall significance of this procedure come mainly from multi-institutional studies, reviews, meta-analyses, and studies conducted in single centres with a high volume of PRT plus HIPEC activity. While taking into account the limitations inherent in such studies, the magnitude of experience gained to date reveals the overall trend of results. The great effort made by surgeons, oncologists, and specialized centers dedicated to treating PSM using PRT plus HIPEC has brought about the possibility of successfully treating aggressive locoregional tumors such as PSMs. It now remains for the inevitable upcoming prospective studies to confirm the promising results obtained thus far with this combined treatment modality and to determine the most appropriate ways to address treatment for PSM.

The purpose of this monograph is to provide a summary of the knowledge base supporting the rationale of associating maximum cytoreduction with HIPEC, pathological assessment and diagnostic workup of patients with PSM, surgical and HIPEC techniques, and management results of the most common forms of PSM. In the world that revolves around PSM management, Italy plays a significant role, as demonstrated by case series treated by the various PSM centers in this country and the vast scientific contribution drawn from the literature and from acts of the major international conventions. Collaboration between many of the most important specialized Italian surgeons and treatment centers has helped provide an overall picture that illustrates the state of the art regarding PSM management. The topics discussed, and the opinions, experiences, and conclusions expressed by the various authors of these chapters, provide an in-depth summary of experiences pertaining to the most critical issues and outline goals to be achieved in the coming years through collective and coordinated efforts.

Rome, September 2014

Angelo Di Giorgio
Enrico Pinto

Contents

Acknowledgments

The volume editors and the publisher gratefully acknowledge the educational contribution offered by Medica S.p.A.

Special thanks to:
Dr. Vittorio Fornasari for the drawings of Chapter 9 and Bernardo Luraschi for the drawings of Chapters 10 and 24;
Section of Iconography of Department of Surgery "Pietro Valdoni", Sapienza University of Rome for technical assistance.

Contributors

Fabio Accarpio Department of Surgery "Pietro Valdoni", Sapienza University of Rome, Rome, Italy

Luca Ansaloni Department of General and Emergency Surgery, "Papa Giovanni XXIII" Hospital, Bergamo, Italy

Joseph Mahler Fouad Atta Department of Surgery "Pietro Valdoni", Sapienza University of Rome, Rome, Italy

Dario Baratti Department of Surgery, National Cancer Institute, Milan, Italy

Daniele Biacchi Department of Surgery "Pietro Valdoni", Sapienza University of Rome, Rome, Italy

Serena Bonomi General Surgery Unit, Bentivoglio Hospital, Bentivoglio (BO), Italy

Antonello D. Cabras Department of Pathology and Laboratory Medicine, National Cancer Institute, Milan, Italy

Maurizio Cardi Department of Surgery "Pietro Valdoni", Sapienza University of Rome, Rome, Italy

Stefano Caruso Department of Medical, Surgical and Neurological Sciences, General and Oncologic Surgery Unit, University of Siena, Siena, Italy

Fausto Catena Department of General Surgery, Parma University Hospital, Parma, Italy

Davide Cavaliere Department of Surgery and Advanced Oncologic Therapies, "G.B. Morgagni – L. Pierantoni" Hospital, Forlì, Italy

Costanza Cavallini Department of Radiology, Oncology, and Human Pathology, Sapienza University of Rome, Rome, Italy

Antonio Ciardi Department of Radiology, Oncology, and Human Pathology, Sapienza University of Rome, Rome, Italy

Maria Ciolina Department of Radiology, Oncology, and Human Pathology, Sapienza University of Rome, Rome, Italy

Tommaso Cioppa Doctoral School of Genetics, Oncology, and Clinical Medicine (GenOMec), University of Siena, Italy

Federico Coccolini Department of General and Emergency Surgery, "Papa Giovanni XXIII" Hospital, Bergamo, Italy

Tommaso Cornali Department of Surgery "Pietro Valdoni", Sapienza University of Rome, Rome, Italy

Giovanni Corso Department of Experimental Oncology, European Institute of Oncology, Milan, Italy

Enrico Cortesi Department of Radiology, Oncology, and Human Pathology, Oncology Unit, Sapienza University of Rome, Rome, Italy

Barbara Costantini Department of Gynecology and Obstetrics, Division of Gynecologic Oncology, Catholic University of Sacred Heart, Rome, Italy

Eugenio Cucinotta Department of Human Pathology, University of Messina, Messina, Italy

Pierandrea De Iaco Department of Oncologic Gynecology, "S. Orsola - Malpighi" University Hospital, Bologna, Italy

Giovanni de Manzoni Department of Surgery, Upper G.I. Surgery Unit, Borgo Trento Hospital, Verona, Italy

Marcello Deraco Department of Surgery, National Cancer Institute, Milan, Italy

Michele De Simone Oncology Surgery Unit, Candiolo Cancer Institute, Candiolo (TO), Italy

Angelo Di Giorgio Department of Surgery "Pietro Valdoni", Sapienza University of Rome, Rome, Italy

Giorgio Ercolani Department of General Surgery, "Sant'Orsola-Malpighi" University Hospital, Bologna, Italy

Anna Fagotti Department of Gynecology and Obstetrics, Division of Gynecologic Oncology, Catholic University of Sacred Heart, Rome, Italy

Giammaria Fiorentini Department of Oncology and Hematology, "Ospedali Riuniti Marche Nord" Hospital, Pesaro, Italy

Francesco Fleres Department of Human Pathology, University of Messina, Messina, Italy

Maria Luisa Framarino dei Malatesta Department of Surgery "Pietro Valdoni", Sapienza University of Rome, Rome, Italy

Franco Iafrate Department of Radiology, Oncology, and Human Pathology, Sapienza University of Rome, Rome, Italy

Simone Giacopuzzi Department of Surgery, Upper G.I. Surgery Unit, Borgo Trento Hospital, Verona, Italy

Sara Giovannoni Department of Radiology, Oncology, and Human Pathology, Oncology Unit, Sapienza University of Rome, Rome, Italy

Antonio Grassi General Surgery Unit, Bentivoglio Hospital, Bentivoglio (BO), Italy

Francesca Guerini Department of Surgery, Upper G.I. Surgery Unit, Borgo Trento Hospital, Verona, Italy

Alessio Impagnatiello Department of Surgery "Pietro Valdoni", Sapienza University of Rome, Rome, Italy

Domenico Rosario Iusco General Surgery Unit, Bentivoglio Hospital, Bentivoglio (BO), Italy

Shigeki Kusamura Department of Surgery, National Cancer Institute, Milan, Italy

Andrea Laghi Department of Radiology, Oncology, and Human Pathology, Sapienza University of Rome, Rome, Italy

Marco Lotti Department of General and Emergency Surgery, "Papa Giovanni XXIII" Hospital, Bergamo, Italy

Antonio Macrì Department of Human Pathology, University of Messina, Messina, Italy

Daniele Marrelli Department of Surgery "Pietro Valdoni", Sapienza University of Rome, Rome, Italy

Alfredo Mellano Oncology Surgery Unit, Candiolo Cancer Institute, Candiolo (TO), Italy

Valentina Mingarelli Department of Surgery "Pietro Valdoni", Sapienza University of Rome, Rome, Italy

Giulia Montori Department of General and Emergency Surgery, "Papa Giovanni XXIII" Hospital, Bergamo, Italy

Enzo Naticchioni Department of Surgery "Pietro Valdoni", Sapienza University of Rome, Rome, Italy

Antonio Daniele Pinna Department of General Surgery, "Sant'Orsola-Malpighi" University Hospital, Bologna, Italy

Enrico Pinto Department of Medical, Surgical, and Neurological Sciences, University of Siena, Siena, Italy

Emanuela Risi Department of Radiology, Oncology, and Human Pathology, Oncology Unit, Sapienza University of Rome, Rome, Italy

Manuela Robella Oncology Surgery Unit, Candiolo Cancer Institute, Candiolo (TO), Italy

Carlo Riccardo Rossi Melanoma and Sarcoma Unit, Veneto Institute of Oncology IOV, Padua; Department of Surgery, Oncology, and Gastroenterology, University of Padua, Padua, Italy

Franco Roviello Department of Medical, Surgical, and Neurological Sciences, General and Oncologic Surgery Unit, University of Siena, Siena, Italy

Edoardo Saladino Department of Human Pathology, University of Messina, Messina, Italy

Paolo Sammartino Department of Surgery "Pietro Valdoni", Sapienza University of Rome, Rome, Italy

Giovanni Scambia Department of Gynecology and Obstetrics, Division of Gynecologic Oncology, Catholic University of Sacred Heart, Rome, Italy

Simone Sibio Department of Surgery "Pietro Valdoni", Sapienza University of Rome, Rome, Italy

Bianca Maria Sollazzo Department of Surgery "Pietro Valdoni", Sapienza University of Rome, Rome, Italy

Antonio Sommariva Melanoma and Sarcoma Unit, Veneto Institute of Oncology IOV, Padua, Italy

Paul H. Sugarbaker Center for Gastrointestinal Malignancies, Washington Cancer Institute, Washington, DC, USA

Patrizia Trenta Department of Radiology, Oncology, and Human Pathology, Oncology Unit, Sapienza University of Rome, Rome, Italy

Marco Vaira Oncology Surgery Unit, Candiolo Cancer Institute, Candiolo (TO), Italy

Carlo Vallicelli Department of Surgery and Advanced Oncologic Therapies, "G.B. Morgagni – L. Pierantoni" Hospital, Forlì, Italy

Giorgio Maria Verdicchia Department of Surgery and Advanced Oncologic Therapies, "G.B. Morgagni – L. Pierantoni" Hospital, Forlì, Italy

Salvatore Virzì General Surgery Unit, Bentivoglio Hospital, Bentivoglio (BO), Italy

Nadia Zaffaroni Department of Experimental Oncology and Molecular Medicine, Molecular Pharmacology Unit, National Cancer Institute, Milan, Italy

Andrea Zanoni Department of Surgery, Upper G.I. Surgery Unit, Borgo Trento Hospital, Verona, Italy

Part I

Background

Peritoneal Surface Malignancies

1

Angelo Di Giorgio

1.1 Definition

The term Peritoneal Surface Malignancies (PSMs) identifies a wide range of epithelial or mesenchymal neoplasms that originate from the primitive structure of the peritoneum or spread over and through the peritoneum membrane as metastases deriving from tumors of intra-abdominal, retroperitoneal, or extra-abdominal organs or viscera (Table 1.1). PSM evolution depends on the degree of aggressiveness of the various neoplastic forms: in contrast with benign or low malignant forms, aggressive forms are able to produce fast and fatal disease progression. The primitive forms are much rarer than secondary forms, and mesotheliomas and serous tumors of the peritoneum are the most common among them. Colorectal, gastric, and ovarian peritoneal carcinomatosis (PC) are the most frequent forms of PSM arising from intraperitoneal viscera. PSMs originating from retroperitoneal tumors, such as the pancreas, kidneys, or adrenals, are rare and even less frequent are those originating from extra-abdominal tumors, such as breast or lung cancer. Epithelial forms are far more frequent than mesenchymal forms. Primary tumors of the peritoneum and carcinomatosis from gynecological or gastrointestinal tumors are overall the most widespread and common PSMs treated in surgery and oncology. Irrespective of histological differences, most PSMs have a common tendency to grow for a relatively long period of time exclusively in the abdominal cavity, thus representing an ideal target for aggressive locoregional treatments.

A. Di Giorgio (✉)
Department of Surgery "Pietro Valdoni", Sapienza University of Rome,
Rome, Italy
e-mail: angelo.digiorgio@uniroma1.it

A. Di Giorgio, E. Pinto (Eds), *Treatment of Peritoneal Surface Malignancies*,
Updates in Surgery
DOI: 10.1007/978-88-470-5711-1_1, © Springer-Verlag Italia 2015

Table 1.1 Peritoneal surface malignancies

	Malignant	Borderline/low grade
Primary	DMPM (Diffuse Malignant Peritoneal Mesothelioma)	WDPM (Well-differentiated Papillary Mesothelioma); MPM (Multicystic Peritoneal Mesothelioma)
	PPSPC (Primary Peritoneal Serous Papillary Carcinoma)	
	DSRCT (Desmoplastic Small Round Cell Tumor)	
Secondary	***Intra-abdominal origin***	
	Colorectal cancer	
	Gastric cancer	
	Ovarian cancer	Ovarian cancer
	PMCA (Peritoneal Mucinous Adenocarcinoma): pseudomyxoma peritonei from mucinous adenocarcinoma of appendix	DPAM (Diffuse Peritoneal Adenomucinosis): pseudomyxoma peritonei from low-grade mucinous tumors of appendix
	Adenocarcinoid of appendix	
	Small-bowel adenocarcinoma	
	GIST (Gastrointestinal Stromal Tumor)	
	Retroperitoneal origin	
	Pancreatic cancer	
	Kidney, ureter, adrenal, bladder cancer	
	Sarcomas	
	Extra-abdominal origin	
	Breast cancer	
	Lung cancer	

Epidemiology: Extent of the Problem

2

Simone Sibio, Joseph Maher Fouad Atta, Alessio Impagnatiello, Bianca Maria Sollazzo, and Daniele Marrelli

2.1 Introduction

Peritoneal carcinomatosis (PC) most commonly represents local or regional evolution of an abdominal carcinoma. Sometimes it can be synchronous with the primary tumor (primary carcinomatosis) but more often is present as recurrent disease (metachronous or secondary) after first-line treatment of the originating tumor. Patients with tumors from colon, ovary, and stomach cancer are more likely to present with PC during their clinical course. Less frequently, other abdominal malignancies, such as uterus, pancreas, small bowel, biliary, or urinary tract, can involve the peritoneum. Tumors originating from the peritoneum itself are definitely rarer: mesothelioma, pseudomyxoma peritonei (PMP), primitive peritoneal carcinoma, and desmoplastic small-round-cell tumor. PC from extra-abdominal tumors, such as lung, breast, melanoma, or peritoneal sarcomatosis, is exceptional, and few epidemiological data are available on them. Statistical analysis of worldwide cancer incidence, prevalence, and mortality rate is available on GLOBOCAN 2012 [1]. In Italy, most epidemiological data are available in the reports from the Italian Association of Tumor Registries (AIRTUM) [2], which collects data regarding incidence, prevalence, and mortality rates from all local and regional tumor registries, covering at least 34% of total population. This data is considered a high-quality regional coverage by and international ranking system (GLOBOCAN 2012 rate B). An overview of available data suggests a global general consideration: mortality related to cancer in general decreased from 75% of global incidence of cancers in 1970 to 47% in 2010 despite a global increased incidence of 25%

S. Sibio (✉)
Department of Surgery "Pietro Valdoni", Sapienza University of Rome, Rome, Italy
e-mail: simone.sibio@uniroma1.it

A. Di Giorgio, E. Pinto (Eds), *Treatment of Peritoneal Surface Malignancies*, Updates in Surgery
DOI: 10.1007/978-88-470-5711-1_2, © Springer-Verlag Italia 2015

in the same 40-year period in Western countries; these data appear related to the strong impact on survival of new treatment strategies and drugs and concur with observations for PC. In Italy 30,000–40,000 new cases of PC from various primary tumors are expected every year. Table 2.1 shows the incidence of PC (primary or secondary) in Italy in 2012 by age [Italian National Institute of Statistics (ISTAT)]. Mortality rate for PC as first cause of death (Table 2.2) or as one of multiple causes of death (Table 2.3) are reported for the previous 6 years in Italy; data are extracted from hospital discharge records by ISTAT and include primary and secondary tumors.

Table 2.1 Incidence of primary (ICD-9-CM 1588–1589) or secondary (ICD-9-CM 1976) peritoneal carcinomatosis in Italy by age

Year 2012						
Description	Age					
	0–44	45–54	55–64	65–74	75+	Total
Malignant neoplasm of peritoneum or retroperitoneum (primary)	133	264	518	665	732	2,312
Malignant neoplasm of peritoneum or retroperitoneum (secondary)	2,862	6,028	10,364	13,605	11,753	44,612

ICD-9-CM International Classification of Diseases, 9th Revision – Clinical Modification

Table 2.2 Mortality for peritoneal carcinomatosis (PC) in Italy (first cause)

ICD-10	Years					
	2006	2007	2008	2009	2010	2011
C48.0	270	222	286	261	257	230
C48.1	15	14	11	17	14	9
C48.2	159	155	198	182	124	125
C48.8	1					
C78.6	272	288	233	276	302	316
Total	717	679	728	736	697	680

ICD-10 International Classification of Diseases, 10th Revision

2.2 Peritoneal Carcinomatosis from Colorectal Cancer

Globally, colorectal cancer (CRC) is the third most common cancer and ranks as the fourth most common cancer-related cause of mortality [1]: it is the third most common cancer in men [746,000 (10 %) cases] and the second most com-

Table 2.3 Mortality for peritoneal carcinomatosis (PC) in Italy (multiple causes)

ICD-10	Years					
	2006	2007	2008	2009	2010	2011
C48.0	297	257	312	289	282	251
C48.1	17	17	15	19	19	11
C48.2	253	252	251	302	210	170
C48.8	1					1
C78.6	8,219	8,648	8,557	9,060	9,505	9,626
Total	8,787	9,174	9,235	9,670	10,016	10,059

ICD-10 International Classification of Diseases, 10th Revision
C48 Malignant neoplasm of peritoneum or retroperitoneum (primary)
C48.1 specified site
C48.2 unspecified site
C48.8 overlapping sites
C78.6 malignant neoplasm of peritoneum or retroperitoneum (secondary)

mon in women [614,000 (9.2%) cases]. Almost 55 % of cases occur in more developed regions. There is wide geographical variation in incidence across the world, and geographical patterns are very similar in men and women: incidence rates vary tenfold in both sexes worldwide, the highest estimated rates being in Australia/New Zealand and the lowest in western Africa (4.5 and 3.8 per 100,000, respectively). Mortality rate is lower [694,000 (8.5 %) deaths] but with more deaths (52 %) in the less developed regions of the world, reflecting a poorer survival in these regions. There is less variability in mortality rates worldwide (sixfold in men, fourfold in women), with the highest estimated mortality rates in both sexes in central and eastern Europe (20.3 per 100,000 for men; 11.7 per 100,000 for women) and the lowest in western Africa (3.5 and 3.0, respectively) [1].

In United States, the incidence of CRC is about 149.000 new cases per year, with a related mortality rate reaching 30 % [3]. A major component of treatment failure is cancer dissemination within the peritoneal cavity appearing as local recurrence of primary tumor or peritoneal metastases, which is estimated to account for 40 % of all patients with CRC [4].

Thomassen et al. [5] studied the incidence of synchronous PC in patients affected by CRC; data were extracted from the Eindhoven Cancer Registry over a period of 15 years; results are reported in Fig. 2.1. In Italy, CRC has an incidence of 38,000–41,000 new cases per year, with a 33 % mortality rate (13,000 deaths per year). Among these patients, about 15 % (6,000 per year) present with primary PC, whereas 35 % of all mortality (4,600 per year) is related to peritoneal recurrence alone, or 11 % of all patients with CRC [2]. Table 2.4 summarizes the more significant experiences in the literature regarding PC incidence and local recurrence from CRC in different series of patients [6–17].

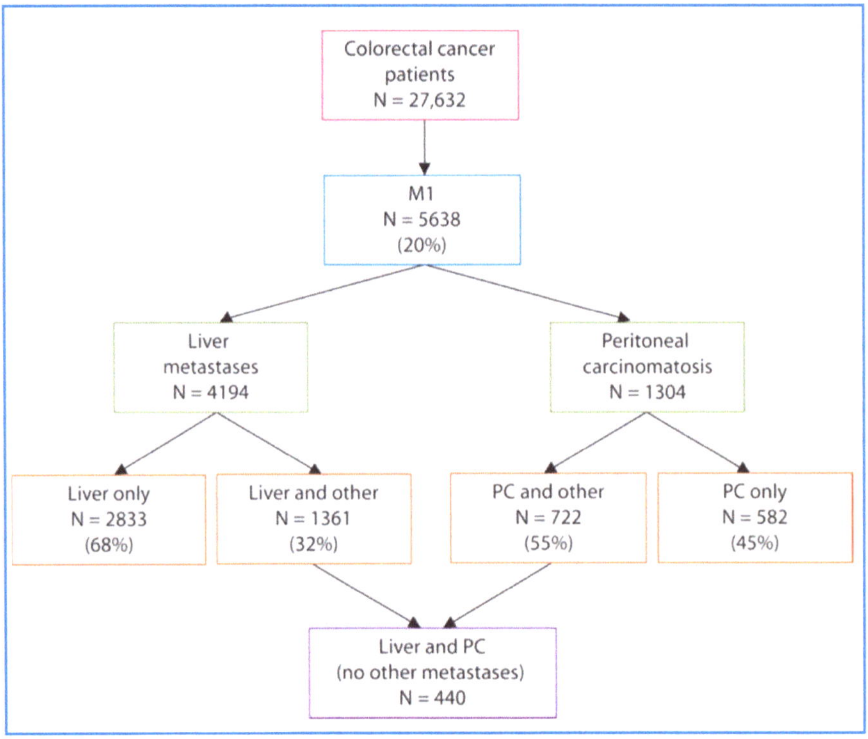

Fig. 2.1 Incidence of synchronous peritoneal carcinomatosis (PC) in patients with colorectal cancer (CRC) in a large, population-based study from Eindhoven Cancer Registry [5]

Table 2.4 Incidence of local recurrence and peritoneal carcinomatosis (PC) from colorectal cancers reported in the literature

Study [Reference]	No. patients	Local recurrence (%)	PC (%)
	Clinical series		
Malcolm et al. [9]	285	3.9	13
Cass et al. [6]	280	23	28
Russell et al. [13]	94	7	12
Mendenhall et al. [10]	140	29	3
Olson et al. [12]	281	9	-
Minsky et al. [11]	294	9	4
Gilbert et al. [8]	31	36	3
Jayne et al. [17]	2,756	-4.9	
	Reoperation series		
Gunderson et al. [14]	91	48	21
Tong et al. [15]	64	48	44
	Autopsy series		
Russell et al. [16]	53	38	36
Gilbert [8]	45	-	40

2.3 Peritoneal Carcinomatosis from Gastric Cancer

Although the incidence of gastric cancer (GC) has decreased in recent years, it is still the fourth most common newly diagnosed cancer worldwide and the second leading cause of cancer-related death [5]. There are major differences in the incidence of GC across countries and continents. Global incidence, as well as primary tumor location and histological type, are constantly changing. In the US and most of western Europe, there has been a marked decline in distal intestinal GC, whereas the incidence of proximal and Barrett's adenocarcinoma of the gastric cardia and esophageal–gastric junction has been increasing. The incidence of diffuse adenocarcinoma, on the other hand, is largely unchanged. Adenocarcinoma of the body of the stomach and antrum predominates in developing countries, among African Americans, and in lower socioeconomic groups, whereas proximal tumors are more common in developed countries, among Caucasians, and in higher socioeconomic classes [18]. Nevertheless, GC is common throughout Europe. In 2000, there were 192,000 new diagnoses, with 158,000 deaths [19].

In Italy, the incidence accounts for 17,000 new patients per year, with higher mortality rates [10,900 (60 %) per year] [1, 2]. Outcome remains poor despite advances in therapy, and an overall 5-year survival rate of about 20% compares very unfavorably with that of 70% achieved in Japan [19]. Peritoneal dissemination is the most frequent pattern of metastasis from GC and commonly occurs via intracoelomic dissemination or tumor spillage during surgery [20]. PC is present at diagnosis in 5–20 % of patients and can affect 60 % after curative treatment [21, 22]. Despite radical surgery and extended lymphadenectomy, 20–50 % of patients will develop peritoneal recurrence during their follow-up. Serosal involvement, Lauren diffuse histotype, and positive peritoneal cytology are the most important risk factors for peritoneal recurrence after radical surgery [23]. Multicenter studies indicate a decrease in locoregional recurrence and an increase in peritoneal recurrence of GC in recent years, with approximately one third having total recurrences after curative surgery [24]. Although there are few data available from cancer registries, PC form GC in Italy is likely to reach 3,500–4,000 cases per year, with a very high mortality rate [3,100 (30 %) of all deaths per year].

2.4 Peritoneal Carcinomatosis from Ovarian Cancer

Epithelial ovarian cancer (EOC) affects > 200,000 women and causes 125,000 deaths annually worldwide [25]. In the USA, the incidence is ~ 22,000 cases per year and is the fifth most common cause of cancer death (15,500). In Italy, there are 4,400 new cases every year, and there is a global mortality rate of 67.7 %. Worldwide, only 40–47 % of patients with EOC can be expected to survive > 5 years. Lifetime risk for OC is one in 70, but some women have a much higher risk, especially those with germ-line mutations of *BRCA1* and *BRCA2* tumor suppressor genes [26]. The incidence is low before menopause, but after this, the incidence rises progressively. Median age at diagnosis is 63 years worldwide [1, 27]. More than 70 % of EOC patients present with peritoneal spread at first diagnosis (82 % in Italy), and > 80 % of deaths are due to PC. Family history is the strongest risk factor for hereditary OC.

Three clinical manifestations of hereditary OC are recognized: site-specific OC, breast and OC syndrome, and the hereditary nonpolyposis CRC (HNP-CC; Lynch II) syndrome. The first two groups are associated with germ-line mutations in the *BRCA1* and *BRCA2* tumor suppressor genes, whereas HNP-CC is associated with germ-line mutations in the DNA mismatch repair (*MMR*) genes, primarily *hMLH1* and *hMSH2*. At least 10 % of all epithelial OC is hereditary, with mutations in the *BRCA* genes accounting for ~ 90 % of cases and most of the remaining 10 % being attributable to HNP-CC [26]. There are no certain risk factors for sporadic EOC, although a study by Peterson et al. of 581 US patients found lower socioeconomic status, estimated by neighborhood socioeconomic status, is associated with OC tumor characteristics indicative of more advanced and aggressive disease; however, reasons for this remain unclear [28]. Interestingly, another study by Bristow et al. demonstrated that prognosis in EOC is highly dependent from epidemiological variables, such as socioeconomic status, and access to high-volume care centers: high-volume physician and annual hospital case volumes are associated with improved OC survival, although access to high-volume care centers is yet limited [29].

2.5 Peritoneal Mesothelioma

Data on descriptive epidemiology of diffuse malignant peritoneal mesothelioma (MPM) are available from many national registries, such as EUROCIM [30], the US Surveillance, Epidemiology, and End Results Cancer Registry (SEER) [27], and in Italy, AIRTUM [2]; diagnostic criteria have changed widely over recent years, which complicates adequate description of epidemiological data. Age-standardized incidence rates range from 0.5 to ~ 3 cases per million worldwide, with 2,500 new cases per year. However, higher rates are reported in smaller areas with widespread past use of asbestos, such as the harbor of Genoa, where the incidence rate is 5.5 per million [31]. In Italy, incidence varies from 0.1 to 6.4 per million, with 1,000 expected new cases per year [2]. Peritoneal mesothelioma must be considered an increasing public health problem because its incidence has been rising worldwide since 1970; an increasing in mortality rate of 5–10 % is expected until 2020 [32]. Mesothelioma is three times more common in men than in women, and incidence increases with age, being tenfold higher in 60–64-year-old individuals than in 30–40-year-olds. Asbestos is the main known cause of the disease, but other risk factors are likely to be involved in its etiology and pathogenesis, such as radiation, viruses, or genetics [31]. SEER median survival data is 10 months, and relative 5-year survival is 16 %. Survival is positively influenced by female gender (related to asbestos exposure), younger age at diagnosis, and epithelioid histology [33].

2.6 Pseudomyxoma Peritonei

In 1884, Werth [34] introduced the term pseudomyxoma peritonei, literally translated as an untrue mucinous tumor of the peritoneum. PMP is a very rare disease, with an incidence of one to two per million per year worldwide; it is characterized by disseminated intraperitoneal mucous and mucinous implants on peritoneal surfaces and omentum and in the subdiaphragmatic space. Global overall 10-year survival is ~ 70 %.

PMP is thought to be associated with appendiceal mucinous neoplasms (AMN). Because ovarian involvement is seen in the majority of female patients, an ovarian primary has long been suggested as the cause of PMP. However, results of several clinical, histopathological, immunohistochemical, and molecular genetic studies strongly suggest that in patient with PMP, ovarian tumor deposits are almost always metastases of an appendiceal primary, although other origins have been described as well [35]. It has also been reported rarely in association with mucinous carcinomas of other organs, such as gallbladder and bile ducts, stomach, pancreas, colon, Fallopian tube, uterine corpus, urachus, urinary bladder, breast, and lung. Although PMP may on rare occasions arise from benign mucinous tumors, it is most commonly associated with well-differentiated malignant tumors or those of borderline malignancy.PMP occurs in approximately two of every 10,000 laparotomies and is more common in women; 75 % of patients are women, with an average age of 53 years [34].

A large population-based study in The Netherlands considered > 167,000 appendectomies performed in that nation in a 10-year period and found 1,482 of them presenting appendiceal neoplastic lesions (nine per 1 million) (Table 2.5), which is higher than worldwide general incidence, with a three- to eight-fold incidence in women compared with men [36]. PMP can be synchronous with the appendiceal lesion (77 %) or metachronous; median evolution time from an appendiceal neoplasm to PMP is ~ 2 years but can be > 10 years.

2.7 Other Secondary Peritoneal Carcinomatosis

Occasionally, every solid tumor originating in the peritoneal cavity can involve the peritoneal surface, such as urinary tract, pancreas, biliary tract, and uterus. Among them, pancreatic carcinoma represents the most frequent histotype. In a large population-based study, Thomassen et al. found 265 (9 %) of 2,924 patients

Table 2.5 Incidence and gender distribution of appendiceal lesions and pseudomyxoma peritonei (PMP) in 167,744 appendectomies in The Netherlands (by age)

Lesion type	Appendiceal		PMP	
	M/F	Ratio	M/F	ratio
Mucocele	186/269	1:1.4	3/8	1:2.7
Mucinous neoplasms	203/371	1:1.8	31/83	1:2.7
Adenoma	153/268	1:1.7	18/52	1:2.9
Adenocarcinoma	50/103	1:2.1	13/31	1:2.4
Nonmucinous neoplasms	219/234	1:1.1	2/11	1:6.0
Adenoma	112/130	1:1.2	1/8	1:8.0
Adenocarcinoma	107/104	1:1.0	1/3	1:3.0
Total	608/874	1:1.4	36/102	1:2.8

M/F, male/female

affected by pancreatic cancer presenting with synchronous PC and observed an increasing trend in patients treated with chemotherapy in more recent years (11 % in 1995–1999 and 22 % in 2005–2009) [37]. PC from extra-abdominal tumors is very rare, and most current literature is based on case reports; among them, breast and lung cancer represent the most frequent tumors associated with PC. In a large study of 1,628 patients with breast cancer, Tuthill et al. identified 44 patients (2.7 %) with PC who had a very poor prognosis (1.57 months) in the UK [38]. Another study of PC from lung cancer in an autopsy series showed a global incidence ranging from 2.7 % to 16 %, together with other sites of metastasis [39].

References

1. WHO GLOBOCAN 2012– Section of cancer information www.iarc.fr
2. Airtum Working Group (2001) La sopravvivenza dei pazienti oncologici in Italia. Epidemiologia e Prevenzione 35:5-6
3. Weir HK1, Thun MJ, Hankey BF et al (2003) Annual report to the nation on the status of cancer, 1975-2000, featuring the uses of surveillance data for cancer prevention and control. J Natl Cancer Inst 95:1276-1299
4. Koppe MJ1, Boerman OC, Oyen WJ, Bleichrodt RP (2006) Peritoneal carcinomatosis of colorectal origin: incidence and current treatment strategies. Ann Surg 243:212-222
5. Thomassen I, van Gestel YR, Lemmens VE, de Hingh IH (2013) Incidence, prognosis, and treatment options for patients with synchronous peritoneal carcinomatosis and liver metastases from colorectal origin. Dis Colon Rectum 56:1373-1380
6. Cass AW, Million RR, Pfaff WW (1976) Patterns of recurrence following surgery alone for adenocarcinoma of the colon and rectum. Cancer 37:2861–2865
7. Eisenberg B, Decosse JJ, Harford F et al (1982) Carcinoma of the colon and rectum: the natural history reviewed in 1704 patients. Cancer 49:1131–1134
8. Gilbert JM, Jeffrey I, Evans M et al (1984) Sites of recurrent tumour after 'curative' colorectal surgery: implications for adjuvant therapy. Br J Surg 71:203–205

9. Malcolm AW, Perencevich NP, Olson RM et al (1981) Analysis of recurrence patterns following curative resection for carcinoma of the colon and rectum. Surg Gynecol Obstet 152:131–136
10. Mendenhall WM, Million RR, Pfaff WW (1983) Patterns of recurrence in adenocarcinoma of the rectum and rectosigmoid treated with surgery alone: implications in treatment planning with adjuvant radiation therapy. Int J Radiat Oncol Biol Phys 9:977–985
11. Minsky BD, Mies C, Recht A et al (1988) Resectable adenocarcinoma of the rectosigmoid and rectum: I. Patterns of failure and survival. Cancer 61:1408 –1416
12. Olson RM, Perencevich NP, Malcolm AW et al (1980) Patterns of recurrence following curative resection of adenocarcinoma of the colon and rectum. Cancer 45:2969 –2974
13. Russell AH, Tong D, Dawson LE et al (1984) Adenocarcinoma of the proximal colon: sites of initial dissemination and patterns of recurrence following surgery alone. Cancer 53:360 –367
14. Gunderson LL, Sosin H, Levitt S. (1985) Extrapelvic colon areas of failure in a reoperation series: implications for adjuvant therapy. Int J Radiat Oncol Biol Phys 11:731–741
15. Tong D, Russell AH, Dawson LE et al (1983) Second laparotomy for proximal colon cancer: sites of recurrence and implications for adjuvant therapy. Am J Surg 145:382–386
16. Russell AH, Pelton J, Reheis CE et al (1985) Adenocarcinoma of the colon: an autopsy study with implications for new therapeutic strategies. Cancer 56:1446 –1451
17. Jayne DG, Fook S, Loi C et al (2002) Peritoneal carcinomatosis from colorectal cancer. Br J Surg 89:1545–1550
18. Goéré D, Gras-Chaput N, Aupérin A, Flament C (2014) Treatment of gastric peritoneal carcinomatosis by combining complete surgical resection of lesions and intraperitoneal immunotherapy using catumaxomab. BMC Cancer 14:148
19. Nissan A, Garofalo A, Esquivel J (2010) Cytoreductive surgery and hyperthermic intra-peritoneal chemotherapy (HIPEC) for gastric adenocarcinoma: why haven't we reached the promised land? J Surg Oncol 102:359-360
20. European Union Network of Excellence (EUNE) for Gastric Cancer Steering Group (2008) astric cancer in Europe. Br J Surg 95:406-408
21. Hioki M, Gotohda N, Konishi M et al (2010) Predictive factors improving survival after gastrectomy in gastric cancer patients with peritoneal carcinomatosis. World J Surg 34:555-562
22. Gunderson LL, Sosin H (1982) Adenocarcinoma of the stomach: areas of failure in a re-operation series (second or symptomatic look) clinicopathologic correlation and implications for adjuvant therapy. Int J Radiat Oncol Biol Phys 8:1-11
23. Roviello F, Marrelli D, de Manzoni G et al (2003) Prospective study of peritoneal recurrence after curative surgery for gastric cancer. Br J Surg 90:1113-1139
24. Marrelli D et al; Italian Research Group for Gastric Cancer (2011) Changing clinical and pathological features of gastric cancer over time. Br J Surg 98:1273-1283
25. Parkin DM, Bray F, Ferlay J, Pisani P (2005) Global cancer statistics, 2002. CA Cancer J Clin 55:74 108
26. Prat J, Ribé A, Gallardo A (2005) Hereditary ovarian cancer. Hum Pathol 36:861-870
27. Surveillance, Epidemiology and End Results (SEER) program. SEER stat Database: Incidence – SEER 9 Regs Public Use. Nov 2003, National Cancer Institute, DCCPS, Surveillance Research Program, Cancer Statistics Branch, April 2004 (http://www.seer.cancer.gov)
28. Peterson CE, Rauscher GH, Johnson TP et al (2014) The association between neighborhood socio-economic status and ovarian cancer tumor characteristics. Cancer Causes Control 25:633-637
29. Bristow RE, Chang J, Ziogas A et al (2014) High-volume ovarian cancer care: Survival impact and disparities in access for advanced-stage disease. Gynecol Oncol 132:403-410
30. European Network of Cancer Registries. Eurocim version 4.0. European incidence database V2.3, C15 Dictionary (2001). Lyon, France: IARC 2001
31. Boffetta P (2007) Epidemiology of peritoneal mesothelioma: a review. Ann Oncol 18:985-990
32. Peto J, Hodgson JT, Matthews FE, Jones JR (1995) Continuing increase in mesothelioma mortality in Britain. Lancet 345:535-539
33. Mirabelli D, Roberti S, Gangemi M et al (2009) Survival of peritoneal malignant mesothelioma in Italy: a population-based study. Int J Cancer 124:194-200

34. Smeenk RM, van Velthuysen ML, Verwaal VJ, Zoetmulder FA (2008) Appendiceal neoplasms and pseudomyxoma peritonei: a population-based study. Eur J Surg Oncol 34:196–201
35. Andréasson H1, Graf W, Nygren P et al (2012) Outcome differences between debulking surgery and cytoreductive surgery in patients with Pseudomyxoma peritonei. Eur J Surg Oncol 38:962-968
36. Sherer DM1, Abulafia O, Eliakim R (2001) Pseudomyxoma peritonei: a review of current literature. Gynecol Obstet Invest 51:73-80
37. Thomassen I, Lemmens VE, Nienhuijs SW et al (2013) Incidence, prognosis, and possible treatment strategies of peritoneal carcinomatosis of pancreatic origin: a population-based study. Pancreas 42:72-75
38. Tuthill M, Pell R, Giuliani R et al (2009) Peritoneal disease in breast cancer: a specific entity with an extremely poor prognosis. Eur J Cancer 45:2146
39. Sereno M, Rodríguez-Esteban I, Gómez-Raposo et al (2013) Lung cancer and peritoneal carcinomatosis. Oncol Lett 6:705-708

Mechanism of Intraperitoneal Spread of Free Cancer Cells

3

Giovanni Corso, Daniele Marrelli, and Franco Roviello

3.1 Introduction

Peritoneal carcinomatosis (PC) from cancer cell dissemination from a primary tumor is considered a local cancer rather than systemic spread. Multiple primary cancers are responsible of peritoneal metastasis (PM). Patients affected by primary epithelial tumors plus PM can benefit from an aggressive surgical approach, such as the cytoreductive surgery (CRS), combined with hyperthermic intraperitoneal chemotherapy (HIPEC), which can result in long-term survival rates in selected patients [1]. Targeted indications are important for the success of these treatments. Patient selection is performed routinely depending on clinical parameters, preoperative tumor staging, and intraoperative findings. However, the origin mechanism of PM underlying specific biological aspects; in fact, some targeted molecules are responsible of tumor spread and peritoneal cancer cells adhesion. These molecular biomarkers are introduced in clinical practice to identify patients eligible for targeted therapies.

This chapter specifically focuses on describing cellular pathogenesis in PM to evaluate its potential role in clinical application.

3.2 Pathophysiology

In PM, three independent mechanisms are responsible for cancer-cell implantation in the peritoneum:

- The primary pathway is dissemination of free cancer cells from a primary

G. Corso (✉)
Department of Experimental Oncology, European Institute of Oncology, Milan, Italy
e-mail: giovanni.corso@ieo.it

A. Di Giorgio, E. Pinto (Eds), *Treatment of Peritoneal Surface Malignancies*, Updates in Surgery
DOI: 10.1007/978-88-470-5711-1_3, © Springer-Verlag Italia 2015

tumor, with exfoliation and direct peritoneal invasion [2]. Free cancer cells cleave to the peritoneal surface via adhesion molecules [3];
- The second mechanism is dissemination of tumor cells through lymphatic or venous vessels within the peritoneal cavity [2];
- The third mechanism is surgical manipulation or trauma [2].

Neoplastic redistribution is a PC that originates from transparietal spread in individuals with low-grade tumors. This diffusion is associated with a nonrandom mechanism of metastasization due to gravity on biological fluids (i.e., ascites). This redistribution plays a preponderant role on the effect of viscosity. Free cancer cells float into the peritoneal space forming cell aggregation in spotted areas as a consequence of gravity and concentration in places of peritoneal fluid absorption. Reabsorption of peritoneal fluids takes place at the omentum and diaphragmatic peritoneum. The most frequently affected locations are pelvis, subphrenic areas, parietocolic grooves, and the Morrison's pouch [3]. In the absence of tumor fluid production, cancer cell motility is limited, implanting close to the primary site. Distant areas are affected when the fluid carrier is presents, such as at the Treitz ligament and the lesser omentum; in the absence of fluid carriers, these sites are unaffected.

In general, in the early stage, the mesenteric surfaces and serosa of the small intestine are spared; the presence of peristaltic motility inhibits cancer cell adhesion. Conversely, fixed areas, such as the duodenum, ileocecal, and rectosigmoid passages, are frequently involved by PM. The association of multiple factors, such as peristalsis, gravity, fluid reabsorption, tumor histotype, and biological features, defined this pattern of peritoneal invasion known as neoplastic redistribution [4].

3.3 Molecular and Cellular Pathology

The pathophysiology of cancer spread, specifically peritoneal dissemination, comprises different stages: (1) detachment of cancer cells from the primary cancer; (2) migration to distant sites, and (3) colonization and adaption in a new microenvironment—in this case, the peritoneum [5]. PM pathophysiology is depicted in Fig. 3.1.

3.3.1 Loss of Cell Adhesion and Increased Motility

After detachment from the primary cancer, free tumor cells show reduced adhesion and increased motility to the peritoneum. In this phase, inactivation of cell–cell adhesion molecules (CAMs) plays a pivotal role in changing the cytoskeletal structure [6]. The CAM group comprises integrins, cadherins, selectins, and some members of the immunoglobulin family. Moreover, among

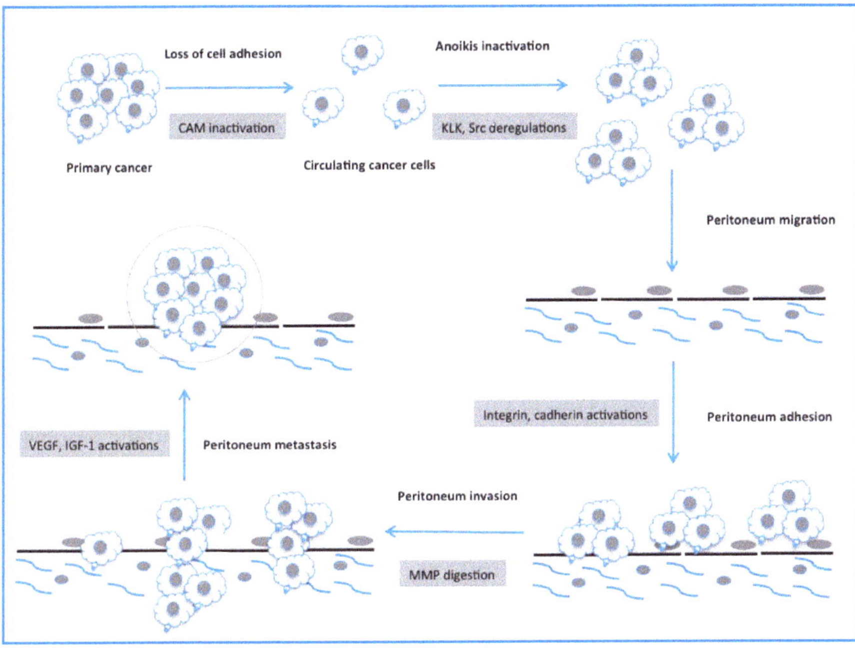

Fig. 3.1 Cellular pathology of peritoneal invasion and colonization and molecular pathways

the mitogen-activated protein kinase (MAPK) cascade, epidermal growth factor receptor (EGFR) and c-MET oncogenes are considered and important pathway in cancer cell spread [7].

3.3.2 Anoikis Resistance

Anoikis is the term that designates the response of nontumor cells to loss of cell-matrix contact due to specific apoptosis programming; metastatic cancer cells are unable to anoikis. This factor causes their survival after detachment from the primary tumor and their spread through vessels to other organs. Anoikis evasion is, in fact, the preliminary step and thus a targeted study for the diffusion of free cancer cells. Interestingly enough, anoikis restoration using targeted therapies is a novel approach in modern medicine, called personalized medicine, for treating patients affected by metastatic cancer [8].

Kallikrein-related peptidase (KLK) and V-Src sarcoma viral oncogene homolog (Src) are involved in the homeostasis of anoikis, and deregulation is responsible of PM.

3.3.3 Migration and Adhesion to the Peritoneum

In this phase, free cancer cells have an increased pathogenic motility. They adhere to the peritoneal surface, where they colonize and invade it. Pivotal molecules—integrin and cadherin proteins—guarantee adhesion between the extracellular matrix (ECM) and tumor cells.

3.3.4 Peritoneal Invasion

For peritoneal invasion, the disruption of ECM by proteolytic enzymes is necessary; cancer cells directly secrete these enzymes. Matrix metallopeptidase (MMP) is a protein involved in this process facilitating cancer cell invasion by ECM digestion [9]. At that stage, cancer cells are able to attach to the basement membrane.

3.3.5 Peritoneal Colonization

Free cancer cells need to survive after detachment from the primary tumor and so produce growth factors and receptors. Peritoneal colonization is associated with stimulation by cancer cells of tumor-associated stroma to produce several growth factors. This phenomenon is called homing; the homing of cancer cells to the peritoneum represents a multistep process that involves malignant progression of the primary tumor, tumor invasion through the ECM, and settling of tumor cells in the peritoneum. In the homing phase, insulin-like growth factor 1 (IGF-1) and vascular endothelial growth factor (VEGF) and their related receptors play a preponderant role [10].

3.4 Conclusions and Remarks

PC remains a clinical entity with and aggressive pattern and unfavorable prognosis, which is evidence of terminal progression in abdominal cavity disease. CRS plus HIPEC represent an aggressive approach to PM treatment that demonstrates favorable perspectives in long-term survival [1]. Targeted genes are involved in the different PM phases, as abovementioned. It is thus reasonable that targeted therapies can be considered in response to cancer cell behavior [10].

Identifying predictive molecular biomarkers at HIPEC is the modern gold standard in the area of cancer research; there are several candidate biomarkers that predict response to antiblastic drugs, but their role in clinical practice is still under investigation, and there is as yet no specific protocol. However, rapid changes in medicine promise novel treatments with targeted therapies for personalized medicine to improve diagnosis, treatment, and care of patients affected by PC.

References

1. Roviello F, Caruso S, Marrelli D et al (2011) Treatment of peritoneal carcinomatosis with cytoreductive surgery and hyperthermic intraperitoneal chemotherapy: state of the art and future developments. Surg Oncol 20:e38-54
2. Stewart JH 4th, Shen P, Levine EA (2005) Intraperitoneal hyperthermic chemotherapy for peritoneal surface malignancy: current status and future directions. Ann Surg Oncol 12:765-777
3. Sugarbaker PH (1996) Observations concerning cancer spread within the peritonealavity and concepts supporting an ordered pathophysiology, Peritoneal carcinomatosis: principles and management. Kluwer Academic Publishers, Boston, pp. 79-100
4. Yonemura Y, Nojima N, Kawamura T (eds) (1998) Principles of the treatment of peritoneal carcinomatosis. Peritoneal Dissemination. Molecular Mechanisms and the Latest Therapy. Maeda Shoten, Kanazawa
5. Nguyen DX, Bos PD, Massagué J (2009) Metastasis: from dissemination to organ-specific colonization. Nat Rev Cancer 9:274-284
6. Yilmaz M, Christofori G (2009) EMT, the cytoskeleton, and cancer cell invasion. Cancer Metastasis Rev 28:15-33
7. Paschos KA, Canovas D, Bird NC (2009) The role of cell adhesion molecules in the progression of colorectal cancer and the development of liver metastasis. Cell Signal 21:665-674
8. Schempp CM, von Schwarzenberg K, Schreiner L et al (2014) V-ATPase inhibition regulates anoikis resistance and metastasis of cancer cells. Mol Cancer Ther in press 2014. doi: 10.1158/1535-7163.MCT-13-0484
9. Hanahan D, Weinberg RA (2011) Hallmarks of cancer: the next generation. Cell 144:646-674
10. de Cuba EM, Kwakman R, van Egmond M et al (2012) Understanding molecular mechanisms in peritoneal dissemination of colorectal cancer: future possibilities for personalised treatment by use of biomarkers. Virchows Arch 461:231-243

Pathology of Peritoneal Surface Malignancies

4

Antonio Ciardi and Angelo Di Giorgio

4.1 Introduction

4.1.1 Role of Pathology in Diagnosis and Staging of Peritoneal Surface Malignancy

The role of the pathologist in a team dealing with patients affected by PSM is crucial. The steps of this work are not merely diagnostic; in fact, before diagnosis is achieved, the pathologist must collect a great deal of information necessary for analyzing the individual case to enable the surgeon to interpret correctly the macroscopic pattern presented by the patient. The majority of patients undergoing surgical procedures for PSM have already been given systemic chemotherapy, and the pathological pattern at the time of the surgical intervention is affected by the grade of therapeutic response. In cases in which lesions are not obvious, it is important to detect and analyze all areas of minimal alteration, both in the serosal surface and in deeper locations (as in visceral specimens such as large- and small-bowel tracts, uterus and adnexa, bladder, gall bladder, and other such areas). It is even more important to apply this protocol in cases in which superficial macroscopic lesions have virtually disappeared. For correct staging, it must be determined with as much certainty as possible that no microscopic residue remains.

For visceral specimens, after accurate exploration of the serosal surface, maximal attention must be given to identifying all suspect deposits in the perivisceral subserosal adipose tissue and all mucosal abnormalities, which may be an indication of a full-thickness, inverse (*ab extrinseco*) infiltration of the vis-

A. Ciardi (✉)
Department of Radiology, Oncology, and Human Pathology, Sapienza University of Rome, Rome, Italy
e-mail: antonio.ciardi@uniroma1.it

A. Di Giorgio, E. Pinto (Eds), *Treatment of Peritoneal Surface Malignancies*, Updates in Surgery
DOI: 10.1007/978-88-470-5711-1_4, © Springer-Verlag Italia 2015

ceral wall. Once again, tissue sampling must be extensive in order detect the true extent of visceral-wall involvement.

Besides analysis of lymph node stations removed from specific sites, a thorough search for other lymph nodes, especially in gastrointestinal (GI) segments, is necessary to exclude metastatic seeding. Other specimens—for example, the round ligament—require systematic sectioning due to the possible presence of very tiny deposits of neoplastic tissue.

The pathologist's actions as a protocol can be summarized in the following steps:

- Detailed macroscopic analysis of all specimens, with particular attention to minimal alterations;
- Thorough examination to detect minimal microscopic neoplastic residues;
- Accurate examination of all visceral tracts removed by the surgeon to identify any area of potential neoplastic infiltration ab extrinseco of the visceral wall;
- Systematic search for perivisceral lymph nodes;

All these actions allow the pathologist to make a final pathological report that:

- Describes the exact nature of the lesion as to histologic type and grading;
- Measures the extent of lesions in all specimens and offers important information regarding staging and prognostic evaluation, such as depth of visceral wall involvement and presence of metastatic seeding in visceral lymph nodes.

The pathologist investigating PSM may be involved in different diagnostic settings. A histocytological diagnosis may follow a laparoscopy/laparotomy procedure performed after an imaging evaluation showing widespread involvement of the peritoneal cavity, curative surgical resection for malignancy elsewhere that during the surgical procedure demonstrates unexpected deposits in the peritoneal serosa, and recurrence of a previously excised tumor. Peritoneal lavage should be performed using a percutaneous closed technique or at the time of laparoscopy or laparotomy. The sensitivity of peritoneal lavage cytology results depends on the ability to completely lavage all regions of the peritoneal cavity and detect cancer cells being shed into the peritoneal cavity by the tumor.

Whether the pathologist is actively involved in a team at a specialized institution treating PSM or discovers the disease incidentally, to obtain an accurate histopathological diagnosis, the main goal is to obtain an adequate amount of tissue in terms of quantity and quality. An inadequate specimen of nonneoplastic tissue may be removed at laparoscopy when the surgeon fails to involve the pathologist in choosing the specimen. Also, tissue size is of utmost importance, as in the majority of cases, multiple immunohistochemical stainings are necessary to clarify the origin of the lesion, particularly when the tumor is microscopically poorly differentiated. Accurate pathological diagnosis is highly important for the oncologist inasmuch as the choice of effective chemotherapy relies on it.

Following curative resection of surgical specimens, searching for the possible presence of microscopic tumor foci revealing previously unsuspected peritoneal diffusion should always be performed. This is particularly true for the omentum in the setting of primary gastrointestinal (GI) or ovarian (OC)/gynecological cancer.

If a correct diagnosis is established preoperatively, different amounts of tissue for pathological examination may be required after cytoreductive surgery (CRS). The surgeon may remove entire organs or part of them, small or wide segments of the peritoneum from different regions, variably sized peritoneal implants, several different lymph node stations, etc. All specimens should be appropriately fixed to allow correct macroscopic and histological examination.

Macroscopic or microscopic tumor foci should be identified, especially in cases in which macroscopic findings are not clearly defined; hence, a careful search for tiny nodules or areas with subtle modifications is essential. If these are not identified, an exhaustive sampling is mandatory to confirm the persistence of or certify the absence of pathology, which is necessary for accurate patient staging.

4.2 Ovarian Carcinomatosis

The histological spectrum of lesions observed in peritoneal carcinomatosis (PC) from OC overlaps that of epithelial tumors of the ovary. Worldwide accepted classification of all ovarian tumors relies on categories referring to the cell/tissue of origin, as follows:

- Epithelial ovarian tumors
- Germ cell tumors
- Sex-cord/stromal tumors
- Borderline epithelial tumors (subdivided in serous, mucinous, and endometrioid)
- Metastatic tumors

Epithelial tumors are by far the most common, accounting for 85–90 % of all OC. The well-characterized subtypes are defined depending on frequency, as follows:

- Serous
- Endometrioid
- Mucinous
- Undifferentiated
- Clear cell
- Brenner type

This classification is based on the classic theory that epithelial tumors originate from the surface epithelium of the ovary, deriving from the embryonic coelom, which differentiate into subtypes via several metaplastic changes that give rise to the typical serous, endometrioid, and mucinous patterns, which resemble fallopian tubal epithelium, endometrium, and cervical mucosa.

The histological hallmark of serous tumors is the predominant presence of tiny papillae with the classic poor or absent stroma and variable grade of cellular lining atypia. The mucinous tumoral area classically comprises mucus-secreting columnar cells, with tubule/tubulopapillary pattern and abundant extracellular mucus. There are two types: classic and intestinal.

Endometrioid tumors are characterized by neoplastic tissue that reproduces the morphology of normal and neoplastic endometrium. Moreover, they are frequently associated with synchronous uterine and ovarian endometrioid tumors. To date, in the tumor/node/metastasis (TNM) classification of the Union Internationale Contre le Cancer (UICC), grading these tumors comprises well-, moderately, and poorly differentiated tumors. However, for serous tumors only, a two-tier grading system has been proposed that divides them in two categories: low-grade serous carcinoma [with no significant atypia and < 12 mitoses per 10 high power field (HPF)], and high-grade serous carcinoma (with significant atypia and > 12 mitoses per 10 HPF).

Since the late 1990s, increasing evidence has challenged the conventional view regarding the origin and development of such tumors [1]. Based on morphologic and molecular genetic evidence, Kurman and Shih [2, 3] proposed a model that groups epithelial OC into two categories: type I and type II. Type I comprises low-grade serous, low-grade endometrioid, mucinous, and clear-cell carcinoma. Type II comprises high-grade tumors of serous or endometrioid pattern, undifferentiated carcinoma, and malignant mixed mesodermal tumors (carcinosarcoma). These two groups differ with regard to clinical behavior, with type I mostly being indolent and confined to the ovary, whereas type II are aggressive and present at an advanced stage. In addition, both groups show different genetic aberrations: Type I tumors are associated with mutations in *KRAS*, *BRAF, PTEN*, *PIK3A*, *CTNNB1*, *ARID1A*, and *PPP2R1A* genes [2, 4–6] that result, via perturbed signalling pathways, in morphologic changes that reflect progression from benign through varying degrees of atypia, to noninvasive and invasive carcinoma. Type II (high-grade tumors) harbor numerous chromosomal aberrations, the most frequent being in *TP53* and *BRCA1/2* genes.

Several studies performed on women at high risk [7, 8] and confirmed subsequently in women with high-grade serous cancers who were not at high risk [9] described the concomitant presence of occult noninvasive and invasive carcinoma of the fallopian tube. These morphological observations prompted some investigators to propose, since 2003 [10], that occult tubal carcinomas may shed malignant cells that then implant and grow on the ovarian surface, simulating primary OC. The occurrence of serous tubal intraepithelial carcinoma (STIC) (Fig. 4.1) is only described in association with high-grade serous carcinoma. STIC are characterized by high nuclear-to-cytoplasmic ratio, pleomorphism, hyperchromasia, lack of ciliated cells, loss of polarity with or without epithelial stratification, and occasional mitotic figures. Nuclei are rounded and enlarged, sometimes with prominent nucleoli. In addition, > 90 % of STIC harbor *TP53* mutation and stain strongly and diffusely with p53, the so-called p53 signature. Strong immunohistochemical staining for p53 is indirect evidence of missense mutation, whereas nonsense mutations correlate with negative staining. Moreover, a high (up to 38 %) Ki-67 labeling index is typical of STIC, a 10 % value being considered the threshold.

Possible explanations for the role of STIC in the development of high-grade serous OC are:

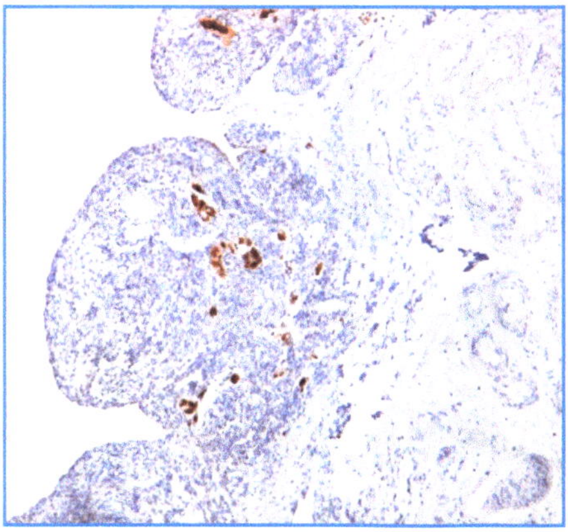

Fig. 4.1 p53-positive staining of small aggregates of neoplastic cells in the fimbria (IHC-P, × 50)

- STIC are detected in > 50 % of all cases of sporadic, high-grade serous pelvic carcinoma and in 10–15 % of fallopian tubes after prophylactic removal from women with germ-line BRCA mutations. In the latter cases, STIC morphologically resembles high-grade serous OC, with no similar lesions found in the ovary;
- Laser-capture microdissection studies showed that 92 % of STIC have TP53 mutations, which are identical to those discovered in concordant OC;
- STIC frequently upregulate oncogene products, such as cyclin E1, Rsf-1, and fatty acid synthase, which are overexpressed in high-grade serous carcinomas;
- The presence of STIC in prophylactic salpingectomy specimens in the absence of carcinoma is among the most important pieces of evidence that argue against the view that STIC represent lateral extension or metastasis from the adjacent high-grade serous carcinoma;
- STIC associated with high-grade serous OC have shortened telomeres compared with those of OC [11]. Shortened telomeres are some of the earliest molecular changes in carcinogenesis; they cause chromosomal instability, a cardinal feature of high-grade pelvic serous carcinomas. A gene-expression study demonstrated that expression profiles of high-grade serous OC more closely resemble fallopian-tube epithelium than ovarian serous epithelium [12].

4.2.1 Pathology

What the pathologist receives after a CRS procedure is a complex puzzle of specimens of different origin. One of them is the peritoneal layer removed because of gross disease. Peritoneal specimens are sampled from the subdiaphragmatic region, left and right abdominal wall, pelvic and prevesical region, and Morrison's pouch. Specimens have different shapes, being quadrangular, triangular, or very irregular with several projections and infoldings. The affected peritoneum usually shows punctiform hemorrhages and is slightly thickened by edema or fibrosis of the subperitoneal connective tissue.

Whitish or pale gray nodules can be observed on the serosal surface, measuring from very tiny spots up to several centimeters in maximum dimension (Fig. 4.2a, b); on the cut section, they are seen to extend deep into the subperitoneal connective tissue or fat (Fig. 4.2c). Macroscopic foci of necrosis are often

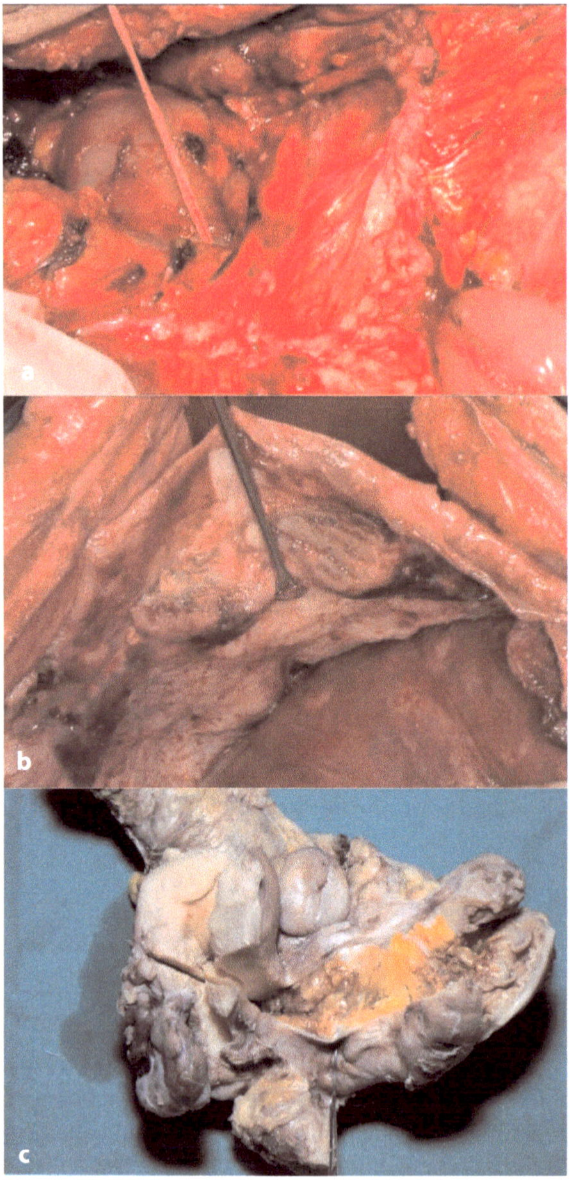

Fig. 4.2a–c **a** Small superficial nodules of the lesser omentum. **b** Plaque-like neoplastic growth in the subdiaphragmatic region. **c** Superficial deposit and deep infiltrating neoplastic tissue in the pouch of Douglas

present in the larger nodules of several centimeters in diameter. Microscopically, nests or sheets of cells growing in a solid pattern, with pleomorphic nuclei and occasionally conspicuous nucleoli are observed. Alternatively, tumor cells may form a papillary growth or microcysts.

In the smaller peritoneal tumor deposits, only tiny papillae or cell aggregates, surrounded by desmoplastic fibrous tissue, are seen. Nodules can have an outgrowth on the peritoneal surface (Fig. 4.3a) or appear in the thickness of the peritoneal sample growing toward the subperitoneal fat tissue (Fig. 4.3b) Often they are multiple and very small (Fig. 4.4a) or are an incidental finding in an apparently noninvolved area of the peritoneum (Fig. 4.4b).

In a minority of cases with very good response to chemotherapy, histology demonstrates subperitoneal foci of desmoplastic tissue with psammoma bodies, with no evidence, or a barely visible aggregate, of malignant cells after a thorough search in multiple samples. In these cases, the psammoma bodies are the distinctive hallmark of the previous solid or papillary neoplastic growth in the subperitoneal tissue (Fig. 4.5).

The omentum (Fig. 4.6a) is always part of surgical resection, and its macroscopic aspect can vary from that of an omental cake to an intermediate multi- and macronodular involvement, to that of very small nodules or irregular thickening in the omental tissue. Omental cake and multimacronodular involvement are associated with massive neoplastic microscopic infiltrates, resulting in diffuse replacement of the omental adipose tissue by whitish, solid, homogenously granular neoplastic tissue. Problems can arise in the macroscopically "normal" omentum, in which an exhaustive sampling must be performed to avoid a misleading diagnosis of absence of neoplastic tissue.

The round ligament (Fig. 4.6b) is also usually sampled and may present superficial nodules or an even surface; however, often on serial sectioning, small nodules can be observed in the subperitoneal fat or in fibrous cord residue of the umbilical vessel. Microscopically, solid or papillary tumor deposits with infiltrating edges are seen within adipose tissue or the fibrous cord.

Several specimens labelled as implant(s) are also received. These can be very small fragments, of irregular shape and with variable texture and color; or they may measure a few centimeters in maximum dimension. They are sampled from the visceral peritoneum (small-bowel tracts, gastric wall, left or right colic angles, large-bowel tracts, liver capsule, lesser omentum, Morrison's pouch). Histologically, all ranges of tumors involvement are possible—from massive infiltration to absence of neoplastic tissue. Small- and large-bowel implants often show tumoral deposits in the subserosa or in the muscle layer, whereas the submucosa and mucosa are frequently involved. Liver-capsule implants are usually exophytic, with no involvement of the underlying liver parenchyma, as the liver capsule can behave as a barrier to liver tissue.

Segments of small and large bowel are often sent for pathological examination and may present multiple micronodules on the serosa or in the subserosa (Fig. 4.7a, b). These can be very small and easily confused with nonneoplastic

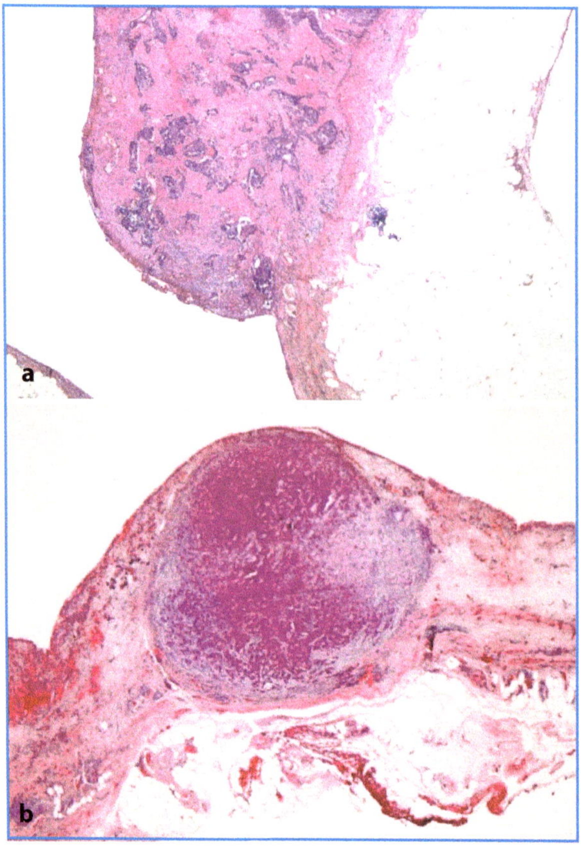

Fig. 4.3a, b **a** Exophytic nodule on the peritoneal surface (H&E, × 12.5). **b** Nodule growing in the thickness of the peritoneal subserosal tissue (periodic acid-Schiff–diastase × 12.5)

fibrous thickening of the subserosal fat; consequently, for this reason, any suspicious whitish gray lesion should be sampled. In the more advanced cases, infiltrating lesions appear as a visible ulcerated thickening of the bowel wall, with deeper growths involving the muscular layer (Fig. 4.7c) and possibly submucosa and mucosa (Fig. 4.8a–c). Perivisceral lymph nodes may be enlarged as the result of metastatic growth. They are not necessarily adjacent or close to neoplastic lesions. The finding of lymph node "metastasis" in these specimens is not because of direct invasion, which prompts the idea that after neoplastic nodule establishment in the pericolic adipose tissue, there is diffusion via lymphatic vessels that mimics diffusion of the advanced primary in the intestinal mucosa. The fact that neoplastic cells shed from pericolic nodules and travel in the lymphatic network along the viscera could be a possible cause of recurrence. In a study conducted at our institution [13] on a cohort of patients who underwent CRS plus HIPEC for primary advanced or recurrent OC, we encountered two interesting findings: First, the depth of colorectal wall invasion is an independ-

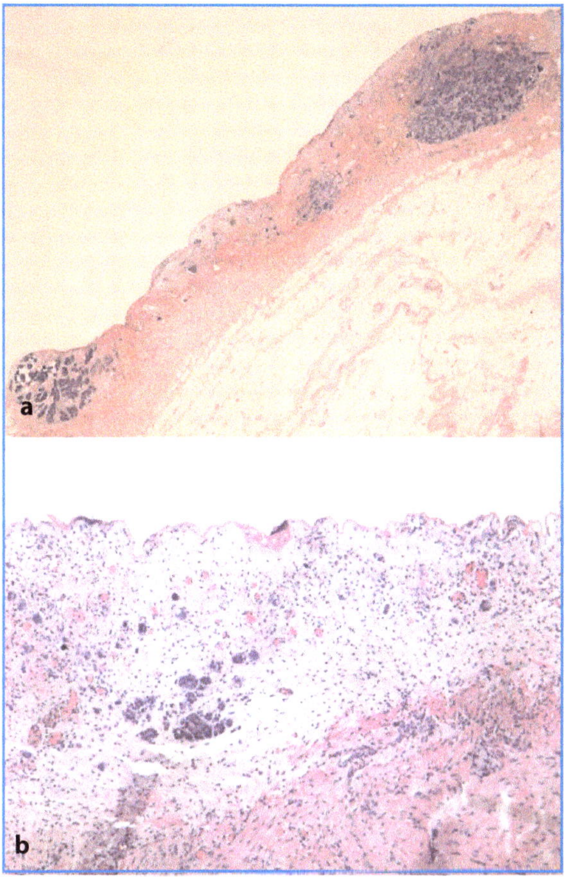

Fig. 4.4a, b **a** Multiple small neoplastic intraperitoneal nodules (H&E, ×12.5). **b** Microfocus of neoplastic cells infiltrating the subperitoneal tissue, with no macroscopic alteration on the peritoneal surface (H&E, × 50)

ent, unfavorable prognostic factor for overall survival (OS) equal to the amount of residual disease; in fact this effect can be explained by multiple regression analysis in which the depth of invasion correlates with more extensive peritoneal spread and overall lymph node metastasis. Two other studies show conclusions that agree, at least partly, with our finding [14, 15]. Second, we found a 42.3 % metastatic spread to mesenteric lymph nodes, in keeping with another study [16]. Other authors report figures that differ significantly from ours [15, 17] and correlate it to certain pathologic variables, such as depth of colorectal-wall invasion [15], spread to retroperitoneal lymph nodes [17], or both [18], or the amount of the large bowel resected [14]. In our experience, whenever metastatic peritoneal spread invades the colorectal wall, one can reasonably expect mesenteric lymph node metastasis equal to or more frequent than that found in the pelvic and interaortocaval (locoregional) stations. Regarding the site of lymph nodes involved, we found that mesorectal lymph node metastasis was

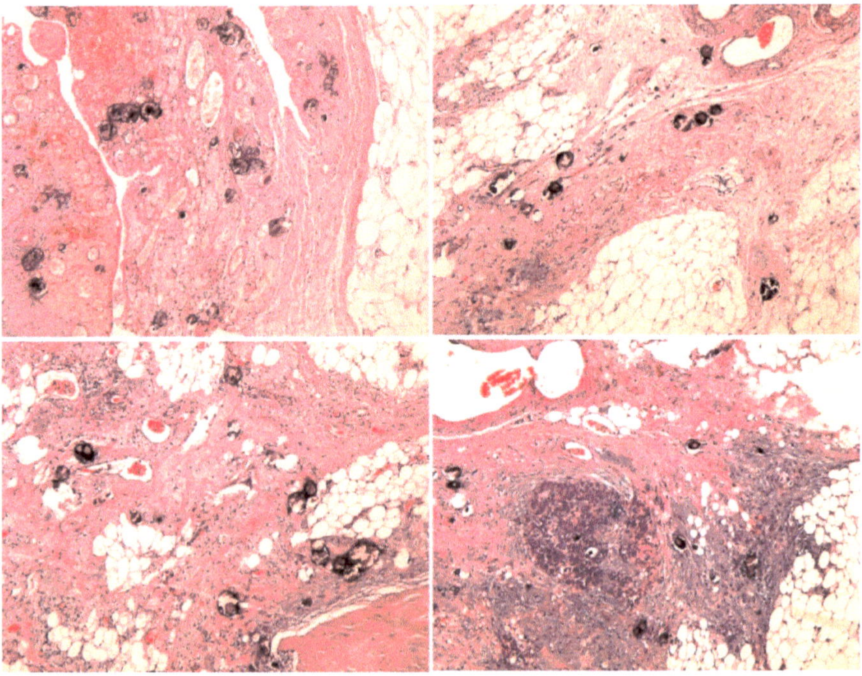

Fig. 4.5 Psammoma bodies inside fibrous desmoplastic tissue, with no or very minimal neoplastic residue (*lower right*) (H&E, × 50)

present in 41.6 % of patients with mesorectal resection, justifying the preferred surgical approach of an almost total mesorectal resection in patients with deep infiltration of the peritoneal pouch and intraperitoneal rectum. Mesenteric lymph node and concurrent locoregional metastases appear to worsen the prognosis, and unsystematic removal of these lymph nodes could result in undiagnosed and residual metastatic disease, a fact that presumably could change this observation, with a less favorable survival for patients with metastatic spread to the mesenteric lymph node [13].

The pouch of Douglas is very frequently involved and shows gross exophytic lesions originating from subperitoneal fat (Fig. 4.9a, b); alternatively lesions are more subtle, and only a thickening of the submesothelial tissue is observed, which corresponds microscopically to small foci of papillary elements or solid paucicellular nests surrounded by desmoplastic fibrous tissue. From the bottom of the pouch of Douglas, lesions can expand to the colic wall or toward the uterus and/or broad ligament. An appropriate sampling of these areas is mandatory when the pathology is not clearly obvious.

The spleen and adipose tissue of the splenic hilus are also typical sites of involvement (*see* Chap. 9, Fig. 9.14). Usually, neoplastic nodules are contained in the hilar adipose tissue, and, if large, may be visible on the peritoneal surface.

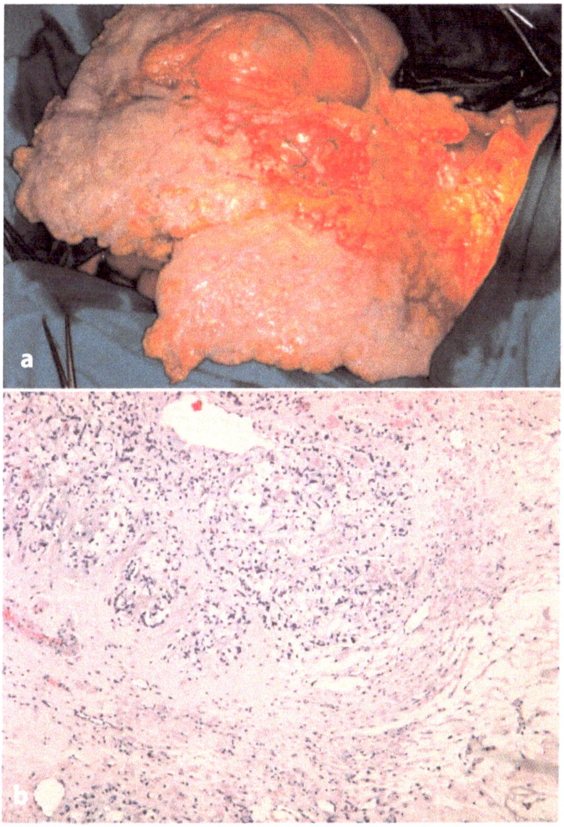

Fig. 4.6a, b **a** Massive involvement of the omentum (omental cake). **b** Signet-ring-cell carcinoma infiltrating fibrous cord of round ligament (H&E, × 50)

Also, the splenic fibrous capsule may present frank nodules or a microscopic nest of neoplastic cells. Very rarely, we have observed neoplastic infiltration of the splenic parenchyma, which in all cases was near the parahilar region, probably where the capsule is thinner and exceptionally we found involvement of an accessory spleen (Fig. 4.10).

Regional lymph nodes for the ovary are located in the pelvis and along the iliac artery. They have a typical elongated shape and usually do not harbor metastasis after systemic chemotherapy. A frequent histological finding is that of fibrous and hyaline tissue—often calcified—in the subcapsular sinuses, which makes the lymph node hard and suspicious for metastasis.

If the uterus and adnexa are part of the surgical resection, the most frequent observation is that of bilateral pathological ovaries, which are variably increased in diameter, with frequent adhesion to the uterus and/or to the large bowel. The surface of the ovary is rough due to the outgrowth of the tumor beyond it. In the majority of cases, lesions are solid, with a variable portion of cystic aspect. In the more florid cases, paratubaric tissues and broad ligaments can harbor the

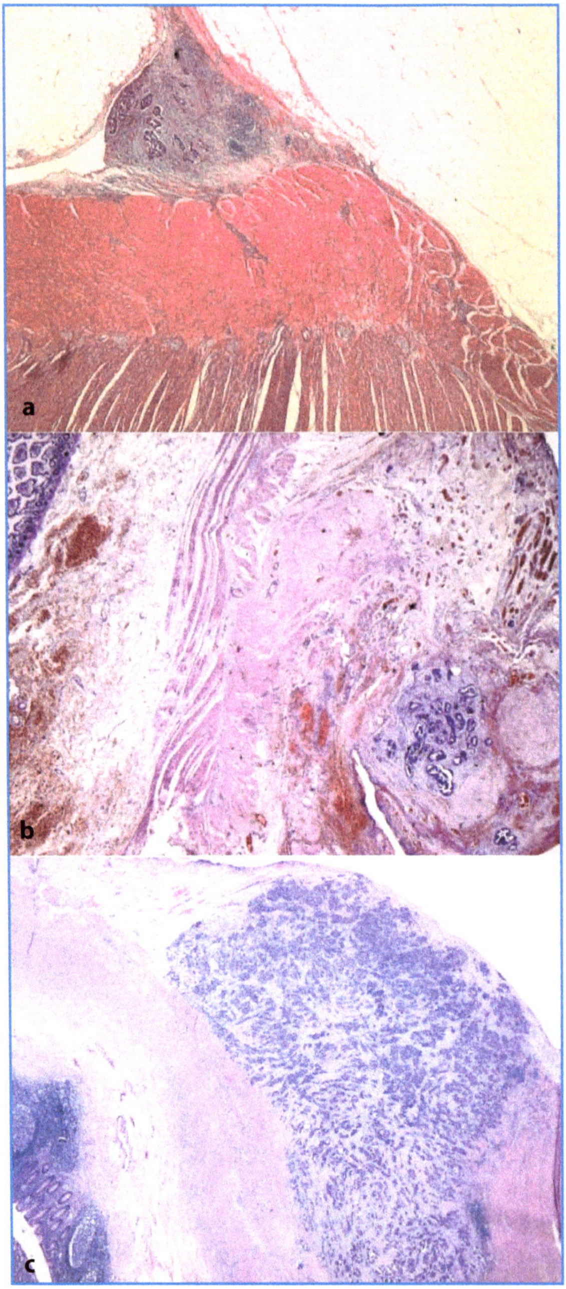

Fig. 4.7a–c Superficial (**a**) and subserosal (**b**) nodules (*ab extrinseco* infiltrative growth) (H&E, × 12.5]. **c** Neoplastic tissue infiltrating up to the muscular layer of the gastrointestinal tract (H&E, × 12.5)

neoplastic tissue. The corpus uteri may show serosal nodules that may or may not extend deep beyond the subserosal tissue to reach the myometrium directly. The latter can be involved lymphatically, as well.

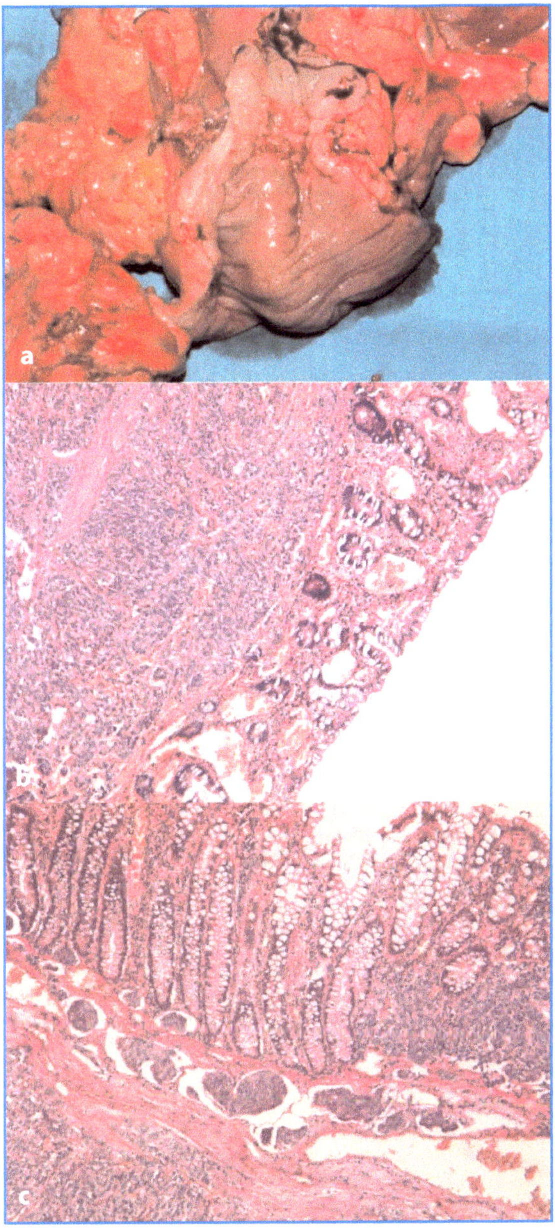

Fig. 4.8a–c **a** Macroscopic evidence of colonic mucosal infiltration. **b** Neoplastic involvement of submucosa and deep mucosa (H&E, × 50). **c** Neoplastic growth in the chorion of the mucosa and mucosal–submucosal lymphatic infiltration (H&E, × 50)

4.3 Peritoneal Carcinomatosis from Colorectal and Appendiceal Tumors

Pseudomyxoma peritonei (PMP), also known as mucinous or gelatinous ascites, is a rare condition, with an incidence of ~ 1/1,000,000 per year [19]. PMP is a

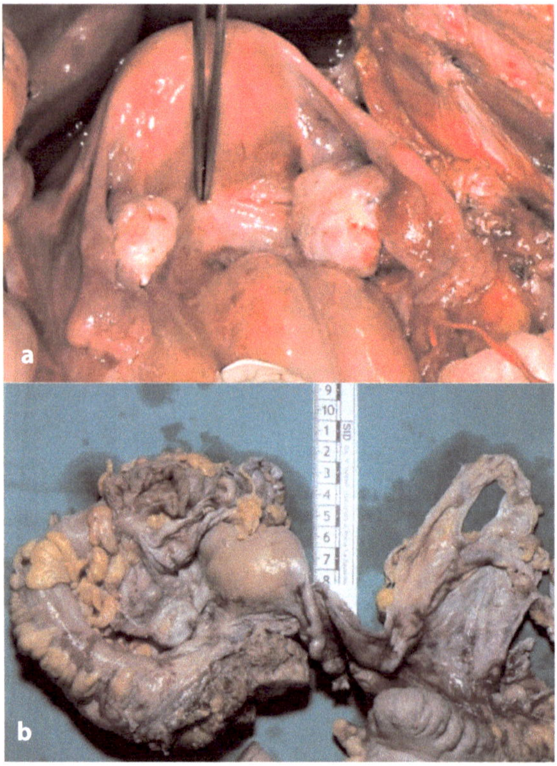

Fig. 4.9a, b **a** Nodules and plaque-like growth in the pouch of Douglas. **b** Nodules in the pouch of Douglas (*left*) and pelvic parietal peritoneum (*right*)

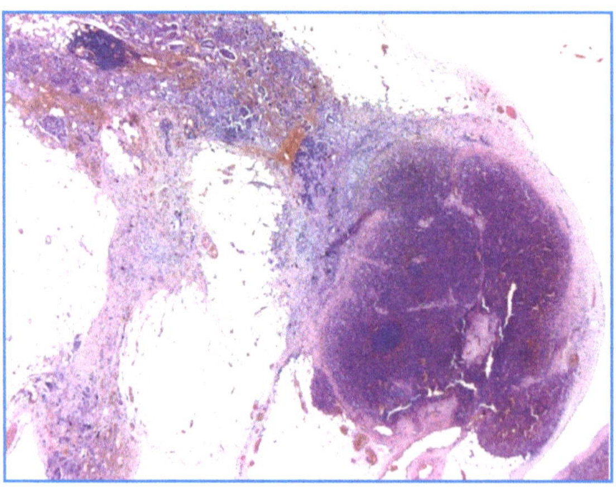

Fig. 4.10 Neoplastic infiltration of accessory spleen (H&E, × 12.5

clinical term and, therefore, should not be used as a pathological diagnosis. It corresponds to the intraoperative clinical finding of mucus or gelatinous fluid in a localized or generalized form occupying the pelvic or abdominal cavity with

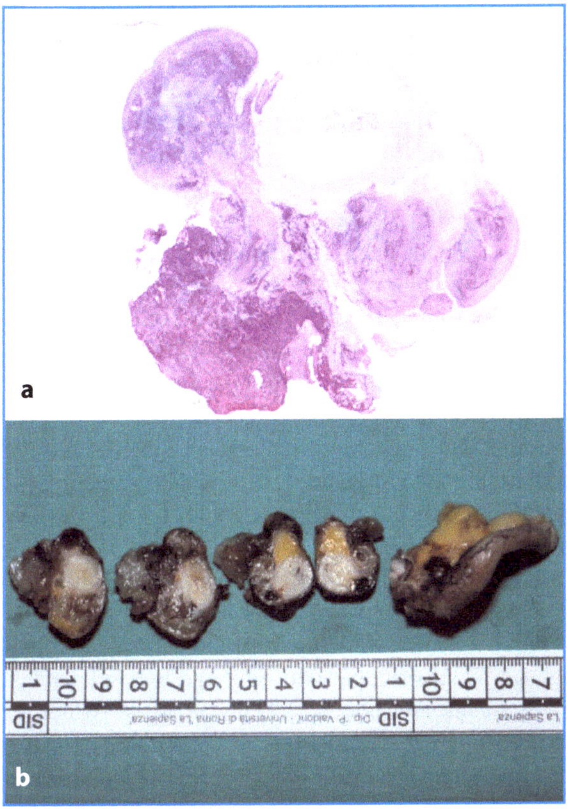

Fig. 4.11a, b **a** Huge mucous deposit on appendix serosal surface (periodic acid-Shiff). **b** Serial sampling of appendix showing neoplastic alteration at different levels

involvement of the omentum. PMP is most probably the result of an appendiceal (Fig. 4.11a) or, more rarely, another type of mucus-secreting tumor in the area of the GI tract other than the appendix. Most cases of PMP originate from ruptured low-grade appendiceal tumors, as shown by molecular genetic and immunohistochemical studies [20, 21]. In many cases, the appendiceal tumor is not easily recognized grossly, and therefore, the entire appendix must be serially sectioned and submitted in its entirety for microscopic examination in order to determine the primary site (Fig. 4.11b).

A proposed classification of mucinous tumors involving the peritoneal cavity recognizes two main categories based solely on pathologic features: disseminated peritoneal adenomucinosis (DPAM), and peritoneal mucinous carcinomatosis (PMCA), the prognostic utility of which has been confirmed by follow-up data with long-term survival for DPAM and very poor prognosis for PMCA patients [22]. Microscopic criteria defining DPAM include disease characterized by histologically bland to low-grade adenomatous mucinous epithelium associated with abundant extracellular mucin and fibrosis, often with an identifiable appendiceal mucinous adenoma or a mucocele. Only rarely are lesions identified within lymph nodes or seen invading the parenchyma of abdominal or pelvic organs. In patients with PMCA, the disease is characterized by peritoneal lesions displaying cytologic and architectural features of mucinous carcinoma associated with extracellular mucin, often with an identifiable invasive mucinous adenocarcinoma of the GI tract. Not infrequently in these cases, parenchymal and lymph node metastases are associated.

A third category has been described and named "peritoneal mucinous carcinomatosis with intermediate or discordant features (PMCA I or D)." This category involves peritoneal lesions that combine DPAM and PMCA-I or markedly atypical appendiceal adenomas associated with peritoneal lesions similar to PMCA-D. However, resection specimens of multivisceral CRS show that in PMP, both low- and high-grade features are seen concurrently at light-microscopy examination. Additionally, several authors reported that despite the low-grade histological features and the long-term prognosis of DPAM, multiple disease relapses always occur, leading eventually to death. A claim for using the term mucinous carcinoma peritonei, either low or high grade, for all cases of PMP was recently made by Bradley et al. [23], who showed that the nomenclature of the condition is still hindered by controversy and confusion.

In our experience, true cases of DPAM show multiple nodular formations—soft, bubble-like, and translucent—covering wide areas of the peritoneum: subdiaphragm right and left (Fig. 4.12a), gastric, parietal right and left, spleen surface, omentum, prevesical peritoneum, and pouch of Douglas areas. At microscopic observation, we found mucus deposits covered by a very thin, fibrous, and transparent capsule harboring neutrophils and plasma cells with a sheet of adenomatous epithelium (Fig. 4.12b). The mesothelium appears hyperplastic, with mesothelial cells showing variable size and shape and being polygonal or elongated. These cells stain positively both with cytokeratin (CK) and vimentin, featuring the immunoprofile of the mesothelium. In no cases have we found infiltration of subserosal tissues.

PMC shows a more infiltrating tendency, and in this setting, we observed an overlap of pathological involvement of the peritoneal cavity either from a known primary tumor from a specific site in the GI tract (small and large bowel, stomach) or from a tumor putatively originating from appendix.

Small, multiple nodular deposits may be observed that remain superficial or subserosal; deeper lesions invade *ab extrinseco* toward the internal layers, reaching the mucosa, with concomitant and progressively severe narrowing of the lumen (Fig. 4.12c). Omentum is a preferred site of neoplastic deposits either from advanced primary tumor or in metachronous PC if not previously removed. There is usually involvement of the parietal peritoneum and the pouch of Douglas, where neoplastic growth can be exophytic or invade the underlying adipose tissue. The bladder and genital organs (uterus and ovaries, less frequently prostate) are usually part of the pathological picture of PC, taking the form of direct infiltration from a sigmoid/rectal large-bowel tumor or as seeding of neoplastic cells from tumors of more proximal tracts (i.e., Krukenberg tumor of the ovaries).

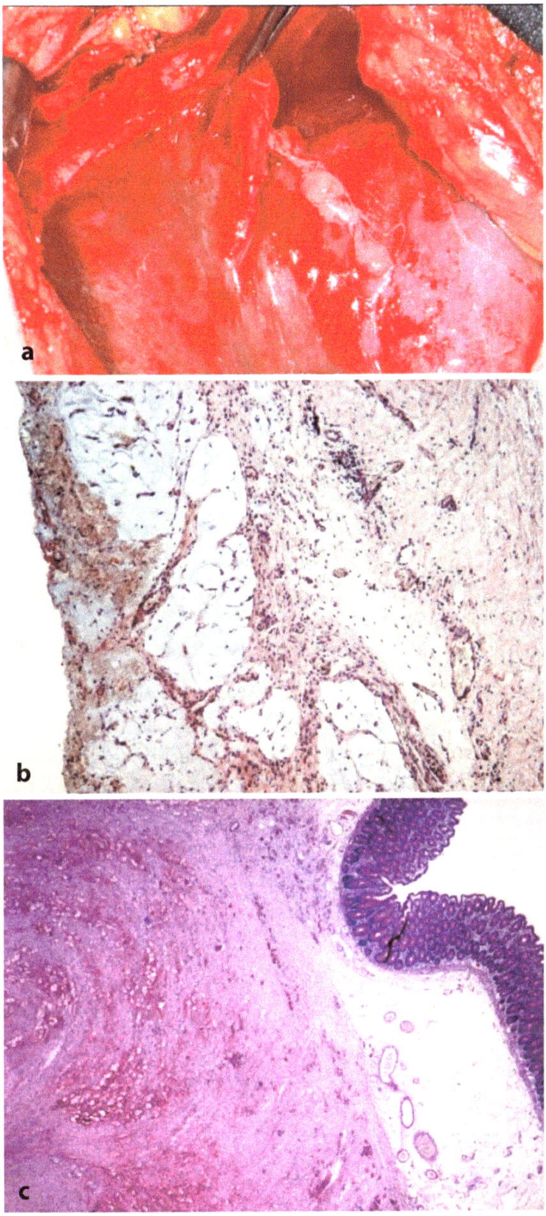

Fig. 4.12a–c **a** Soft, bubble-like lesion on the liver–subdiaphragmatic surface typical of disseminated adenomucinosis. **b** Mucous deposits with subtle fibrous lobulation and inflammatory cells (H&E, × 50). **c** Signet-ring cells and mucous infiltration of gastrointestinal wall (muscle layer and submucosa) (periodic acid-Schiff–diastase, × 12.5)

Ovarian mucinous adenocarcinomas associated with PC from GI cancer may be erroneously considered as primary ovarian neoplasms, particularly if they are discovered during the first operative procedure, but molecular analysis demonstrates identical *KRAS* mutations in the large bowel/appendiceal tumor and synchronous ovarian tumors. Ovarian metastases result from neoplastic mucinous cells being deposited on the ovarian surface or having penetrated the ovarian stroma.

4.4 Peritoneal Carcinomatosis from Gastric Cancer (GC)

In the Far East, the most common pattern of disease failure after curative resection of GC is PC [24]. However, little is known about the actual incidence of PC in the setting of GC. A study based on the Eindhoven Cancer Registry population of 2,029 patients diagnosed with GC in The Netherlands found a 39 % rate of metastatic disease, of which 35 % developed PC in the metastatic setting; in 24 %, the peritoneum was the only site of metastasis [25]. Prognosis of patients with PC from GC is very poor, with median survival (MS) of 4.6 months for patients with PC only and 3.3 months for patients with PC plus other metastatic sites. Taking the hypothesis that PC is caused by serosal infiltration by the primary tumor and subsequent shedding of malignant cells into the peritoneal cavity, it is acceptable to consider advanced T and N stages as risk factors for patients with GC developing PC; risk appears to be greater if they are of younger age. Other risk factors for both synchronous and metachronous PC are signet-ring-cell histology of the primary tumor or linitis plastica [25].

Diagnostic laparoscopy with peritoneal cytology is the best procedure for staging advanced GC, and peritoneal cytology has been included as a staging procedure, regardless of how it is obtained (peritoneal lavage, usually during staging laparoscopy; ascitic fluid tapping if ascites is present). Positive peritoneal cytology makes the disease stage IV. Peritoneal cytology has yet to gain integration into the clinical practice of surgeons, and with missing peritoneal cytology, surgeons are accustomed to operating on GC cases without proper staging.

Cytology workup should include both Giemsa [Romanowsky, Diff Quick, May-Grunwald Giemsa (MGG), or similar methods] and Papanicolaou stains, as well as cell-block preparation (hematoxylin and eosin staining). In doubtful cases, immunohistochemical stains can be performed—usually monoclonal carcinoembryonic antigen (CEA). Real-time polymerase chain reaction (RT-PCR) to detect CK-20 and CEA messenger RNA (mRNA) expression as signs of metastasis may also help in the routine workup [26].

The pathological picture of PC from GC differs in the setting of primary advanced gastric lesion from that of PC following previous gastric resection. In the first case, the main area of neoplastic deposits is the omentum, with possible direct infiltration of the spleen or pancreas and lesser omentum, depending on location of the primary tumor. Parietal, visceral, and pelvic implants are part of the picture. Not infrequently, we have observed metastatic seeding at the ovaries (Krukenberg tumor). We also observed two cases of PC from diffuse-type GC involving the residual gastrocolic ligament and the transverse portion of the large bowel, with the dominant pathological feature represented by diffuse perineural neoplastic infiltration of the mesocolon and bowel wall (transparietal).

4.5 Peritoneal Carcinomatosis from Endometrial Cancer

PC from endometrial cancer (EC) has been rarely reported. A MEDLINE search retrieved only three articles: one concerned a wound recurrence of endometrial cancer, and two consisted of a small series of patients with PC. All patients were treated with complete CRS plus HIPEC [27–29]. The most recent series [27] involved 13 patients, of whom seven were alive after a follow-up ranging from 1.56 to 124.83 months: three had recurrence and four did not. The other published series was a small group of five patients, two of whom survived without recurrence after 2 and 3 years, and two of whom were living with recurrence after 1 and 3 years [28]. No reference was made in these articles to the overall incidence of advanced EC. However, treatment resulted in an apparent beneficial effect on survival of these patients with advanced disease. Eight cases of PC from EC have been treated in our institution with peritonectomy (PRT) plus HIPEC, with survival ranging from 12 to 95 months (*see* Chap. 22, Table 22.2).

Peritoneal involvement from endometrial neoplasms has a spectrum ranging from limited peritoneal areas with tiny nodules to multiple sites of neoplastic growth with nodular or plaque-like shape. Nodules can be of small or medium size and often are observed in the mesocolon, mesosigmoid, adipose tissue of splenic hilus and round ligament, and liver capsule. Plaque-like thickening is frequently seen in the subdiaphragmatic peritoneum, small- and large-bowel serosa, and subserosal adipose tissue, although nodular growth can be observed, as well. These plaque-like formations induce partial stenosis of the intestinal lumen. Macroscopic evidence of metastatic diffusion to the pericolic lymph nodes is a frequent finding, and regional lymph node stations can show metastatic nodules.

Microscopically, cases with low neoplastic burden are characterized by multiple foci of a small number of neoplastic cells, accompanied by desmoplastic stroma, and sparse in the subserosal tissue of the parietal or visceral peritoneum. Nodular and plaque-like formations show solid, papillary, cystic–papillary and, less frequently, a tubular pattern. Fibrous septa of variable thickness are present. These formations can be exophytic or invade subserosal adipose tissue. Differently from OC, involvement of muscular or more inner layers of the bowel is less frequent. Metastatic involvement of pericolic lymph nodes is usually an epiphenomenon of extensive neoplastic growth in the subserosal adipose tissue.

4.6 Peritoneal Carcinomatosis from Breast Cancer

Peritoneal involvement from previous breast cancer (BC) is a rare event. It can develop many years after the original diagnosis, with the longest reported interval being 30 years (median 18 years). Most papers in the literature are case reports. In one study [30], only 73 of 12,001 patients diagnosed with metastatic disease secondary to BC were found to have histologically confirmed metastatic disease to the GI tract and peritoneum. Twenty-three patients had GI metastasis only, with no involvement of the peritoneum. Lobular BC is prevalent in peritoneal metastasis, with rates as high as 54 % of patients compared with the 10–12 % overall percentage of lobular type in breast primaries. MS in this setting is very short, ranging from 1.5 months after treatment with chemotherapy or hormonal therapy [31] up to 26 months after surgery (mostly palliation for obstruction). A small group of five patients treated at our institution with CRS plus HIPEC achieved long-term survival, with one patient surviving up to 10 years [32].

Ductal BC is associated with a less evident macroscopic involvement. Small nodules (< 2cm in diameter) can be observed in the omentum (lesser and greater), hilus of the spleen, round ligament, parietal (parietocolic right cleft) and pelvic (pouch of Douglas) peritoneum, and subserosal adipose tissue of the left colon and mesosigmoid; single implants may be present in the cecum, mesorectum, mesentery, appendix vermiform, myometrium, paratubaric, and paraovarian tissue, with penetration of ovarian stroma.

Lobular BC shows a macroscopic picture of multiple stenosis of the large and small bowel, with tubular narrowing of the lumen due to deeper involvement of the parietal layers up to the mucosa, which appears ulcerated; round ligament, parietal peritoneum, and splenic capsule are also sites of neoplastic seeding, as are the ovaries and Fallopian tubes (ovaries show massive involvement, as in the Krukenberg type of tumor).

A panel of immunohistochemical stains is needed to confirm the diagnosis, with positive stains for CK-7 and gross cystic disease fluid protein-15 (GCDFP-15), whereas stains for Wilms' tumor 1 (WT1), cancer antigen 125 (CA-125), and CK-20 is negative. E-cadherin assessment is helpful in differential diagnosis between lobular and ductal BC.

4.7 Peritoneal Carcinomatosis from Pancreatic Cancer

Data regarding incidence, prognosis, and treatment opportunities of PC following pancreatic cancer are sparse in the literature. Very few studies focus on this topic. The most recent investigation is from The Netherlands [33]. The authors searched for the diagnosis of nonendocrine pancreatic cancer in the Eindhoven Cancer Registry over a period of 15 years. They found 2,924 cases, of which 265 presented with synchronous PC (mean incidence 9 %, increasing to 11 % in the last 5 years of the study). Most cases presented with metastasis in other locations. The reported MS in patients with synchronous PC was only 6 weeks. Other studies—an autopsy-based study [34] and a group of patients treated with palliative chemotherapy [35]—report incidences as high as 31 %. Another paper on disease recurrence after surgical treatment for pancreatic cancer found a PC incidence of 30 % (21/69 patients), with a grim prognosis witnessed by an actuarial 5-year survival of only 6.8 %. The main pathological characteristic independently associated with PC was invasion of the portal vein. The authors stated that PC cannot be excised surgically because cancer cells are distributed randomly across a large area of the peritoneum [36].

On the basis of results obtained in PC from CRC, Farma et al. [37] treated seven patients with pancreatic carcinoma with radical surgery plus HIPEC, achieving a mean survival of 16 (range 2–62) months but with a high incidence of severe complications, from which they conclude that such treatment should currently not be offered. A case report focused on successful combined IP and systemic chemotherapy, with disappearance of peritoneal deposits and consequent radical resection [38]. The main avenues of progression of pancreatic cancer outside the organ are liver metastasis, local retroperitoneal extension, including periaortic lymph nodes, and peritoneal dissemination. This has been evaluated as being as frequent as 31 % in postmortem studies of patients with pancreatic cancer [34]. The main areas of deposits in peritoneal spread of pancreatic cancer are the omentum and tracts of the large and small bowel. Many of these cases present with synchronous, often multiple, metastases in the liver, which is an exclusive criterion for surgical treatment of PC from pancreatic cancer. PC is not a rare event in the course of digestive endocrine tumors, especially in patients with carcinoid tumors, with a prevalence of 27 % (8/30) [39].

4.8 Primary Tumors of the Peritoneum

4.8.1 Malignant Peritoneal Mesothelioma

Mesotheliomas are rare, aggressive tumors arising from serous surfaces: pleura (65–70 %), peritoneum (30 %), tunica vaginalis testis [3 5%], and pericardium (1–2 %). Malignant peritoneal mesothelioma (MPM) is the second rarest form of the disease and accounts for approximately 20–25 % of all mesothelioma cases each year. It generally affects men between the ages of 50 and 69 years. First described in 1908 by Miller and Wynn [40], it is a rare neoplasm with a rapid, fatal course (MS 6–12 month). Only 50 % of patients with MPM of peritoneal origin have a history of asbestos exposure. However, latency between exposure to asbestos and the development of MPM symptoms can be anywhere from 20–50 years. There are two main theories regarding how asbestos exposure leads to the development of MPM: (1) asbestos fibers are ingested, and these fibers work their way from digestive organs into the peritoneal membrane; (2) asbestos fibers are inhaled and travel to the peritoneal membrane via the lymphatic system. Most people with years of asbestos exposure never develop mesothelioma, yet others with very brief exposure may develop the disease. This indicates that other factors may be involved in the pathogenesis of this disease. Some research indicates a link between mesothelioma and Simian virus 40. Other possible risk factors include prior radiation exposure, exposure to thorium, talc, erionite, or mica, as well as in patients affected by familial Mediterranean fever and diffuse lymphocytic lymphoma.

MPM can arise both from visceral and parietal peritoneum. It is diagnosed in advanced stages in most cases, and it often takes considerable time to arrive at the correct diagnosis, as the mean time from symptoms to diagnosis is 122 days [41]. It may present as multiple tiny masses or as one dominant, localized mass and generally little or no ascites, or shows widespread small nodules, no dominant mass, and presence of ascites. The widespread progression of malignant cells on peritoneal surfaces results in copious fluid production, which can be attributed to retention of a functional property of normal mesothelial cells. Neoplastic growth can involve the wall of several viscera (Fig. 4.13 upper panel).

Cytologic analysis of ascites has a low diagnostic potential due to high cytologic diversity of tumor cells and to the small number of malignant cells within the fluid. When there is no effusion, sampling by fine-needle aspiration of the tumor can be used to reach a diagnosis. Normally, a definitive diagnosis is obtained through tissue biopsy obtained at peritoneoscopy or diagnostic surgery.

Mesotheliomas have three basic histologic forms: epithelioid (the most frequent), sarcomatoid, and mixed (biphasic). More often, areas showing features and admixtures of these three types may be encountered within a single tumor; a sarcomatoid component is observed in 25 % of cases, but a pure sarcomatoid variety is extremely rare. The epithelioid MPM can grow with four different patterns: tubular, papillary (the most common, often found in association with other patterns), diffuse, and deciduoid (cells with abundant, glassy-looking eosinophilic cytoplasm). Atypia is a frequent feature but is typically mild; only a few cases have moderate or severe atypia.

Immunohistochemistry is also useful to distinguish MPM from primary papillary serous carcinoma of the peritoneum, serous OC, colorectal adenocarcinoma diffusely involving the peritoneum, and borderline serous tumors. In particular, calretinin, CK (Fig. 4.13, middle and lower panels), and thrombomodulin are typically positive in patients with mesotheliomas and negative in those with serous carcinomas. MPM usually remains confined to the peritoneal cavity for most of its natural history, and the typical growth pattern is locally expansive masses. Hematogenous or lymphatic metastasis is unusual.

Multicystic mesothelioma and well-differentiated peritoneal mesothelioma typically occur in the peritoneum of women with no history of asbestos exposure and show low malignant potential. Multicystic mesothelioma predominantly affects the pelvic peritoneum of young women, has a high tendency to recur locally, but shows no tendency to metastasize, and consequently requires only surgical treatment.

4.8.2 Primary Peritoneal Serous Papillary Carcinoma

Primary peritoneal serous papillary carcinoma (PPSPC) is a papillary serous-surface carcinoma affecting cells lining the peritoneum or abdominal cavity and

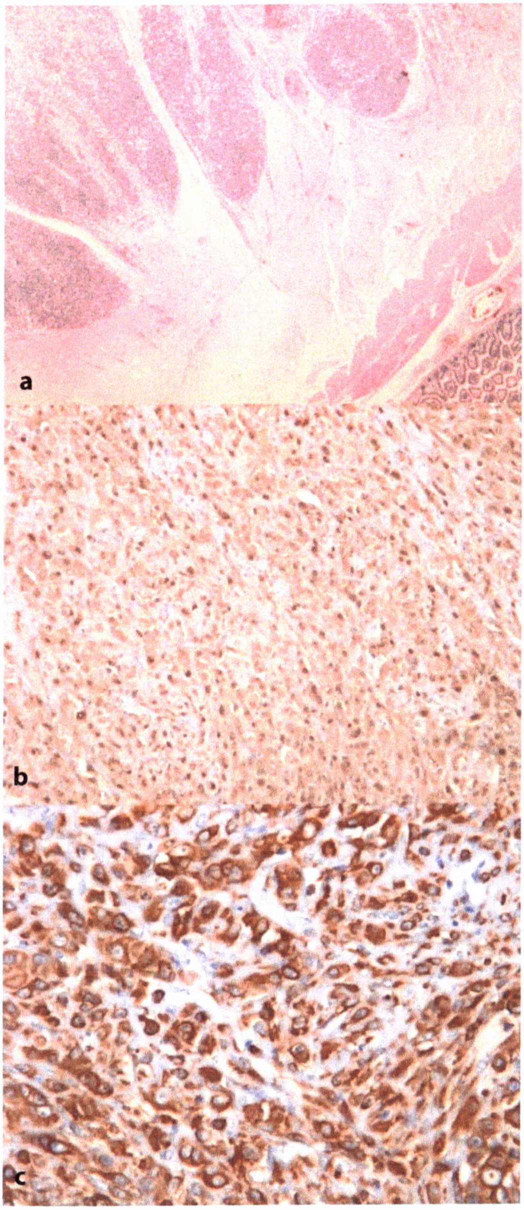

Fig. 4.13 Malignant mesothelioma (**a**) infiltrating the muscle layer of the gastrointestinal tract (H&E, × 12.5); (**b**) for anticalretinin antibody showing nuclear and cytoplasmic staining [IHC (P), × 50]; typical perinuclear circular pattern (**c**) of cytokeratin in mesothelioma cells [IHC (P), × 100]

develops almost exclusively in postmenopausal women. Since the establishment in 1959 of extraovarian peritoneal serous papillary carcinoma as a clinical entity, only a limited number of cases have been described, and its clinicopathologic features remain obscure. In early studies, it was thought to arise from the mesothelium of the peritoneum [42]. However, since ovarian and peritoneal epithelium share common embryonal origin from the coelomic epithelium, it is believed that serous carcinomas of the ovaries, uterus, fallopian tubes, and cervix, as well as PPSPC, actually represent one entity; the fallopian tube may be another source of PPSPC [43]. Expression of Müllerian-specific markers, such as *PAX8*, and lack of coexisting precursors on the ovarian surface, also support an origin in the fallopian fimbriated end or Müllerian inclusions. Women with *BRCA1/2* mutation have a 5 % risk of developing PPSPC, even after prophylactic oophorectomy. Schorge et al. [44] described *BRCA1* mutations in 48 % of patients with PPSPC. However, only 10 % of ovarian and primary peritoneal cancers are genetically linked.

PPSPC and serous OC appear identical microscopically. Tumor distribution pattern in the abdominal cavity often differentiates PPSPC from OC. Patients with PPSPC present with PC without evident gross tumoral disease and usually have normal ovaries and tubes or only superficial involvement of the ovaries. Criteria for PPSPC stipulated by the World Health Organization (WHO) and the Gynecologic Oncology Group (GOG) are the following: (1) ovaries must be normal in size or enlarged by a benign process only; (2) extraovarian tumors must exceed the ovarian tumors in size; (3) microscopic carcinoma in the ovary must be superficial and $< 5 \times 5$ mm.

Because of the similarities to OC, most scientists are applying the Fédération Internationale de Gynécologie et Obstétrique (International Federation of Gynecology and Obstetrics) FIGO staging criteria for epithelial OC to determine PPSPC stage. Patients with PPSPC tend to be older and have higher-grade tumors compared with patients with primary ovarian serous carcinoma, leading to a shorter OS for PPSPC patients. Nearly all patients diagnosed will have stage III or higher, because warning signs are typically few until cancer is widespread.

In our institution, 12 patients underwent PRT plus HIPEC for PPSPC, as described (*see* Chap. 21, Table 21.1).

4.8.3 Desmoplastic Small Round-cell Tumor

First described in 1989, desmoplastic small round-cell tumor (DSRCT) is a rare but highly aggressive neoplasm that typically occurs in adolescent boys and young men. The male-to-female ratio is approximately five to one, and mean age at diagnosis is 22 years [45]. DSRCT generally develops in the abdomen and has a tendency toward peritoneal spread, with subsequent metastasis to distant lymph nodes, liver, and lungs, as recorded in the vast majority (80 %) of patients. Abdominal or pelvic tumors show sizes ranging from 3.5 to 23 cm. Extra-abdominal sites, although rare, are described and involve prostate, testis, shoulder, and thigh. Eighty percent of patients have evidence of metastasis at presentation, with lungs and liver being the commonest sites. The reported MS of DSRCT varies from 17 to 25 months, indicating a very poor outcome.

Chemotherapy is the most frequently used therapeutic modality, but multimodal treatment with chemotherapy, surgery, and radiotherapy appears to represent optimal management. Moreover, two studies found that aggressive surgical debulking of DSRCT is of prognostic significance [46, 47], and another reported achievement of a longer MS [48]. The use of CRS plus HIPEC has also been reported (heated cisplatin is given IP at a dose of 100–150 mg/m^2) [49–51].

At our institution we treated a young male patient with diffuse peritoneal disease with no extra-abdominal sites of involvement. Specimens from abdominopelvic cytoreduction showed diffuse involvement of multiple sites: right and left colon (ileocolic angle), sigmoid colon (including mesosigmoid), rectum, bladder (adipose tissue), iliac fossa right and left, periappendicular adipose tissue, obturatoria fossa bilaterally, liver capsule, splenic capsule, Morrison's pouch, omentum at the inferior border, subdiaphragmatic right and left tissue, diffuse lymphadenopathy [paracaval, interaortocaval, retroinguinal, iliac right and left, iliac bifurcation (interiliac), paraortic, left inguinal]. Macroscopic observations revealed mainly nodules, with smooth external surface, whitish in color, and of firm consistency (Fig. 4.14a). The cut surface had a fascicular appearance, nodule size ranged from 0.5 to 22 cm, and—in particular—we observed multinodular disease in perivesical adipose tissue, where the single maximum diameter measured 2 cm, with merging nodule reaching up to 8 cm. The periappendicular adipose tissue (Fig. 4.14b) and epiploic appendages (at their apex) harbored small nodules (from 0.5 to 5 cm) of neoplastic tissue. The omentum (7.5 cm), mesosigmoid (13 cm), and pararectal/pelvic site (22 cm) showed the biggest nodular or mass-like deposition of the neoplastic process. At subdiaphragmatic sites, we found wide plaque-like neoplastic growth. Microscopically, the lesion is characterized by a nest, island, or anastomosing ribbons of medium-sized cells with round or oval nuclei and scanty cytoplasm with indistinct border immersed in abundant desmoplastic stroma. Neoplastic tissue is mainly exophytic or infiltrating subserosal or perivisceral adipose tissue, with focal involvement of the muscle layer of the large bowel (Fig. 4.14c). Areas of necrosis are present, but not in all nodules, and often accompanied by evident apoptosis. Immunohistochemical stains were positive for epithelial membrane antigen (EMA), CK, synaptophysin, neuron-specific enolase, *MNF116*, and *WT1* (clone c19), whereas negative stain was recorded for CD99, smooth-muscle actin (SMA), desmin, vimentin, human melanoma black 45 (HMB45), S100 protein, CD57, CD15, CEA; chromogranin A, and glial fibrillary acidic protein (GFAP), confirming that the cells of this tumor coexpress epithelial, mesenchymal, myogenic, and neural markers [52]. A peculiar characteristic is represented by diffuse metastasis in extraintestinal lymph nodes (pericolic, ileocolic, transverse, and mesocolic were negative); usually, lymph nodes are enlarged and massively occupied by neoplastic tissue, often with multiple foci of necrosis.

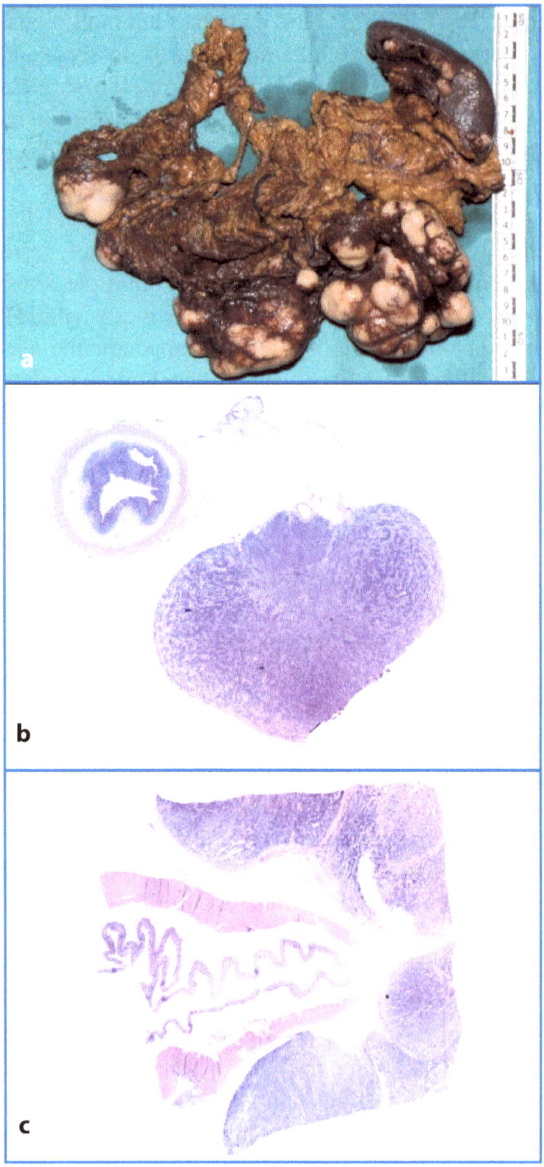

Fig. 4.14a–c **a** Desmoplastic small round-cell tumor (DSRCT), macroscopic pattern of growth with multiple smooth, whitish, and firm nodules (omentum, splenic). **b** Macroslide showing nodule of DSRCT in adipose tissue surrounding the appendix. **c** DSRCT involving subserosal and external muscle layer of the gastrointestinal tract

4.9 Peritoneal Sarcomatosis

Peritoneal sarcomatosis (PS) is a rare, recently described, entity and can be defined as the recurrence or spread of a soft-tissue sarcoma throughout the abdomen in the absence of any extra-abdominal dissemination, or at least other sites of disease of major clinical concern. This gives rise to presentations in which abdominal spread of disease is the dominating clinical factor, thus the main therapeutic challenge [53]. Soft-tissue sarcomas comprise 0.8 % of all cancers and frequently metastasize to the lung, followed by bone and liver [54]. Of all soft-tissue sarcomas, 30 % are located in the abdomen, with a recurrence rate after therapy of 50–70 % [55]. Almost all tumors that evolve toward PS have high-grade histology.

Sarcomatosis may arise from recurrent intra-abdominal sarcomas or may be metastatic from extremity sarcomas. The possible explanations for the former modality are tumor multifocality, ill-defined borders (an anatomic characteristic that can affect completeness of resection), tumor rupture during its removal, and—for uterine lesions—tumor "morcellation," especially when the suspected diagnosis is that of a benign leiomyoma. Over the years, PS has been treated with surgery, chemotherapy, and radiotherapy with very poor results and often only with palliative intent. The prognosis of PS is very dismal, and MS is < 1 year [55]. An exception to this rule is GI stromal tumors (GISTs), because the natural history of these tumors is greatly affected by targeted medical therapy based on imatinib.

The encouraging results of CRS plus HIPEC treatment in the setting of PC have prompted some authors to investigate the impact of this method for treating PS. There are several reports on this topic, but the majority is observational studies [56–59], and only one is a randomized trial [60]. The common feature to all these studies is the small number of patients, with the Italian Society of Locoregional Treatment in Oncology (SITILO) study having the highest number of patients. MS range varies from 20 to 34 months [57], and the impact of HIPEC/early postoperative intraperitoneal chemotherapy (EPIC) seems to be irrelevant, as per conclusions of the randomized study by Bonvalot et al. [60]. In addition, MS values did not differ significantly from those reported by Bilimoria et al. [53], who treated PS with surgery and conventional chemoradiotherapy. The interpretation of these results is affected by: (1) heterogeneity of histological types across the case series, (2) different inclusion criteria, and (3) different treatment modalities (HIPEC, EPIC) [61]. One possible explanation for these poor results in PS might lie in the natural history of sarcomas, which tend to spread across anatomical structures such as nerves and vessels, which in the abdomen are retroperitoneal and are therefore not accessible to peritoneal bathing [62]. It may be concluded that, at present, there is no sufficient evidence to support treating patients with peritoneal sarcomatosis with HIPEC or EPIC, and thus it should be all the more considered investigational for patients with multiple peritoneal implants (true peritoneal sarcomatosis).

In general, PS does not manifest a specific clinical picture; however, unlike carcinomatosis, the presence of ascites is variable in sarcomatosis [62]. Peritoneal lesions from recurrent or metastatic sarcomas are more often spherical and deforming and often vascular, whereas carcinomatosis implants tend to be flat or ovoid and conform to adjacent structures. Bowel obstruction and hydronephrosis are less frequently seen with sarcomatosis.

Tumors that most frequently give rise to peritoneal sarcomatosis are leiomyosarcomas [63-65], GISTs [66-68], and liposarcomas [69, 70]. Case series published hitherto are heterogeneous inasmuch as they include different histology with very small sample sizes. In the literature, in addition to the cited histology, we found cases of hemangiopericytoma, solitary fibrous tumor, clear-cell sarcoma of soft tissue, rhabdomyosarcoma, synovial-cell sarcoma, spindle-cell sarcoma, fibrosarcoma, and desmoplastic round-cell sarcoma.

References

1. Nik NN, Vang R, Shih IM, Kurman RJ (2014) Origin and pathogenesis of pelvic (ovarian, tubal, and primary peritoneal) serous carcinoma. Ann Rev Pathol Mech Dis 9:27–45
2. Shih I, KurmanRJ (2004) Ovarian tumorigenesis: a proposed model based on morphological andmolecular genetic analysis. Am J Pathol 164:1511–1518
3. Kurman RJ, Shih I (2011) Molecular pathogenesis and extraovarian origin of epithelial OC shifting the paradigm. Hum Pathol 42:918–931
4. Jones S, Wang TL, Shih I et al (2010) Frequent mutations of chromatin remodeling gene ARID1A in ovarian clear cell carcinoma. Science 330:228–231
5. Wiegand KC, Shah SP, Al-Agha OM et al (2010) ARID1A mutations in endometriosis associated ovarian carcinomas. N Engl J Med 363:1532–1543
6. Cho KR, Shih I (2009) Ovarian cancer. Annu Rev Pathol Mech Dis 4:287–313
7. Piek JM, van Diest PJ, Zweemer RP et al (2001) Dysplastic changes in prophylactically removed fallopian tubes of women predisposed to developing OC. J Pathol 195:451–456
8. Medeiros F, Muto MG, Lee Y et al (2006) The tubal fimbria is a preferred site for early adenocarcinoma in women with familial OC syndrome. Am J Surg Pathol 30:230–236
9. Kindelberger DW, Lee Y, Miron A et al (2007) Intraepithelial carcinoma of the fimbria and pelvic serous carcinoma: evidence for a causal relationship. Am J Surg Pathol 31:161–169
10. Piek JM, Verheijen RH, Kenemans P et al (2003) BRCA1/2-related OCs are of tubal origin: a hypothesis. Gynecol Oncol 90:491
11. Kuhn E, Meeker A, Wang TL et al (2010) Shortened telomeres in serous tubal intraepithelial carcinoma, an early event in ovarian high-grade serous carcinogenesis. Am J Surg Pathol 34:829–836
12. Marquez RT, Baggerly KA, Patterson AP et al (2005) Patterns of gene expression in different histiotypes of epithelial OC correlate with those in normal fallopian tube, endometrium, and colon. Clin Cancer Res 11:6116–126
13. Di Giorgio A, Cardi M, Biacchi D et al (2013) Depth of colorectal-wall invasion and lymph-node involvement as major outcome factors influencing surgical strategy in patients with advanced and recurrent OC with diffuse peritoneal metastases. World J Surg Oncol 11:64-72
14. Scarabelli C, Gallo A, Franceschi S et al (2000) Primary cytoreductive surgery with rectosigmoid colon resection for patients with advanced epithelial ovarian carcinoma. Cancer 88:389–397
15. Park JY, Seo SS, Kang S et al (2006) The benefits of low anterior en bloc resection as part of cytoreductive surgery for advanced primary and recurrent epithelial OC patients outweigh morbidity concerns. Gynecol Oncol 103:977–984
16. Dvoretsky PM, Richards KA, Angel C et al (1988) Distribution of disease at autopsy in 100 women with OC. Hum Pathol 19:57–63
17. Salani R, Diaz-Montes T, Giuntoli RL, Bristow RE (2007) Surgical management of mesenteric lymph node metastasis in patients undergoing rectosigmoid colectomy for locally advanced ovarian carcinoma. Ann Surg Oncol 14:3552–3557

18. Baiocchi G, Cestari LA, Macedo MP et al (2011) Surgical implications of mesenteric lymph node metastasis from advanced OC after bowel resection. J Surg Oncol 104:250–254
19. Baratti D, Kusamura S, Nonaka D et al (2008) Pseudomyxoma Peritonei: Clinical Pathological and Biological Prognostic Factors in Patients Treated with Cytoreductive Surgery and Hyperthermic Intraperitoneal Chemotherapy (HIPEC). Ann Surg Oncol 15:526–534
20. Szych C, Staebler A, Connolly DC et al (1999) Molecular genetic evidence supporting the clonality and appendiceal origin of pseudomyxoma peritonei in women. Am J Pathol 154:1849–1855
21. Carr NJ, Emory TS, Sobin LH (2002) Epithelial neoplasms of the appendix and colorectum: an analysis of cell proliferation, apoptosis and expression of p53, CD44, bcl-2. Arch Pathol Lab Med 126:837–841
22. Ronnett BM, Yan H, Kurman RJ et al (2001) Patients with pseudomyxoma peritonei associated with disseminated peritoneal adenomucinosis have a significantly more favorable prognosis than patients with peritoneal mucinous carcinomatosis. Cancer 92:85–91
23. Bradley RF, Stewart JH, Russell GB et al (2006) Pseudomyxoma peritonei of appendiceal origin: a clinicopathological analysis of 101 patients uniformly treated at a single institution, with literature review. Am J Surg Pathol 30:551–559
24. Maehara Y, Hasuda S, Koga T Y (2000) Postoperative outcome and sites of recurrence in patients following curative resection of GIC. Br J Surg 87:353–357
25. Thomassen I, van Gestel YR, van Ramshorst B et al (2014) Peritoneal carcinomatosis of gastric origin: A population-based study on incidence, survival and risk factors. Int J Cancer 134:622–628
26. Kodera Y (2013) Gastric cancer with minimal peritoneal metastasis: is this a sign to give up or to treat more aggressively? Nagoya J Med Sci 75:3-10
27. Delotte J, Desantis M, Frigenza M et al (2014) Cytoreductive surgery with hyperthermic intraperitoneal chemotherapy for the treatment of endometrial cancer with peritoneal carcinomatosis. Eur J Obstet Gynecol Reprod Biol 172:11-114
28. Bakrin N, Cotte E, Sayag-Beaujard A et al (2010) Cytoreductive surgery with hyperthermic intraperitoneal chemotherapy for the treatment of recurrent endometrial carcinoma confined to the peritoneal cavity. Int J Gynecol Cancer 20:809–814
29. Santeufemia DA, Lumachi F, Basso SM (2013) Cytoreductive surgery with hyperthermic intraperitoneal chemotherapy as salvage treatment for a late wound recurrence of endometrial cancer. Anticancer Res 33:1041-1044
30. Mc Lemore EC, Pockaj BA, Reynolds C et al (2005) Breast cancer: presentation and intervention in women with gastrointestinal metastases and carcinomatosis. Ann Surg Oncol 12:886–894
31. Tuthill M, Pell R, Giuliani R et al (2009) Peritoneal disease in breast cancer: a specific entity with an extremely poor prognosis. Eur J Cancer 45:2146–2149
32. Cardi M, Sammartino P, Framarino ML et al (2013) Treatment of peritoneal carcinomatosis from breast cancer by maximal cytoreduction and HPEC: A preliminary report on 5 cases. The Breast 22:845-849
33. Thomassen I, Lemmens VEPP, Nienhuijs SW et al (2013) Incidence, Prognosis, and Possible Treatment Strategies of Peritoneal Carcinomatosis of Pancreatic Origin. Pancreas 42:72-75
34. Blastik M, Plavecz E, Zalatnai A (2011) Pancreatic carcinomas in a 60-year, institute-based autopsy material with special emphasis of metastatic pattern. Pancreas 40:478-480
35. Morizane C, Okusaka T, Morita S et al (2011) Construction and validation of a prognostic index for patients with metastatic pancreatic adenocarcinoma. Pancreas 40:415-421
36. Shibata K, Matsumoto T, Yada K et al (2005) Factors Predicting Recurrence After Resection of Pancreatic Ductal Carcinoma. Pancreas 31:69–73
37. Farma JM, Pingpank JF, Libutti SK et al (2005) Limited Survival in Patients With Carcinomatosis From Foregut Malignancies After Cytoreduction and Continuous Hyperthermic Peritoneal Perfusion. J Gastrointest Surg 9:1346–1353
38. Kimura H, Fushida S, Mukawa A et al (2009) A resected case of effective treatment with S-

1/gemcitabine and paclitaxel combination chemotherapy for advanced pancreatic cancer with peritoneal and liver metastases]. Gan To Kagaku Ryoho 36:1191-1194
39. Vasseur B, Cadiot G, Zins M et al (1996) Peritoneal Carcinomatosis in Patients with Digestive Endocrine Tumors. Cancer 78:1686-1692
40. Raptopoulos V (1985) Peritoneal mesothelioma. Crit Rev Diagn Imaging 24:293–328
41. De Pangher Manzini V (2005) Malignant peritoneal mesothelioma. Tumori 91:1–5
42. Raju U, Fine G, Greenawald KA, Ohorodnik JM (1989) Primary papillary serous neoplasia of the peritoneum: a clinicopathologic and ultrastructural study of eight cases. Hum Pathol 20:426–436
43. Seidman JD, Zhao P, Yemelyanova A et al (2011) "Primary peritoneal" high-grade serous carcinoma is very likely metastatic from serous tubal intraepithelial carcinoma: assessing the new paradigm of ovarian and pelvic serous carcinogenesis and its implications for screening for OC. Gynecol Oncol 120:470–473
44. Schorge JO, Muto MG, Lee SJ et al (2000) BRCA1-related papillary serous carcinoma of the peritoneum has a unique molecular pathogenesis. Cancer Res 60:1361–1364
45. Gerald WL, Ladanyi M, de Alava E et al (1998) Clinical, pathologic, and molecular spectrum of tumors associated with t(11;22)(p13;q12): desmoplastic small round-cell tumor and its variants. J Clin Oncol 16:3028–3036
46. Schwarz RE, Gerald WL, Kushner BH et al (1998) Desmoplastic small round cell tumors: prognostic indicators and results of surgical management. Ann Surg Oncol 5:416–422
47. Lal DR, Su WT, Wolden SL et al (2005) Results of multimodal treatment for desmoplastic small round cell tumors. J Pediatr Surg 40:251–255
48. Hassan I, Shyyan R, Donohue JH et al (2005) Intraabdominal desmoplastic small round cell tumors: a diagnostic and therapeutic challenge. Cancer 104:1264–1270
49. Subbiah V, Viny AD, Anderson PM et al (2012) Optimizing the therapy of desmoplastic small round cell tumor: combined experience from the two major cancer centers. J Clin Oncol 30:10021
50. Hayes-Jordan A, Anderson P, Curley S et al (2007) Continuous hyperthermic peritoneal perfusion for desmoplastic small round cell tumor. J Pediatr Surg 42:E29–E32
51. Hayes-Jordan A, Green H, Fitzgerald N et al (2010) Novel treatment for desmoplastic small round cell tumor: hyperthermic intraperitoneal perfusion. J Pediatr Surg 45:1000–1006
52. Chang F (2006) Desmoplastic small round cell tumors: cytologic, histologic, and immunohisto-chemical features. Arch Pathol Lab Med 130:728–732
53. Bilimoria MM, Holtz DJ, Mirza NQ et al (2002) Tumor volume as a prognostic factor for sarcomatosis. Cancer 94:2441–2446
54. National Cancer Institute, U.S. National Institutes of Health (2009) Surveillance epidemiology and end results. Available at http/www.seer.cancer.gov. Accessed May 31, 2014
55. Munene G, Mack LA, Temple WJ (2011) Systematic review on the efficacy of multimodal treatment of sarcomatosis with cytoreduction and intraperitoneal chemotherapy. Ann Surg Oncol 18:207-213
56. Berthet B, Sugarbaker TA, Chang D et al (1999) Quantitative methodologies for selection of patients with recurrent abdominopelvic sarcoma for treatment. Eur J Cancer 35:413–419
57. Rossi CR, Deraco M, De Simone M et al (2004) Hyperthermic intraperitoneal intraoperative chemotherapy after cytoreductive surgery for the treatment of abdominal sarcomatosis: Clinical outcome and prognostic factors in 60 consecutive patients. Cancer 100:1943–1950
58. Baumgartner JM, Ahrendt SA, Pingpank JF et al (2013) Aggressive Locoregional Management of Recurrent Peritoneal Sarcomatosis. J Surg Oncol 107:329–334
59. Salti GI, Ailabouni L, Undevia D (2012) Cytoreductive Surgery and Hyperthermic Intraperitoneal Chemotherapy for the Treatment of Peritoneal Sarcomatosis. Ann Surg Oncol 19:1410–1415
60. Bonvalot S, Cavalcanti A, Le Pe´choux C et al (2005) Randomized trial of cytoreduction followed by intraperitoneal chemotherapy versus cytoreduction alone in patients with peritoneal sarcomatosis. Eur J Surg Oncol 31:917–923

61. Rossi CR, Casali P, Kusamura S (2008) The Consensus Statement on the Locoregional Treatment of Abdominal Sarcomatosis. J Surg Oncol 98:291–294
62. Oei TN, Jagannathan JP, Ramaiya N, Ros PR (2010) Peritoneal Sarcomatosis Versus Peritoneal Carcinomatosis: Imaging Findings at MDCT. AJR 195:W229–W235
63. Licht JD, Weissmann LB, Antman K (1988) Gastrointestinal sarcomas. Semin Oncol 15:181–188
64. Miettinen M, Virolainen M, Sarlomo-Rikala M (1995) Gastrointestinal stromal tumors - Value of CD34 antigen in their identification and separation from true leiomyomas and schwannomas. Am J Surg Pathol 19:207–216
65. Katz SC, DeMatteo RP (2008) Gastrointestinal stromal tumors and leiomyosarcoma. J Surg Oncol 97:350–359
66. Miettinen M, Monihan JM, Sarlomo- Rikala M et al (1999) Gastrointestinal stromal tumors/smooth muscle tumors (GISTs) primary to the omentum and mesentery. Am J Surg Pathol 23:1109–1118
67. Burkill GJ, Badran M, Thomas JM (2003) Malignant gastrointestinal stromal tumor: distribution, imaging features, and pattern of metastatic spread. Radiology 226:527–532
68. Kindblom LG, Remotti HE, Aldenborg F, Meis-Kindblom JM (1998) Gastrointestinal pacemaker cell tumor (GIPACT). Gastrointestinal stromal tumors show phenotypic characteristics of the interstitial cell of Cajal. Am J Pathol 152:1259–1269
69. Cheng EY, Springfield DS, Mankin HJ (1995) Frequent incidence of extrapulmonary sites of initial metastasis in patients with liposarcoma. Cancer 75:1120–1127
70. Pearlstone DB, Pisters PW, Bold RJ et al (1999) Patterns of recurrence in extremity liposarcoma: implications for staging and follow-up. Cancer 85:85-92

5 Classification of Intraperitoneal Spread

Simone Giacopuzzi, Francesca Guerini, Andrea Zanoni,
and Giovanni de Manzoni

5.1 Introduction

An accurate staging system for cancer diseases aims at providing a prognostic indication that is as accurate as possible. It also aids in treatment planning, evaluating therapeutic results, and interchanging information between different treatment centers. Peritoneal carcinomatosis (PC), once considered as an end stage of neoplastic disease, now can and should be staged: the better understanding of the biology and pathways of tumor dissemination with intraperitoneal spread has, in fact, prompted the concept that PC is not a manifestation of a systemic diffusion of the disease but is a locoregional entity. In particular, when we speak about PC, we do not refer to a metastasis in the common sense of the word because, as previously illustrated, this disease does not follow hematogenous or lymphatic dissemination but spreads via different pathways. Furthermore, Sugarbaker's research [1] created a new mindset toward surgical treatment of PC, the approach to which now has curative intent. In Sugarbaker's discussion, PC from different cancers is considered: gastrointestinal neoplasms, such as gastric cancer (GC), colorectal cancer (CRC), and appendiceal cancer [pseudomyxoma peritonei (PMP)]; gynecological cancers, such as ovarian cancer (OC); and malignant peritoneal mesothelioma (MPM). All these pathologies have a frequent peritoneal spread, and all follow different diffusion patterns. The classification of peritoneal metastasis considers three factors: (1) extension of peritoneal involvement (2) type of primary, (3) residual disease. These are the cornerstones of the staging system.

S. Giacopuzzi (✉)
Department of Surgery, Upper G.I. Surgery Unit, Borgo Trento Hospital,
Verona, Italy

A. Di Giorgio, E. Pinto (Eds), *Treatment of Peritoneal Surface Malignancies*,
Updates in Surgery
DOI: 10.1007/978-88-470-5711-1_5, © Springer-Verlag Italia 2015

5.2 Extension of Peritoneal Involvement

PC staging is difficult, even with imaging methods. Therefore, intraoperative exploration is an important factor, and quantitative prognostic indicators play an important role in guiding treatment selection. There remain many concerns related to diagnostic descriptive methods, which are first of all based on the fact that calculations are made by different surgeons. Nonetheless, studies in this direction show good agreement. Two quantitative staging systems are currently in use: the Gilly PC staging system, and the Peritoneal Cancer Index (PCI).

5.2.1 Gilly Peritoneal Carcinomatosis Staging

The Gilly PC staging format was first described in Lyon, France [2] in 1994. This prognostic tool accounts for size and partially for distribution, localized or diffuse, of malignant granulations (Table 5.1). Two advantages of this system are ease of use and reproducibility. It also has an important prognostic role: it allows identification of four different classes on the basis of different median survival rates, and only patients with stages 1 and 2 are candidate to surgery [3]. The usefulness of this technique was shown in the multicentric prospective Evolution of Peritoneal Carcinomatosis (EVOCAPE) study [4], which gathered data from 370 patients with PC from nongynecologic malignancies. Studies [5] focusing on GC, moreover, observed that in a resectable neoplasia with carcinomatosis stages 1 and 2, the 1-year survival rates was 80 % versus 10 % for patients with unresectable primary tumors in carcinomatosis stages 3 and 4.

A limit of the Gilly staging system is that it does not clarify whether peritoneal spread is potentially resectable or not [6]. A second weakness concerns failure to quantify the distribution of peritoneal surface implants in stages 3 and 4 because in these categories, nodule distribution is not taken into account; only size is considered. In fact, a different prognosis can be expected if carcinomatosis is confined to one portion of the abdomen, regardless of tumor implant size. Despite these limitations, the Gilly staging system was proven to be an important prognostic indicator in several clinical trials [7-9].

Table 5.1 Gilly peritoneal carcinomatosis staging system. (Modified from [2])

Stage	Peritoneal carcinomatosis description
0	No macroscopic disease
1	Malignant granulations < 5 mm in diameter; localized in one part of the abdomen
2	Malignant granulations < 5 mm in diameter; diffuse to the whole abdomen
3	Malignant granulations from 5 mm to 2 cm in diameter
4	Localized or diffuse large malignant masses (> 2 cm in diameter)

5.2.2 Peritoneal Cancer Index

The PCI was first described by Jacquet and Sugarbaker [10] and established at the Washington Cancer Institute. This classification system scores lesion distribution on the peritoneal surface on the basis of their size, producing a quantitative score. First, the abdomen is divided in nine regions by two transverse and two sagittal straight lines. The upper transverse plane is located beneath the costal margin, and the lower transverse plane is placed at the anterior superior iliac spine; the sagittal planes divide the abdomen into three equal sectors. The regions are then numbered starting from the umbilical area, which is assigned 0, proceeding in a clockwise direction from space 1, under the right hemidiaphragm, to space 8, located in the right side. Regions from 9 to12 divide the small bowel into upper and lower jejunum and upper and lower ileum. To make the indexing tool more quantitative and reproducible, each region is also defined by the anatomic structures located in each region (Table 5.2).

Second, the Lesion-Size (LS) score is determined to assess the diameter of the largest tumor implant (Table 5.3). A confluence of disease is automatically scored as LS-3; primary tumors or recurrences localized at the primary site and that can be removed definitively are excluded from the assessment.

Lesion sizes are then added to obtain a number ranging from 0 to 39. In invasive cancers in which cytoreductive surgery (CRS) and perioperative intraperitoneally administered chemotherapy (IP-CHT) are used as treatment,

Table 5.2 Peritoneal Cancer Index (PCI). (Modified from [10])

Regions	Anatomic structures
0	Central: Midline abdominal incision; entire greater omentum; transverse colon
1	Right upper: superior surface of the right lobe of the liver; undersurface of the right hemidiaphragm; right retrohepatic space
2	Epigastrium: epigastric fat pad; left lobe of the liver; lesser omentum; falciform ligament
3	Left upper: undersurface of the left hemidiaphragm; spleen; tail of pancreas; anterior and posterior surfaces of the stomach
4	Left flank: descending colon; left abdominal gutter
5	Left lower: pelvic sidewall lateral to the sigmoid colon; sigmoid colon
6	Pelvis: female internal genitalia with ovaries, tubes, and uterus; bladder, pouch of Douglas; rectosigmoid colon
7	Right lower: right pelvic sidewall; cecum; appendix
8	Right flank: right abdominal gutter; ascending colon
9	Upper jejunum
10	Lower jejunum
11	Upper ileum
12	Lower ileum

Table 5.3 Lesion-size (LS) score in Peritoneal Cancer Index (PCI). (Modified from [10])

Score	Description
LS-0	No implants seen
LS-1	Implants < 0.5 cm
LS-2	Implants between 0.5 and 5 cm
LS-3	Implants > 5 cm or a confluence of disease

PCI gives a threshold value for favorable versus poor prognosis and moreover allows estimation of the probability of complete cytoreduction.

There are two important limits: Sugarbaker and Jablonski [11] indicated that PCI was a meaningful score for colon cancer but not for mucinous appendiceal tumors, such as PMP, and for minimally aggressive mesothelioma. These diseases are, in fact, noninvasive, and a PCI of 39 can easily be converted to 0 using CRS. Furthermore, there is a low probability of recurrences after complete cytoreduction in these pathologies with perioperative intraperitoneal chemotherapy; therefore, the PCI has no prognostic implication in such cases [12]. A second limit of PCI staging is that it does not give a qualitative score of the regions, considering the invasion of the hepatoduodenal ligament and small-intestine mesentery, at the same level of other regions. Rather, invasion of these structures is considered a contraindication to surgery.

5.3 Type of Primary

Several preoperative scoring systems have been advocated to predict the optimal resectability of PC. Different classification systems have been developed for different neoplastic pathologies in order to provide a detailed picture of locoregional disease.

5.3.1 Peritoneal Carcinomatosis in Colon Cancer

In the sixth edition of the *AJCC Cancer Staging Manual* [13,15], stage pT4a indicates tumors invading adjacent structures or organs, whereas pT4b indicates tumors involving visceral peritoneum. In order to better classify this stage, the PCI is used. This was, in fact, described for the first time in colon cancer. At The Netherlands Cancer Institute [16], however, the Simplified PCI (SPCI) has also been established, which has also been used for PMP staging. As with the PCI, this system calculates tumour load, quantitatively scoring the volume of localizations in each region; however, it considers only seven regions, reaching a maximum score of 21 (Table 5.4). The SPCI was developed for prac-

Table 5.4 Simplified Peritoneal Cancer Index (SPCI). (Modified from [16])

Tumor size and abdominal regions Tumor measured as	
Large	> 5 cm
Moderate	1–5 cm
Small	< 1 cm
None	–
Abdominal regions	
1	Pelvis
2	Right lower abdomen
3	Greater omentum, transverse colon and spleen
4	Right subdiaphragmatic area
5	Left subdiaphragmatic area
6	Subhepatic and lesser omental area
7	Small bowel and small-bowel mesentery

tical convenience to maximize simplicity and proved useful in patients with CRC. Using the seven anatomic regions, Verwaal et al. and Swellengrabe et al. [17, 18] observed that in patients in whom five of the seven regions were affected or in whom SPCI > 12 was found, the possibility of treatment benefits were significantly diminished. They also attempted to correlate SPCI and postoperative course: patients with a high SPCI have greater morbidity and mortality. However, there are two defects: First, the epigastric region–important because it may influence the Completeness of Cytoreduction score (CC)–is not considered separately. Second is the Dutch group's misuse of their own tool: in their recent publications, they report a survival analysis and toxicity assessment with SPCI, but regions only were evaluated, and tumor size was not indicated.

A separate consideration of prior surgical score (PSS) [19] is required. According to Sugarbaker, who designed this simple scoring system, prior surgical exeresis plays a role in tumor cell diffusion over the peritoneum. PSS has been identified as a prognostic factor in several studies, but its value resulted in being of little interest. This classification system quantifies surgical extent prior to definitive treatment: the first operation is equivalent to a prior attempt at complete cytoreduction without using perioperative IP-CHT. The assessment uses a diagram similar to that for PCI but excludes abdominopelvic regions 9–12 (Table 5.5). The PSS is of prognostic value in PC secondary to PMP and primary ovarian tumors and MPM. In PMP treated using combined therapy, survival of patients with a PSS 0–2 was 70% at 5 years; with a prior surgical score of 3, the 5-year survival was 51 % ($p = 0.001$) [20]. When managing carcinomatosis, the

Table 5.5 Prior Surgical Score (PSS). (Modified from [19])

Score	Description
0	No prior surgery or biopsy only
1	One region with prior surgery
2	Two to five regions previously dissected
3	More than five regions previously dissected

extent of prior resection before definitive cytoreduction with IP-CHT has, in fact, a negative impact on survival. Essentially, PSS "shows that the greater the surgery the poorer the results of carcinomatosis treatment" [19]. This occurs because of the cancer-cell-entrapment phenomenon: cancer imbedded in scar tissue is difficult or impossible to remove by peritonectomy or to eradicate using IP-CHT.

5.3.2 Peritoneal Carcinomatosis in Gastric Cancer

In the most widely used staging system, the TNM, carcinomatosis is still associated with stage M. In the latest (seventh edition) of the *AJCC Cancer Staging Manual* [21], positive peritoneal lavage is considered an M1 (stage IV), similar to macroscopic PC.

The Japanese Research Society for Gastric Cancer originally classified peritoneal disease from primary gastric tumors according to location; they also perform a cytological examination using peritoneal washing fluid. For the original classification, a "P factor" is given to patients with carcinomatosis from GC, which are then classified into five categories [22] (Table 5.6). The classification is very simple, validated for gastric malignancy, frequently applied, and also used in patients with carcinomatosis from recurrent GC. It was shown to be an important prognostic factor in Japanese studies [23-26], which reported a significantly lower survival rate after treatment in patients with P3 carcinomatosis versus those with P2 or P1. One criticism is perhaps that PC size is not

Table 5.6 Peritoneal Carcinomatosis (PC) staging, Japanese Research Society for Gastric Cancer. (Modified from [22])

Stage	Description
P0/Cy0	No carcinomatosis seen by the surgeon or established at the time of surgery
P0/Cy1	No macroscopic PC but a positive peritoneal wash cytology
P1	PC in the upper abdomen, immediately adjacent to the stomach and above the transverse colon
P2	Scattered implants; countable pc in peritoneal cavity but few in number
P3	Numerous implants throughout the abdomen and pelvis

taken into consideration. Furthermore, a major limit of the staging system is its inability to describe carcinomatosis accurately by failing to indicate its distribution within the different regions of the abdominal cavity. We believe, however, that in a context of aggressive and difficult unresectable carcinomatosis, such as PC from GC, obtaining a photograph of intraperitoneal diffusion is not so important: the fundamental distinction is the difference between carcinomatosis confined to adjacent organs and diffuse and/or dotted carcinomatosis.

5.3.3 Peritoneal Carcinomatosis in Ovarian Cancer

Incomplete TNM staging in assessing peritoneal dissemination of OC, despite it being a frequent occurrence of the disease, led to the development of different carcinomatosis staging systems. Fagotti et al. [27] developed a laparoscopy-based score for predicting surgical resectability. Eight laparoscopic features were investigated as potential indicators of surgical outcome:

- Presence of ovarian masses (unilateral or bilateral)
- Omental cake
- Diaphragmatic carcinomatosis
- PC
- Mesenteric retraction
- Bowel invasion
- Stomach infiltration
- Liver metastases

These satisfied the basic inclusion criteria, and a final predictive index value of 2 was assigned to each one. In the final model, a predictive index score ≥ 8 identified patients undergoing suboptimal surgery with a specificity of 100 %.

Brun et al. [28] modified this score (Fagotti-modified score) and evaluated its relevance in identifying patients appropriate for optimal CRS. It was at least as accurate as the original Fagotti score in selecting patients with advanced-stage OC who could possibly undergo optimal CRS. A modified score was constructed by selecting four of the seven parameters:

- Diaphragmatic carcinomatosis
- Mesenteric retraction
- Stomach infiltration
- Liver metastases

A modified score ≥ 4 was associated with suboptimal cytoreduction, with a specificity of 100 % and an accuracy of 56 %. Chereau et al. [29, 30] presented a comparative analysis of different evaluation scores applied to a series of patients who were candidates for interval debulking surgery. They found an 86 % success rate using the Fagotti score and 91 % with the Fagotti-modified score, demonstrating a strong correlation between these scores and so justifying their relevance in evaluating the spread of carcinomatosis. A prognostic role was not an aim of that study.

The numeric ranking system developed by Eisenkop et al. [31] is also applicable for carcinomatosis from OC. It reflects the continuum of tumor involvement from stage IIIC OC of five anatomic regions: right upper quadrant, left upper quadrant, pelvis, retroperitoneum, and central abdomen. Disease in each anatomic region is intraoperatively ranked according to the findings and awards a numeric score from 0 to 15 to indicate disease extent. There were significant differences in survival for patients with a total score ranging from 0 to 5 compared with those ranging from 6 to 10 or 11. Moreover, the Eisenkop ranking system provides valuable information regarding the exact distribution of carcinomatosis and furthermore reveals that cytoreduction to a visibly disease-free outcome has a more significant influence on survival than does the extent of metastatic disease present before surgery. A criticism is that numerical ranking has similar findings with similar survival rates in patients with intermediate (6–10) and high (> 10) scores and is thus better at discriminating outcomes in patients with low scores with respect to those with higher scores. The Aletti Score [32], unlike others, reflects surgery extent, not disease extent. All patients are classified using the Surgical Complexity Score (SCS), where 1 corresponds to simple, 2 to intermediate, and 3 to complex.

The PCI and Fagotti-modified scores are the most important for predicting the feasibility of a complete resection.

5.3.4 Peritoneal Carcinomatosis in Pseudomyxoma Peritonei and Mesothelioma

In the seventh edition of the AJCC TNM staging system [33], appendiceal tumors are classified separately from CRC. Peritoneal invasion within the right lower quadrant is classified as stage T4a, whereas PC beyond it or PMP is classified as M1a. Precisely, these stages are modified because of the particular nature of mucinous carcinomas. In patients with carcinomatosis from GC, invasive implants are disseminated within the peritoneal cavity, but in two conditions, biological aggressiveness of the disease has a broad spectrum: mucinous appendiceal malignancies (oftentimes clinically designated PMP syndrome) and MPM. In these diseases, a noninvasive process may be widely disseminated on peritoneal surfaces. For PMP syndrome, histologic classification described by Ronnett et al. [34, 35] has been the most widely used. The histopathologic examination distinguishes between a disseminated peritoneal adenomucinosis (DPAM) and peritoneal mucinous carcinomatosis (PMCA) or a hybrid type. The primary appendiceal tumor was described as a cystadenoma; intermediate type showed predominantly adenomucinosis but was combined with focal areas of mucinous adenocarcinomas, which showed invasion and atypia. Survival differences between patients with adenomucinosis and those with intermediate type or mucinous adenocarcinoma were significant, with a P value of < 0.0001. This result could be explained by the specific character of PMP, which is a minimally aggressive peritoneal tumor despite a large amount of mucous ascites production [36, 37]. The natural history of appendiceal malignancies is, in fact, characterized by early peritoneal dissemination, but the mucinous localization has a low biological aggressiveness and spreads in anatomic sites that are easily resectable by peritonectomy [38, 39]. A noninvasive histopathology is extremely important in selecting patients who are most likely to benefit from this treatment strategy [40-42]. PCI is now the most frequently used scoring system.

5.4 Pathological Staging

Similarly to staging every disease, carcinomatosis evaluation should consider the pathological aspect. In fact, each method described above provides clinical staging based only on intraoperative observations, without considering pathological findings. We therefore proposed pathological staging of the disease, verifying in a retrospective study its correspondence with clinical observations. We took into account patients suffering from PC diffusion or at risk of developing this condition who were treated with hyperthermic intraperitoneal chemotherapy (HIPEC) at our department. Our population consisted of patients with PC from GC, CRC, OC, PMP, or MPM who underwent HIPEC and peritonectomy, which was performed as described by Sugarbaker [1]. Tumor load was intraoperatively described by PCI. After CRS, every surgical specimen was sent for pathologic evaluation, specifying the region from which it was removed. In the pathological report, location and size of resected specimens were specified.

We identified 48 patients suffering from OC, 20 from CRC, 24 with PMP, and 20 with GC. We excluded patients undergoing prophylactic treatment or palliation, i.e., in whom residual disease was > 2.5 cm (CC2–CC3). Furthermore, because of the small sample size, we excluded patients with PC from GC treated with therapeutic intent. We divided cases into PC from OC (40) and PC from intestinal cancer, colonic, or appendiceal tumors (28).

Histological examinations were reviewed for each case, and a histopathological PCI (pPCI) was calculated using the same criteria of clinical PCI (cPCI) construction: localization according to the classic division of the abdomen into 13 quadrants and the size of every surgical specimen was specified.

We then compared the pPCI assigned with the cPCI. The first observations led us to create some subgroups: within the group of OC patients, we considered separately those who received neoadjuvant chemotherapy (NACT) and those who underwent other treatment modalities. Another group comprised patients with intestinal PC, i.e., all those with PC from CRC (18); the remaining group comprised patients with PC from PMP (21). In colorectal cases, we distinguished mucinous neoplasia (8) from other histological type.

Thus, within the ovarian PC group, the NACT group comprised 19 patients; the second group comprised 21 patients treated upfront who relapsed or underwent second-look examination (non-NACT group). In patients with PC from

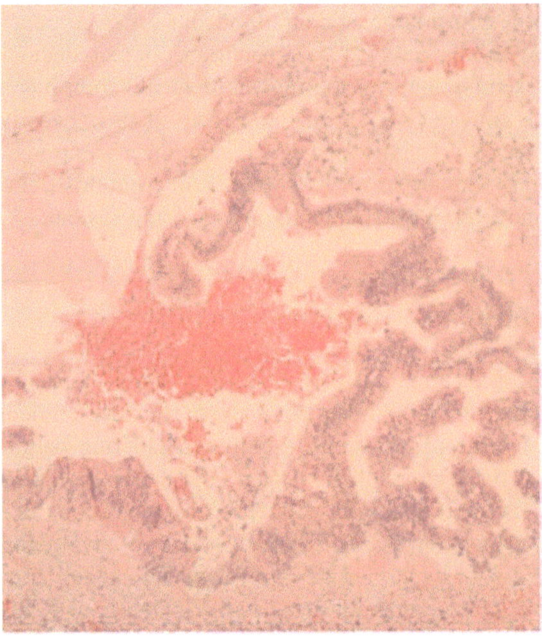

Fig. 5.1 Mucinous neoplastic tissue

OC, there was good correspondence between cPCI and pPCI in 18/21 treated with different protocols, except those who underwent NACT. We observed poor correspondence in11/20 who underwent NACT.

Within the intestinal PC group, the first subgroup comprised 29 patients with mucinous adenocarcinoma and the second comprised ten patients with nonmucinous adenocarcinoma. In the latter subgroup, there was matching between cPCI and pPCI in 8/10 patients; in the former, there was a correspondence in only 6/29. Our observations reinforced doubts regarding the use of PCI in mucinous colonic tumors or appendiceal neoplasms. In fact, the mismatch between clinical observation and pathological findings does not quantify the disease, because many lesions removed are pure lakes of mucin without cells (Figs. 5.1 and 5.2). Thus, PCI does not have a prognostic value or role in intraoperative planning when approaching this kind of pathology.

The other finding was the result obtained in relation to patients undergoing cytoreduction after NACT or perioperative chemotherapy. In such cases, in fact, many lesions removed are the result of a fibrotic process and do not represent solid neoplastic lesions. The possibility of confounding with a fibrotic lesion should be avoided when the observed amount of disease is a contraindication to surgery. Intraoperative evaluation for surgical planning requires an extemporary pathologic finding, using a sampling, in order to guide the surgeon accurately.

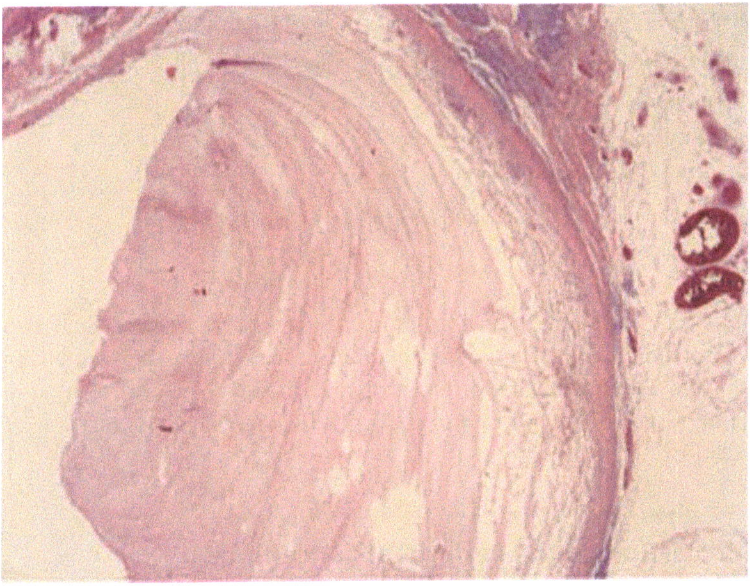

Fig. 5.2 Lakes of mucin without cells

5.5 Residual Disease

The PCI guides the surgeon because it provides an indication for resection. This occurs because of the intuitive and documented correlation described in the literature between the spread of disease and the possible benefit of its removal. The size of tumor nodules remaining after cytoreduction is therefore important because predicts prognosis by estimating the possibility of cancer eradication. Results of several studies [43] show a direct correlation between CC score and survival in patients with carcinomatosis from all primary cancer types. In clinical practice, the *R* parameter identifies the absence or presence of residual tumor after surgical treatment: the Lyon group [44, 45] successfully used complete (R0) or incomplete (R1–R2) cytoreduction to assess completeness of surgical clearance. In detail, R0 indicates the absence of residual tumor, R1 the presence of microscopic residual tumor, and R2 the presence of macroscopic residual tumor. R0 corresponds to a curative resection, and the prognosis is to be considered unfavorable for R1–R2. Similarly but more specifically, Jacquet and Sugarbaker [10] used the CC score to assess surgical clearance of carcinomatosis. The CC score assesses residual disease after maximal surgical effort, classifying residual disease extent after CRS into four categories (Table 5.7). CC score is a prognostic indicator in both noninvasive and invasive peritoneal-surface malignant disease; it has been used to accurately predict PMP and CRC

Table 5.7 Completeness of Cytoreduction (CC) score. (Modified from [10])

Score	Description
CC0	No visible residual tumor
CC1	Residual tumor ≤ 2.5 mm in diameter
CC2	Residual tumor between 2.5 mm and 2.5 cm
CC3	Residual tumor > 2.5 cm or confluence of disease present at any site

prognosis, but prognosis was worse in more diffuse disease (more than two quadrants), no matter how good a cytoreduction procedure was performed. In OC, CRS appears as the most important prognostic factor: survival results, in fact, are mainly affected by CC score: CC0 resulted in a median survival of 44–66 months [46, 47].

5.6 Clinical Role of the Peritoneal Cancer Index

The PCI is the most widely validated and precise quantitative prognostic indicator and is a factor associated in determining whether or not complete CRS can be achieved. It is used worldwide to assess PC from different tumors: for patients with high-grade CRC, PMP, OC, or GCs, a PCI > 20 is a relative contraindication. In reality, however, every disease has a different behavior in carcinomatosis that must be assessed at the time of classification. The PCI, therefore, can be applied to all the above-mentioned pathologies but assumes a different role for each one: the cutoff PCI beyond which surgical intervention is not recommended depends on tumor histology.

5.6.1 Colon Cancer

The PCI was first described for CRC, in which survival results were significantly better when the PCI was < 16 [48]. Elias and colleagues [49] reported that survival results were significantly better when the PCI was < 16 compared with ≥ 16. Sugarbaker [50] suggested that carcinomatosis from CRC with a PCI > 20 should be treated only with palliative intent. In a series of patients with CRC, Sugarbaker reported a 5-year survival rate of 50 % when PCI was < 10, a rate of 20 % for an index of 11–20, and a rate of 0 % for an index > 20 [51].

5.6.2 Ovarian Cancer

A few years after PCI introduction, Tentes et al. [52] evaluated the score for OC. OC with intraperitoneal dissemination can be effectively treated with CRS, even with a PCI score up to 30. The history of ovarian disease, which spreads frequently to the peritoneum, moves the surgical cutoff. In particular, the disease-free survival, the high chemosensitivity, and the possibility of obtaining a radical surgery [53, 54] play an essential role in surgical planning.

5.6.3 Gastric Cancer

GC is believed to have a more aggressive biological behavior than CRC. Glehen et al. and Canbay et al. [55, 56] suggest that carcinomatosis from GC with a PCI score > 12, or even > 7, should be treated with palliative intent without peritonectomy. They report, in fact, that the survival of GC patients with a PCI score ≤ 6 was significantly better than those with a PCI score ≥ 7. These important studies show that regardless of CC, PCI affects survival, confirming its unique prognostic value in the multivariate analysis. In the description of carcinomatosis from GC, spread beyond local mesenteric infiltration or over the annexes (Krukenberg) is enough to exclude patients from surgical treatment.

5.6.4 Pseudomyxoma Peritonei

In less invasive mucinous appendiceal cancers or in PMP, CRS quality appears to be the key for successful treatment. When considering such frameworks, is also appropriate to consider the absence of therapeutic alternatives.

5.7 Conclusions

Every PC scoring system is an attempt to assess quantitatively tumor spread over parietal and visceral peritoneum with the aim of standardized evaluation criteria and allowing better comparison between studies. All scores discussed in this chapter provide an intraoperative recommendation to the surgeon, but because of a lack of objectivity toward disease variability and absence of pathological findings, these tools are insufficient to dictate the indication for surgery. A classification of peritoneal metastasis should also consider primary tumor type and attempt to provide a clear cutoff for each type; it should, moreover, clearly indicate the possibility of performing radical resection, which is the most important prognostic factor. For this reason, a staging system cannot leave histology out of consideration.

References

1. Sugarbaker PH (1989) Management of peritoneal carcinomatosis. Acta Med Austriaca 16:57-60

2. Gilly FN, Carry PY, Sayag AC et al (1994) Regional chemotherapy (with mitomycin C) and intra-operative hyperthermia for digestive cancers with peritoneal carcinomatosis. Hepatogastroenterology 41:124-129
3. Sayag-Beaujard AC1, Francois Y, Glehen O et al (1999) Intraperitoneal chemo-hyperthermia with mitomycin C for gastric cancer patients with peritoneal carcinomatosis. Anticancer Res 1375-82
4. Sadeghi B, Arvieux C, Glehen O et al (2000) Peritoneal carcinomatosis from non-gynaecologic malignancies. Results of the EVOCAPE 1 multicentric prospective study. Cancer 88:358-363
5. Glehen O, Schreiber V, Cotte E et al (2004) Cytoreductive surgery and intraperitoneal chemohyperthermia for peritoneal carcinomatosis arising from gastric cancer. Arch Surg 139:20–26
6. Harmon RH, Sugarbaker PH (2005) Prognostic indicators in peritoneal carcinomatosis from gastrointestinal cancer. Int Semin Surg Oncol 2:3
7. Glehen O, Mithieux F, Osinsky D et al (2003) Surgery combined with peritonectomy procedures and intraperitoneal chemohyperthermia in abdominal cancers with peritoneal carcinomatosis: A phase II study. J Clin Oncol 21:799-806
8. Beaujard AC, Glehen O, Caillot JL et al (2000) Intraperitoneal chemohyperthermia with mitomycin C for digestive tract cancer patients with peritoneal carcinomatosis. Cancer 88:2512–2519
9. Rey Y, Porcheron J, Talabard JN et al (2000) Carcinoses péritonéales traitées par chirurgie de cytoréduction et chimiohyperthermie intrapéritonéale. Ann Chir 125:631–642
10. Jacquet P, Sugarbaker PH (1996) Clinical research methodologies in diagnosis and staging of patients with peritoneal carcinomatosis. In: Sugarbaker PH (ed) Peritoneal carcinomatosis: principles of management. Kluwer Academic Publishers, Boston, USA, pp 359–374
11. Sugarbaker PH, Jablonski KA (1995) Prognostic features of 51 colorectal and 130 appendiceal cancer patients with peritoneal carcinomatosis treated by cytoreductive surgery and intraperitoneal chemotherapy. Ann Surg 221:124-132
12. Sugarbaker PH (1999) Review Management of peritoneal-surface malignancy: the surgeon's role. Langenbecks Arch Surg 384:576-587
13. Compton C, Fenoglio-Preiser CM, Pettigrew N, Fielding LP (2000) American Joint Committee on Cancer Prognostic Factors Consensus Conference: Colorectal Working Group. Cancer 88:1739-1757
14. Compton CC, for the Members of the Cancer Committee, College of American Pathologists (2005) Colon and rectum. College of American Pathologists http://www.cap.org/apps/docs/cancer_protocols/2005/colonrectum05_ckw. pdf
15. Ishida H, Kumamoto K, Ishibashi K et al (2013) Should isolated peritoneal carcinomatosis from colorectal cancer be sub-classified into stage IVB in era of modern chemotherapy? Tech Coloproctol 17:647-652
16. Witkamp AJ, de Bree E, Kaag MM et al (2001) Extensive cytoreductive surgery followed by intra-operative hyperthermic intraperitoneal chemotherapy with mitomycin-C in patients with peritoneal carcinomatosis of colorectal origin. Eur J Cancer 37:979–984
17. Verwaal VJ, van Tinteren H, Ruth SV, Zoetmulder FAN (2004) Toxicity of cytoreduction and hyperthermic intra-peritoneal chemotherapy. J Surg Oncol 85:61-67
18. Swellengrebel HA1, Zoetmulder FA, Smeenk RM et al (2009) Quantitative intra-operative assessment of peritoneal carcinomatosis - a comparison of three prognostic tools. Eur J Surg Oncol 35:1078-84
19. Harmon RH, Sugarbaker (2005) Prognostic indicators in peritoneal carcinomatosis from gastrointestinal cancer. Int Semin Surg Oncol 2:3
20. Sugarbaker PH (1999) Results of treatment of 385 patients with peritoneal surface spread of appendiceal malignancy. Ann Surg Oncol 6:727–731
21. Kay Washington (2010) 7th Edition of the AJCC Cancer Staging Manual: Stomach. Ann Surg Oncol 17:3077–3079
22. Japanese research Society for Gastric Cancer (1993) The general rules for the gastric cancer study in surgery and pathology, 12 edn. Kanehara Shuppan, Tokyo

23. Ouchi K, Sugawara T, Ono H et al (1998) Therapeutic significance of palliative operations for gastric cancer for survival and quality of life. J Surg Oncol 69:41–44
24. Hagiwara A, Togawa T, Yamasaki J et al (1999) Extensive gastrectomy and carbon-adsorbed mitomycin C for gastric cancer with peritoneal metastases: case reports of survivors and their implications. Hepatogastroenterology 46:1673–1677
25. Fujimura T, Yonemura Y, Fushida S et al (1990) Continuous hyperthermic peritoneal perfusion for the treatment of peritoneal dissemination in gastric cancers and subsequent second-look operation. Cancer 65:65-71
26. Fujimoto S, Shrestha RD, Kokubun M et al (1990) Positive results of combined therapy of surgery and intraperitoneal hyperthermic perfusion for far-advanced gastric cancer. Ann Surg 212:592-596
27. Fagotti A, Ferrandina G, Fanfani F et al (2006) A laparoscopy-based score to predict surgical outcome in patients with advanced ovarian carcinoma: a pilot study. Ann Surg Oncol 131156–11561
28. Brun JL, Rouzier R, Uzan S, Daraï E (2008) External validation of a laparoscopic-based score to evaluate resectability of advanced ovarian cancers: clues for a simplified score. Gynecol Oncol 110:354-359
29. Chéreau E, Ballester M, Selle F et al (2010) Comparison of peritoneal carcinomatosis scoring methods in predicting resectability and prognosis in advanced ovarian cancer. Am J Obstet Gynecol 202:178.e1-178.e10
30. Chereau E, Lavoue V, Ballester M et al (2011) External validation of a laparoscopic-based score to evaluate resectability for patients with advanced ovarian cancer undergoing interval debulking surgery. Anticancer Res 31:4469–4474
31. Eisenkop SM1, Spirtos NM, Friedman RL et al (2003) Relative influences of tumor volume before surgery and the cytoreductive outcome on survival for patients with advanced ovarian cancer: a prospective study. Gynecol Oncol 90:390-396
32. Aletti GD1, Podratz KC, Moriarty JP et al (2009) Aggressive and complex surgery for advanced ovarian cancer: an economic analysis. Gynecol Oncol 112:16-21
33. Edge SB, Byrd DR, Compton CC (2010) The American Joint Committee on Cancer: the 7th edition of the AJCC cancer staging manual and the future of TNM. Compton CC et al., AJCC Cancer Staging Manual, 7 edn, Springer, Berlin, New York
34. Ronnett BM, Shmookler BM, Sugarbaker PH, Kurman RJ (1997) Pseudomyxoma peritonei: New concepts in diagnosis, origin, nomenclature, relationship to mucinous borderline (low malignant potential) tumors of the ovary. Chicago Anatomic Pathology: ASCP Press 197–226
35. Ronnett BM, Zahn CM, Kurman RJ et al (2005) Disseminated peritoneal adenomucinosis and peritoneal mucinous carcinomatosis. A clinicopathologic analysis of 109 cases with emphasis on distinguishing pathologic features, site of origin, prognosis, and relationship to "pseudomyxoma peritonei". Am J Surg Pathol 19:1390-1408
36. Sugarbaker PH (1994) Pseudomyxoma peritonei: a cancer whose biology is characterized by a redistribution phenomenon. Ann Surg 219:109–111
37. Esquivel J, Sugarbaker PH (2000) Clinical presentation of the Pseudomyxoma peritonei syndrome. Br J Surg 87:1414-1418
38. Sugarbaker PH (1999) Management of peritoneal surface malignancy: The surgeon's role. Langenbeck's Arch Surg 384:576–587
39. Sugarbaker PH (2001) Cytoreductive surgery and peri-operative intraperitoneal chemotherapy as a curative approach to pseudomyxoma peritonei syndrome. Eur J Surg Oncol 27:239–243
40. Jacquet P, Sugarbaker PH (1996) Current methodologies for clinical assessment of patients with peritoneal carcinomatosis. J Exp Clin Cancer Res 15:49–58
41. Sugarbaker PH (1996) Chang D, Koslowe P. Peritoneal carcinomatosis from appendiceal cancer. A paradigm for treatment of abdomino pelvic dissemination of gastrointestinal malignancy. Acta Chir Austriaca 28:4–87
42. Sugarbaker PH, Chang D (1999) Results of treatment of 385 patients with peritoneal surface spread of appendiceal malignancy. Ann Surg Oncol 6:727–731
43. Yonemura Y, Kawamura T, Bandou E (2005) Treatment of peritoneal dissemination from gas-

tric cancer by peritonectomy and chemohyperthermic peritoneal perfusion. Br J Surg 92:370-375
44. Cho BC, Jeung HC, Choi HU et al (2007) Prognostic impact of resection margin involvement after extended (D2/D3) gastrectomy for advanced gastric cancer: a 15-year experience at a single institute. J Surg Oncol 95:461-468
45. Biondi A, Persiani R, Cananzi F et al (2010) R0 resection in the treatment of gastric cancer: room for improvement. World J Gastroenterol 16:3358-3370
46. Munkarah AR, Coleman RL (2004) critical evaluation of secondary cytoreduction in recurrent ovarian cancer. Gynecol Oncol 95:273-280
47. Glehen O, Gilly FN (2007) Current Clinical Oncology: Intraperitoneal Cancer Therapy 9:131-145
48. Sugarbaker TA, Chang D, Koslowe P, Sugarbaker PH (1996) Patterns of spread of recurrent intraabdominal sarcoma. In: Sugarbaker PH, editor. Peritoneal Carcinomatosis: Principles of management. Boston: Kluwer Academic; pp. 65–78
49. Elias D, Blot F, El Otmany A et al (2001) Curative treatment of peritoneal carcinomatosis arising from colorectal cancer by complete resection and intraperitoneal chemotherapy. Cancer 92:71–76
50. Sugarbaker PH (1998) Intraperitoneal chemotherapy and cytoreductive surgery for the prevention and treatment of peritoneal carcinomatosis and sarcomatosis. Semin Surg Oncol 14:254–261
51. Sugarbaker PH (1999) Successful management of microscopic residual disease in large bowel cancer. Cancer Chemother Pharmacol 43 Suppl:S15–S25
52. Tentes AAK, Tripsiannis G, Markakidis SK et al (2003) Peritoneal cancer index: a prognostic indicator of survival in advanced ovarian cancer. Eur J Surg Oncol 29:69-73
53. Vergote I, Tropé CG, Amant F et al; European Organization for Research and Treatment of Cancer-Gynaecological Cancer Group; NCIC Clinical Trials Group (2010) Neoadjuvant chemotherapy or primary surgery in stage IIIC or IV ovarian cancer. N Engl J Med 363:943-953
54. Eisenkop SM, Spirtos NM, Friedman RL et al (2003) Relative influences of tumor volume before surgery and the cytoreductive outcome on survival for patients with advanced ovarian cancer: a prospective study. Gynecol Oncol 90:390-366
55. Glehen O, Gilly FN, Arvieux C et al; Association Française de Chirurgie (2010) Peritoneal carcinomatosis from gastric cancer: a multi-institutional study of 159 patients treated by cytoreductive surgery combined with perioperative intraperitoneal chemotherapy. Ann Surg Oncol 17:2370-2377
56. Canbay E, Mizumoto A, Ichinose M et al (2014) Outcome data of patients with peritoneal carcinomatosis from gastric origin treated by a strategy of bidirectional chemotherapy prior to cytoreductive surgery and hyperthermic intraperitoneal chemotherapy in a single specialized center in Japan. Ann Surg Oncol. 21:1147-1152

Diagnostic Imaging and Laparoscopy

6

Franco Iafrate, Maria Ciolina, Costanza Cavallini,
Daniele Biacchi, Enzo Naticchioni, and Andrea Laghi

6.1 Introduction

Pretreatment and preoperative assessment of peritoneal carcinomatosis (PC) can be very challenging in the field of imaging, and a comprehensive study could require integration of multidetector computed tomography (MDCT), magnetic resonance imaging (MRI) with conventional and diffusion-weighted sequences, and positron emission tomography (PET) or PET/CT [1, 2]. These imaging tools are able to provide accurate information on morphology, size, and location of peritoneal implants, lymph node enlargement, and presence of ascites. A detailed preoperative assessment of PC is essential to provide the surgeon with a detailed preoperative map of carcinomatosis and allow evaluation of the radiological Peritoneal Cancer Index (PCI) [3, 4]. This score correlates with patient prognosis, and the ability to calculate it using CT and MR with diffusion-weighted imaging (DWI) before any treatment is begun can guide therapeutic management of the patient. It can differentiate patients who are candidates for surgical intervention with hyperthermic intraperitoneal chemotherapy (HIPEC) from those with a high radiological PCI and who are therefore candidates for systemic chemotherapy [5]. The principal diagnostic techniques for accurate evaluation of peritoneal malignancy are represented by MDCT, MRI, PET, and combined PET/MDCT or PET/MRI. The role of ultrasound (US) imaging is limited in peritoneal imaging. However, this imaging modality is often the first one used when peritoneal disease is discovered incidentally, and it remains one of the diagnostic techniques for image-guided biopsy to obtain a histological diagnosis [1].

F. Iafrate (✉)
Department of Radiology, Oncology, and Human Pathology, Sapienza University of Rome, Rome, Italy
e-mail: francoiafrate@gmail.com

A. Di Giorgio, E. Pinto (Eds), *Treatment of Peritoneal Surface Malignancies*, Updates in Surgery
DOI: 10.1007/978-88-470-5711-1_6, © Springer-Verlag Italia 2015

6.2 Multidetector Computed Tomography

6.2.1 Imaging Technique

CT imaging is routinely performed using MDCT, particularly a 64-detector row scanner. Patient preparation comprises fasting for 6 h, oral administration of at least 500 ml of water 15–20 min prior to the study, and IV administration of hyoscine butylbromide (Buscopan) can be considered. CT scanning is performed with the patient in the supine position from the diaphragm to the ischial tuberosities before and after IV administration of contrast media. The arterial phase is preferred if hypervascular primary tumors (i.e., hypervascular metastases from breast cancer, neuroendocrine tumors such as carcinoid) are suspected and to better depict vascular infiltration of implants located adjacent to vascular structures. A delayed phase, acquired from 5 to 10 min after contrast injection, can increase contrast resolution in some small implants. Axial and other multiplanar reformatted (MPR) images are useful to detect peritoneal disease and check the common peritoneal site of pathological involvement and different patterns of appearence (see Box 6.1 on page 18).

6.2.2 Advantages of Computed Tomography

MDCT represents the more versatile diagnostic method in evaluating peritoneal disease due to its wide availability, rapid execution time, absence of misregistration artifacts, and the possibility of acquiring thin sections to obtain MPR images covering a large volume of tissue [6] and detecting subcentimetric implants. Using an adequate diagnostic technique (both section thickness and reconstruction interval of 3 mm), the reported mean sensitivity for detecting implants ≥ 5 mm is 89 %, with a specificity of 92 % [7]. CT examination allows exploration of the entire abdomen, especially certain sites that are difficult to evaluate at surgery, such as diaphragm, splenic hilum, mesenteric root, and para-aortic nodes [8, 9], which is clinically helpful for planning surgical intervention.

The use of MPR enables assessment of disease above the peritoneal surface. In particular, in the pelvis, sagittal scans allow assessment of the vaginal cuff, cul-de-sac, bladder, and rectosigmoid colon [10], whereas coronal images enable better evaluation of paracolic gutters (Fig. 6.1), extension of omental disease, and number and location of implants over hepatic and splenic surfaces (Fig. 6.2). IV injection of contrast material may also identify the enhancing degree of masses [11] and depict the relationship of nodules to viscera and blood vessels as it would appear at surgery, especially using 3D data display. Moreover, on the basis of CT data, the radiologist can develop a radiologic scoring systems for predicting surgical success based on the PCI, as proposed by Sugarbaker, and to eventually determine whether patients are candidates for neoadjuvant chemotherapy (NACT) prior to surgery [12–15].

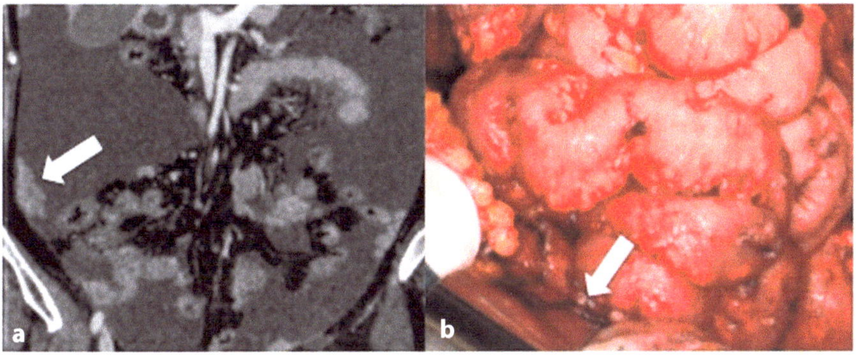

Fig. 6.1 Coronal contrast-enhanced computed tomography (CT) image showing (**a**) multiple nodules with a diameter > 5 mm diffusely involving the tunica serosa over bowel loops and paracolic gutters (*arrows*), (**b**) as documented during surgical intervention (*arrow*)

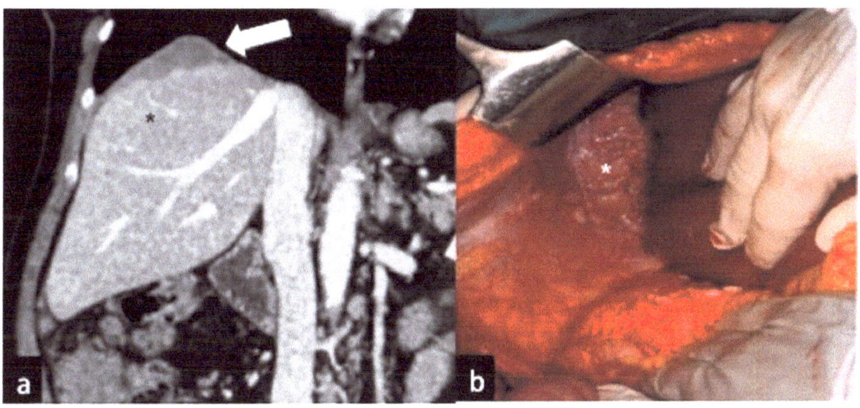

Fig. 6.2 Coronal computed tomography (CT) image showing (**a**) irregular soft tissue (*arrow*) of inconstant extension formed by the confluence of multiple nodular implants in the right subdiaphragmatic space scalloping the liver surface and presenting a lower density than the parenchyma (*black asterisk*) on contrast-enhanced scan. **b** During surgical intervention, the pathological subdiaphragmatic tissue was confirmed (*white asterisk*)

6.2.3 Disadvantages of Computed Tomography

In the literature, overall sensitivity and specificity of contrast-enhanced (CE) MDCT in identifying peritoneal deposits vary substantially, ranging from 25 % to 93 % [6, 16] and from 78 % to 98 %, respectively [6, 17]. The reason for this wide variability is multifactorial, including differences in tumor characteristics (size or density), patient features (CT assessment of peritoneal metastases is more difficult in very thin patients), radiologist expertise, diagnostic criteria used in CT interpretation, and CT techniques. Coakley et al. reported an overall sensitivity of 85–93 % for implants > 10 mm that decreased to 25–50 % for implants < 10 mm [16]. However, there was no information about the type of spiral scanner used and section collimation was 5 mm, 7–8 mm, or 10 mm [16]. Even using an advanced CT technique, for small peritoneal nodules, detection rate for peritoneal metastases is not greatly improved. In particular, when malignant peritoneal deposits have a low volume (< 5 mm), reported CT sensitivity tends to decrease [6, 18]. Marin et al., using a 64-row CT scanner with a more accurate technique (effective section thickness and reconstruction interval 3 mm), assessed preoperatively PC in 18 patients with different neoplasm types. They found a mean sensitivity of 89 % for lesions ≥ 5 mm but a sensitivity of only 43 % for lesions < 5 mm in diameter [7]. Identifying neoplastic implants in challenging anatomic sites represents another disadvantage of CT. In the literature, the reported per-site sensitivity for the exact location of peritoneal implants is only 25–37 % [14].

6.3 Magnetic Resonance Imaging

6.3.1 Imaging Technique

MRI for peritoneal malignancies is performed using a high-field system (1.5–3.0 Tesla). Larger phased-array surface coils or the use of two-array coils combined provides simultaneous coverage of the abdomen and pelvis [2]. The protocol includes patient fasting for 8 h, oral administration of water (500 ml), and intramuscular administration of hyoscine butylbromide (Buscopan) before pelvic scans. Abdominal imaging comprises T2-weighted fast spin-echo (SE) axial and coronal imaging and for the pelvis comprises high-resolution T2-weighted fast SE sequences in axial, coronal, and sagittal planes. Gadolinium administration IV is not mandatory for implant detection, but if it is administrated, postenhanced acquisitions should be performed with a delay of ~ 5 min. DWI should be performed for both abdomen and pelvis, acquiring axial scans using breath-hold, single-shot SE planar sequences. Sensitivity of DWI sequences for hypercellular tissue can be increased by increasing the b value; acquisition using a b value of 0 s/mm^2, 800 s/mm^2, and 1,000 s/mm^2 is usually satisfactory. All axial DWI images can also be depicted with black-and-white reverse-contrast display, and apparent diffusion coefficient (ADC) maps are usually available to provide quantitative assessment [2].

6.3.2 Advantages of Conventional Magnetic Resonance with Diffusion-weighted Imaging

Over the last decade, the role of MRI in peritoneal malignancy has significantly increased, primarily due to technical improvements and wider availability. Using

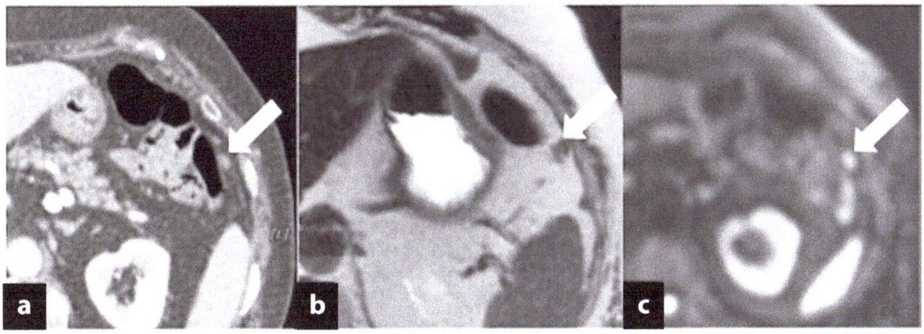

Fig. 6.3 Axial computed tomography (CT) image showing (**a**) a solid nodule < 5 mm near the splenic flexure (*arrow*) suspected to be fibrotic tissue in a patient with sigmoid cancer (pT3N+) treated with surgical intervention and adjuvant chemotherapy 6 months earlier. **b** Axial T2-weighted magnetic resonance image (MRI) better depicts the small, solid nodule (*arrow*) due to the high-contrast resolution. **c** At diffusion-weighted imaging (DWI), the nodule shows hypercellularity and is strongly suspected to be a peritoneal metastasis

conventional sequences with DWI is comparable with MDCT for detecting peritoneal deposits (> 1 cm) and in certain cases surpasses that of CT sensitivity and specificity [19–21]. The reported sensitivity and specificity of conventional MRI with DWI is 90 % and 95.5 %, respectively [20]. Combining traditional MR sequences and DWI increases accuracy for peritoneal implants measuring < 10 mm and for peritoneal implants located in sites difficult to evaluate on CT. In particular, conventional MRI with DWI seems to improve detection of malignant deposits over subdiaphragmatic spaces, hepatic hilum, Treitz ligament, small-bowel wall, and mesenteric root [22–25], which are crucial sites to definitely or temporarily exclude patient candidacy for surgery (Fig. 6.3). Moreover, using high-resolution MR sequences to study the pelvis is the better imaging modality for predicting primary or metastatic gynecological malignancies due to its superior spatial and contrast resolution [21, 22].

DWI is a functional magnetic resonance imaging (fMRI) technique in which the signal comes from the restricted water mobility typically present within hypercellular tumors. This high signal intensity of neoplastic nodules increases the contrast between the site of neoplastic disease and surrounding tissue [20]. Increased contrast between malignant tissue and around normal tissue makes it easier to detect smaller implants, which appear as hyperintense spots surrounded by hypointense normal tissue, due to signal suppression of surrounding ascites, bowel contents, and fat, with an increased contrast-to-noise ratio (CNR).

DWI also allows quantitative assessment by calculating the ADC of each voxel, which occurs automatically on current MRI systems by assuming a monoexponential model of signal decay between two or more b values. Therefore, once the ADC value is determined, the MR system can displayed a parametric map that essentially reflects differences in tissue diffusivity at different b values [22]. Integration between conventional MRI, dimensional criteria, and DWI

seems also to improve the ability to assess metastatic lymph nodes by 17–21 %. Many studies found that inflammatory lymph nodes present higher value on ADC maps than metastatic nodes [26].
In the early posttreatment period, conventional MRI and DWI can be helpful in distinguishing between inflammatory tissues and residual disease. In fact, high-intensity signal on T2-weighted sequences, unrestricted signal on DWI, and high value on ADC mapping is frequently related to postsurgical edema and inflammation, whereas restriction on DWI and low ADC value is suggestive of active tumor cells [26].

The correct way to quantify and assess tumor response to treatment is evaluation of tumor dimensional changes on CT or MRI and laboratory tests for tumor markers. Furthermore, a high value on ADC mapping is related to a positive treatment response. That is because chemotherapy causes necrosis inside the tumor, resulting in increased diffusion of water molecules and consequently increased ADC value.

6.3.3 Disadvantages of Conventional Magnetic Resonance with Diffusion-weighted Imaging

Disadvantages of MRI are represented by high cost, long acquisition time, and motion and susceptibility artifacts. Disadvantages of DWI are mainly related to low spatial resolution and some possible pitfalls. Sometimes, tissues presenting long T2 relaxation time, such as cysts or postsurgery edema that may appear hyperintense on high b values, is a phenomenon called T2 shine through. That artifact can cause misinterpretation of radiological images, inducing false positive findings; ADC mapping can rectify this problem. On the other hand, a low ADC value suggests real restriction of water diffusion [22], which indicates neoplastic disease.

As mentioned earlier, the increased cell density on DWI permits recognition of neoplastic tissues due to restriction of water movement represented by high signal intensity on high b value and low signal intensity on ADC mapping. However, some types of tumor, such mucinous tumors and well-differentiated adenocarcinomas, have a lower cell density and therefore may show low signal intensity on high b values [22]. Moreover, some densely cellular normal tissue, such as bowel mucosa, endometrium, and normal lymph nodes, present restricted diffusion appearing hyperintense in DWI with low ADC values. In posttreatment follow-up, anatomical modification in the postoperative abdomen and the small size of recurrent tumors decrease diagnostic accuracy due to formation of fibrotic tissue that can present restricted diffusion and low ADC values [22]. Necrosis and abscesses also have high values on DWI sequences with high b values but generally present higher values on the ADC map [22] and different enhancement after contrast administration. Therefore, interpretation of DW images needs to be performed in conjunction with conventional MRI.

6.4 Positron Emission Tomography/Computed Tomography

6.4.1 Imaging Technique

In clinical practice, PET with [^{18}F]-fluorodeoxyglucose (FDG) PET has significantly improved in diagnostic accuracy and now exerts a major impact on patient management, in particular for diagnosis, staging, therapy monitoring, and restaging recurrent disease. [^{18}F]-FDG-PET is based on identifying the increase in glycolytic activity in malignant cells, which preferably concentrate glucose due to increased membrane transporters of glucose (GLUT-1). Imaging systems that combine [^{18}F]-FDG-PET and CT allow simultaneous evaluation. Anatomical and functional total-body [^{18}F]-FDG-PET/CT imaging is routinely performed using the Hamacher method of injecting patients with 5 MBq/kg of [^{18}F]-FDG hydrated with 500 ml of saline solution. PET/CT acquisition in 2D mode begins 60 min after IV administration. The axis of both systems is mechanically aligned to move the patient from the CT into the PET gantry by moving the examination table by 60 cm. Finally, PET and CT images are coregistered on hardware. Patients are usually scanned in the supine position, starting from the head and moving to just above the first scanning position on the CT scanner. Before scanning the patient, a scout view is obtained to define axial imaging range. Acquisition parameters are 120 kV, 80 mA, tube-rotation time 0.8 s, pitch 1.5).

PET/CT is performed after CT, covering the same field of view (FOV) and with acquisition time ~ 4 min per table position. Axial and other MPR images can be used to detect peritoneal disease and check the common peritoneal site of pathological involvement.

6.4.2 Advantages of Positron Emission Tomography/Computed Tomography

Combining morphological and functional imaging has clear advantages in oncological imaging, particularly for evaluating peritoneal malignancies. The role of PET in diagnosing malignant neoplastic disease in the ovary remains controversial. A recent study demonstrates good diagnostic accuracy in differentiating malignant and benign ovarian tumors; [^{18}F]-FDG-PET shows 87–100 % sensitivity, 74–100 % specificity, and 92–97 % accuracy [27]. Detecting ovarian cancer (OC) depends on lesion the size. This may be due to resolution limitations with PET despite the availability of integrated PET/CT systems, for which diagnosing microscopic lesions remains barely feasible.

The key role of [^{18}F]-FDG-PET in PC evaluation is the presurgical evaluation of abdominal and retroperitoneal lymph node and distant metastases (N/M), in which functional imaging may have a higher morphology. Kitajima et al. reported that in detecting pelvic metastases and para-aortic lymph nodes, CT sensitivity, specificity, and accuracy were, respectively, 37.5 %, 100 % and 86.5 %, whereas those of PET/CE-CT were 81.3 %, 96.6 %, and 93.2 % [27, 28].

Morphological imaging, however, is limited in detecting early response to therapy because anatomical changes are usually visible only 2–3 months after therapy, whereas metabolic changes appear after two to three sessions of chemotherapy. Functional imaging using PET/CT is somewhat crucial in identifying nonresponsive patients, thus improving patient management, avoiding the use of ineffective therapies, helping avoid adverse effects, and reducing delay before administering a more effective treatment, thus decreasing costs.

Nishiyama et al. shown that reducing the standard uptake value (SUV) after the first cycle of chemotherapy can predict response to chemotherapy or chemoradiotherapy in patients with gynecological cancers (uterine, $n = 13$; ovarian, $n = 8$) [29]: on the basis of histopathological analysis of surgical samples, 10 patients were responsive and 11 nonresponsive. Considering a cutoff SUV of 3.8 to differentiate between responsive and nonresponsive patients, [^{18}F]-FDG-PET showed a sensitivity of 90 %, a specificity of 63.6 %, and an accuracy of 76.2 %; considering SUV variation of 65 %, [^{18}F]-FDG-PET showed a sensitivity of 90 %, a specificity of 81.8 %, and an accuracy of 85.7 %.

In the course of restaging after initial debulking surgery and chemotherapy in first-line treatment, it is important to assess the possible presence of residual or recurrence of disease during follow-up. Approximately 20–30 % of patients with early-stage disease and 50–75 % with advanced disease who obtain complete response after first-line therapy may experience subsequent relapse. The clinical follow-up generally includes serum CA 125, physical examination, and conventional imaging tests.

CT and MRI are the imaging methods most commonly used in patients with suspected recurrence of OC; however, they have limitations in distinguishing residual tumor from necrosis or fibrosis and in characterizing distant lymph node, bone, and muscle metastases. [^{18}F]-FDG-PET compared with physical examination and CT scan shows a sensitivity of 73–100 %, a specificity of 71–100 %, and accuracy of 83–100 % [30], primarily due to the high-contrast resolution (Fig. 6.4). However, compared with [^{18}F]-FDG-PET plus histopathology obtained during a second-look laparotomy evaluation, the diagnostic accuracy of [^{18}F]-FDG-PET alone tends to be lower, with a reported sensitivity, specificity, and accuracy of 53–83 %, 40–86 %, and 63–82 %, respectively [30]. These discrepancies are attributable to the fact that small lesions may not be seen due to the lower resolution of [^{18}F]-FDG-PET. Therefore, [^{18}F]-FDG-PET is a noninvasive imaging methodology that is more accurate for restaging, especially for assessing peritoneal spread and lymph node, bone, and muscle metastases because it allows imaging of the entire body in a single examination.

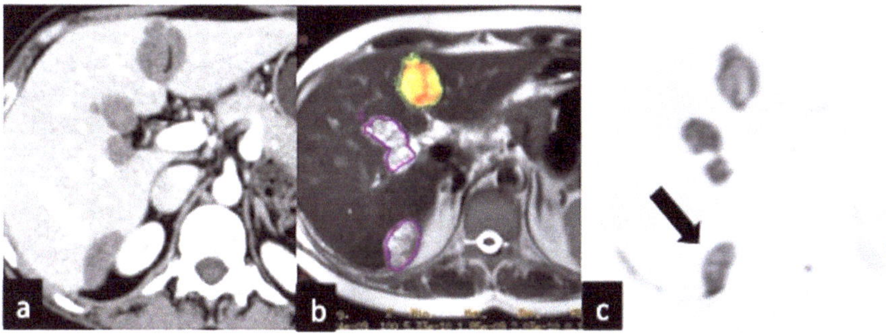

Fig. 6.4 Peritoneal cystic implants (*arrows*) above the liver surface (at the hilum, near the falciform ligament, and within Morison's pouch) on (**a**) axial computed tomography (CT), (**b**) axial magnetic resonance imaging (MRI), and (**c**) on positron emission tomography (PET/CT) in a patient with metastatic ovarian cancer. PET/CT shows the highest contrast resolution

6.4.3 Disadvantages of Positron Emission Tomography/Computed Tomography

The disadvantages of PET/CT imaging are mainly related to high costs and poor availability of the equipment around the world, which often prevents its routine use. Another important drawback of PET/CT is its lower spatial resolution and lower sensitivity for lesions < 1 cm, resulting in reduced sensitivity in detecting small implants, particularly during the first staging.

6.5 Preoperative Staging of Peritoneal Disease

The task of preoperative imaging is to determine accurate extension of peritoneal disease, stratifying patients who are good surgical candidates from those who may be candidates for NACT in an attempt to reduce tumor burden. The PCI, introduced by Jacquet and Sugarbaker [13], is considered the most accurate system for staging PC from different primary tumor types based on quantification and distribution of peritoneal implants found at laparotomy. According to this method, the abdominopelvic area is subdivided into 13 sections (nine areas plus relating to the small bowel) (Fig. 6.5). PC lesion size is rated on a four-point scale ranging from 0 to 3 points, with a possible maximum score of 39: LS 0, no tumor detected; LS 1, tumor up to 0.5 cm maximum diameter, LS 2, tumor > 0.5 cm up to 5 cm in maximum diameter; LS 3, tumor or confluent lesions > 5 cm in maximum diameter [31].

The PCI score also represents a widely validated and precise quantitative prognostic indicator [2, 3], predicting whether complete resection of peritoneal implants can be achieved after cytoreductive surgery plus hyperthermic

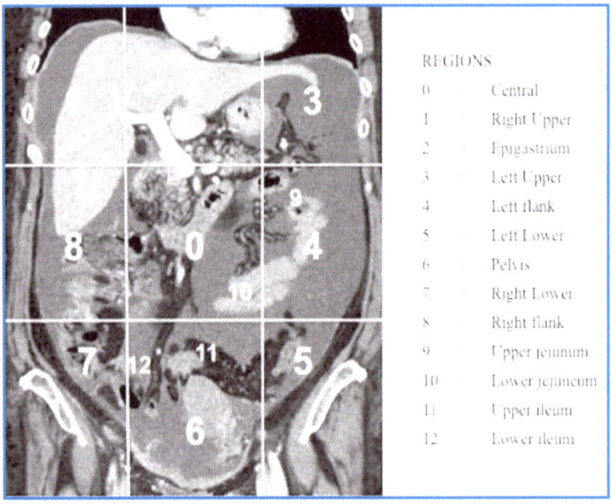

Fig. 6.5 Preoperative staging of peritoneal carcinomatosis (PC). The abdomiopelvis is virtually subdivided into 13 areas: nine areas plus four relating to the small bowel

intraperitoneal chemotherapy (CRS plus HIPEC). Assessing potentially nonresectable or nonoptimally cytoreducible disease that can contraindicate CRS plus HIPEC comprises the following diagnostic criteria [32]:

- Extensive involvement of the small bowel or mesenteric root
- Involved lymph node superior to the celiac axis
- Pleural infiltration
- Pelvic sidewall invasion
- Bladder trigone involvement
- Hepatic parenchymal metastases or implants near the right hepatic vein or the porta hepatis
- PCI > 12 for gastric and > 20 for colorectal cancer [21, 31]; > 30 for less-invasive mucinous appendiceal and OC [33–36]

6.5.1 Preoperative Assessment of Peritoneal Cancer Index: Comparison between Imaging Modalities

6.5.1.1 Multidetector Computed Tomography

MDCT, using an adequate diagnostic technique, has a high mean sensitivity of 89 % for implants measuring ≥ 5 mm but a sensitivity of 43 % for implants with a diameter < 5 mm [7].

Main advantages:

- Wide availability
- Short execution time
- Lower cost
- Multiplanar imaging
- Thin section (1–3 mm)

- High spatial resolution
- Few or absent artifacts

Main disadvantages:

- Low contrast resolution
- Moderate sensitivity for implants < 5 mm
- Diagnostic accuracy strictly depending on CT technique and radiologist experience

MDCT remains the modality of choice for primary staging, especially in patients with poor compliance for diagnostic examinations, providing a great deal of information about a large volume of tissue in just a few minutes and permitting assessment of metastatic extraperitoneal disease.

6.5.1.2 Magnetic Resonance Imaging

MRI offers excellent soft-tissue contrast to depict small-volume peritoneal tumors using both conventional and DWI sequences. The reported overall sensitivity of conventional MRI with DWI for PC assessment is 90 % [21], and sensitivity for lesions < 10 mm remains satisfactory, corresponding to 85 %, which is higher than that of CT, which ranges from 25 % to 50 %.

Main Advantages:

- High-contrast resolution
- High sensitivity also for implants < 10 mm
- Free from radiation exposure
- Multiplanar imaging
- Higher spatial resolution in the studies of pelvic malignancies
- DWI with morphological unenhanced sequences offers an accurate alterative method in case of reported allergy or renal failure, which contraindicate enhanced MDCT

Main Disadvantages

- Every contraindication to MRI must be considered
- Lack of relative availability
- Not recommended in patients with poor compliance
- Higher costs in some centers
- Imaging artifacts
- Longer acquisition time
- Metastatic extra-abdominal disease is not evaluated
- Difficulties in differentiating between postsurgery edema, cysts, and other benign findings
- Diagnostic accuracy strictly depends on MRI technique and radiologist experience

MRI with conventional and DWI should be always considered the modality of choice for primary staging of abdominal disease, especially in young and tolerant patients. In those cases, additional CT to study the thorax should be also considered.

MRI with conventional and DWI can be performed after MDCT in cases in which CT is executed with a suboptimal technique or if equivocal CT findings requiring a superior diagnostic method to achieve detailed surgical planning or determine whether the patient needs neoadjuvant chemotherapy.

6.5.1.3 [^{18}F]-Fluorodeoxyglucose Positron Emission Tomography/Computed Tomography

[^{18}F]-FDG-PET/CT provides metabolic information enabling the identification of malignant lesions with high-contrast resolution due to their augmented glucose consumption. Klumpp et al. reported sensitivity and specificity values for PET/CT of 92–93 % and 94–96 %, respectively, which is higher than MRI (sensitivity 87 %, specificity 86–92 %) [37]. In a meta-analysis, Chang et al. reported an overall pooled estimated sensitivity and specificity of FDG-PET or PET/CT scans in PC detection of 72.4 % and 96.7 %, respectively [38].

Main advantages:
- High sensitivity and specificity
- Higher contrast resolution than conventional MDCT
- Multiplanar imaging
- Few or absent artifacts
- Better interobserver agreement in comparison with MDCT and MRI, as well as better correlation

Main Disadvantages:
- Poor availability
- High cost
- Lower spatial resolution
- Long execution time

6.5.2 Personal Experience

In June 2008, our team created a tight connection with a group of surgeons from the Department of Surgery, "Sapienza" University, Rome, who seldom use HIPEC, in an attempt to evaluate MDCT accuracy in the preoperative definition of the PCI in patients with advanced OC, colonic, and gastric cancer who underwent peritonectomy (PRT) plus HIPEC. In our series, we evaluated up 120 patients affected by ovarian, gastric, and colonic carcinomatosis, attaining very good sensitivity (up to 90 %) in evaluation of the 13 abdominopelvic areas, with overall sensitivity of ~ 85 % and acceptable overall specificity for all regions except for mesenteric root, pelvic sidewall invasion, and Treitz ligament region, in which specificity values varied between reader experience from 40–65 %. Due to the poor results in the latter instances, in 2012, we began using DW-MRI for patients in whom results were unclear. In some patients, we obtained better specificity in the mesenteric root, porta hepatis, and pelvic sidewall in comparison with MDCT. Of the 13 abdominopelvic areas, the best results were obtained in the splenic hilum (region 3), with sensitivity 91 % and specificity 90 %, and overall positive (PPV) and negative (NPV) predictive values of 95 % and 88 %, respectively. This was also the case for both hemidiaphragms, with 94 % and 95 % sensitivity and specificity and PPV and NPV 90 % and 90 %, respectively

We found that there is a learning curve in radiological evaluation using the PCI that is clearly related to the level of radiologist experience. This is true for interpretation time as well as for sensitivity and specificity results.

6.5.3 Conclusions

MDCT, MR with DWI and CT/PET are accurate and complementary diagnostic tools to recognize and report in detail spread of peritoneal disease offering a map of neoplastic implants, and an accurate calculation of PCI score with final aim to plan the optimal patient treatment.

6.6 Laparoscopy

Laparoscopy is increasingly being used among the many available diagnostic tools as a promising means in diagnostic workup of patients with peritoneal surface malignancies (PSM), providing direct access to the peritoneal cavity and therefore allowing better evaluation of disease. There is as yet no general agreement regarding its routine use, although it may be appropriately performed in selected cases in which the other clinical and imaging techniques fail to provide accurate assessment of intra-abdominal and pelvic disease spread. The main indications for video laparoscopic surgery (VLS) are:

- Diagnosis:
  - To confirm the presence of peritoneal metastases when other imaging techniques give uncertain results
  - To obtain tissue samples for histopathological study for diagnosing the primary tumor
- Staging:
  - To evaluate intra-abdominal tumor spread, assess resectability, and predict optimal CRS in primary and recurrent PC
  - To assess response to neoadjuvant/adjuvant chemotherapy

While no there are no reported negative consequences of laparoscopy when histological confirmation is needed, some controversy exists about its routine use for staging purposes, especially regarding the possibility of providing more information about actually disease extent compared with noninvasive diagnostics. In the majority of patients, clinical data and imaging techniques (CT, MRI, PET/CT) normally provide enough information for accurate staging and excluding patients with unresectable disease.

In high-volume specialized centers, optimal cytoreduction is achieved even without laparoscopy in ~ 80–90 % of cases, with complete cytoreduction (CC) in 60–70 % [39–41]. These data seem to suggest that current preoperative diagnostic workup, in which laparoscopy is not routine, allows appropriate resectability evaluation and the possibility of optimal cytoreduction in most cases selected for surgery. These data concur with literature reports in which laparoscopy is included in the preoperative workup of patients with PSM in < 10 % of cases [42]. In our personal experience, we performed a laparoscopic procedure in 43 (13.2 %) patients scheduled for CRS plus HIPEC.

In 2006, results of a survey reported at the Fifth International Workshop on Peritoneal Surface Malignancy regarding consensus on preoperative investigations [43] showed that laparoscopy was fundamental in 9.4 %, useful in 78.1 %, and useless in 12.5 % of cases by a worldwide expertise panel. More recently, a Cochrane Review by Rutten et al. [44] on the role of laparoscopy to establish resectability in patients with advanced OC concluded that "…laparoscopy should not be a standard procedure in clinical practice" and that "…no statement can be made on whether laparoscopy is more accurate than clinical and radiological diagnostic workup." Nevertheless, some recent reports emphasize the efficacy of diagnostic laparoscopy to predict resectability and optimal CRS, achieving a PPV for resectability ranging from 87.5–97 % of cases. Regarding optimal CRS predictability, Fagotti et al. reported a 100 % accuracy for anticipating possible optimal CRS using a Predictive Index Score (PIS) in ovarian PC [45–49] (Table 6.1).

6.6.1 Personal Experience

In our personal experience with CRS plus HIPEC, we performed diagnostic laparoscopy in 43 patients (Table 6.2). In two patients with recurrent disease, laparoscopy could not be performed or completed due to adhesions or massive abdominal invasion. Eleven patients underwent laparoscopy to achieve histological confirmation, and four patients where investigated to assess results of NACT and confirm indication and timing of CRS plus HIPEC. VLS to assess resectability was performed in nine primary PSM and 19 recurrent PSM patients. Regardless of indications, laparoscopic PCI evaluation was obtained for all patients and compared with the PCI evaluated at open surgery (Table 6.3). Results were substantially similar, confirming the accuracy of VLS in evaluating the extent of intra-abdominal disease; it was also able to predict resectability in 95 % of cases, even if in patients with recurrent disease results were somewhat conflicting. In 39 patients, we could reach optimal cytoreduction (CC-0, CC-1); two patients were unresectable, one due to massive tumor infiltration of the first jejunal loop and the other of the porta hepatis.

To draw definitive conclusions when comparing VLS with other commonly used and less invasive diagnostic tools, a cost–benefit analysis should be carefully evaluated considering:

Table 6.1 Staging laparoscopy reported in the literature

Study [Reference]	Patients (*N*) and PSM	Operative time (min)	Complications and morbidity	Hospital stay (days)	Resectability PPV (%)	Resectability NPV (%)	Nonoptimal CRS PPV (%)	Laparoscopy accuracy (%)
Pomel et al. [45]	11 mixed	Median 38 (range 23-57)	18 % 1 serosal injury 1 postoperative trocar ascitic leakage	Median 1.7	87.5	NA	NA	NA
Garofalo and Valle [46]	197 mixed	Mean 35 (range 15-45)	2 % 1 trocar infection 1 intraoperative bleeding 1 diaphragm perforation	NA	96	NA	NA	NA
Laterza et al. [47]	33 Mesothelioma	Mean 40 (range 20-60)	None	NA	97	97	NA	NA
Fagotti et al. [49]	113 Ovarian	NA	None	NA	NA	NA	100[a]	77.3–100

PPV, positive predictive value; *NPV*, negative predictive value
[a]Predictive index value > 8 according to Fagotti score [48]

Table 6.2 Video laparoscopic surgery (VLS) in patients selected for cytoreductive surgery plus hyperthermic intraperitoneal chemotherapy (CRS plus HIPEC) (43/326 patients)

No. patients	VLS indications	Histology	Complications
11	Cyto-histological typization	4 ovarian 2 mesothelioma 2 PMP 3 other	1 postoperative trocar ascitic leakage
Preoperative Assessment			
4	Post-NACT	3 ovarian 1 gastric	None
9	Primary PSM	5 gastric 2 colorectal 2 ovarian	None
19	Recurrence PSM	11 ovarian 4 colorectal 4 other	2 VLS unfeasible

PSM, peritoneal surface malignancy; *NACT*, neoadjuvant chemotherapy

- Rate of VLS-related complications
- Intra-abdominal tumor spread influencing VLS feasibility
- Trocar-site metastases

Complication grade and rates are low in literature reports, even if invasiveness, need for general anesthesia, and the sometimes poor clinical conditions of patients have to be considered, especially when an early second major surgical procedure is scheduled (CRS plus HIPEC).

Trocar-site metastasis after a laparoscopic approach for removing various intra-abdominal tumors is reported in many papers [50]. However, no clear data are available regarding trocar-site metastases after a diagnostic or staging laparoscopy in patients with PSM for whom a higher incidence would be expected due to the presence in 60 % of cases of malignant ascites, which is considered a predisposing factor for their development [51–53]. Of the 53 patients in our series who underwent a diagnostic or staging laparoscopy (41 done in our institution and 12 performed elsewhere during previous hospitalizations), 22 (41.5 %) developed trocar-site metastases. Time interval between procedure and metastases is highly variable and seems to be correlated with tumor type [51]; incidence seems also related to the number of trocars used. As excision of port-site metastases is difficult, is therefore be recommended to use the least possible number of trocars and, if possible, place them all in the midline [54].

The general impression is that literature reports tend to minimize adverse effects while emphasizing advantages in terms of diagnostic accuracy and predictivity of optimal cytoreduction. However, in specialized centers relying on preoperative PCI or similar classifications to select patients for CRS plus HIPEC, the use of laparoscopy seems to be growing and is routinely used in

Table 6.3 Peritoneal Cancer Index (PCI) comparing laparoscopy versus laparotomy and resectability (41 patients)

Indications	No. patients	Laparoscopic PCI			χ^2	CRS PCI			Resectability (%)
		0–13	14–26	27–39		0–13	14–26	27–39	
Cyto-histological typization	11	2	7	2	← ns →	1	7	3	90.9
Preoperative assessment:									
Post-NACT	4	3	1	0	← ns →	3	1	0	100
Primary	9	1	5	3	← ns →	0	6	3	100
Recurrence	17	5	9	3	← ns →	5	11	1	94.1
Total	41	11	22	8		9	25	7	
Unresectability						0	2	0	

NACT, neoadjuvant chemotherapy; *CRS*, cytoreductive surgery; *ns*, not significant

many centers, even if no clear data or prospective randomized trials are available to support its use in patients with peritoneal metastases from many primary tumor types. VLS seems, instead, to play a relevant role in predicting resectability in PSM from primary gastric cancer and to evaluate the efficacy of the increasing use of aggressive neoadjuvant intraperitoneal and systemic chemotherapy (NIPS) [55].

6.6.2 Conclusions

In conclusion, laparoscopy can play an important role in diagnosing PSM, particularly for histological confirmation and resectability evaluation. For preoperative staging, further prospective controlled studies are needed to confirm the potential indications and efficacy of VLS compared with other noninvasive diagnostic tools while considering risks and complications.

BOX 6.1 Different patterns of appearance of Peritoneal Carcinomatosis at Multidetector CT

Pattern	Findings	Image
Micronodular	Tiny 1- to 5-mm milky spots of peritoneal implants (*arrow*) diffusely involving the tunica serosa and subserosal fat. Greater omentum, lesser omentum, and mesentery are typically involved, as shown in this axial contrast-enhanced image	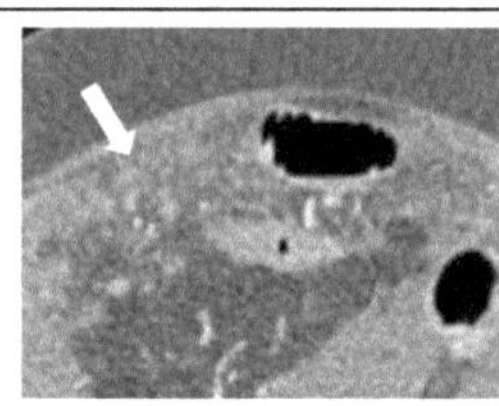
Nodular	Nodules with a diameter > 5 mm diffusely involving the tunica serosa and subserosal fat. Nodules may have an oval shape with rounded contours or present a stellate pattern, with star-shaped appearance and spiculated margins (axial contrast-enhanced computed tomography image *arrow*)	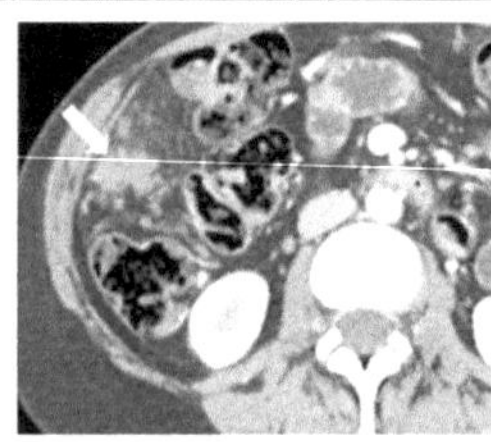
Omental cake	Omental cake can be defined as a stratified consolidation of the omental fat due to diffuse nodular involvement of the greater omentum combined with a fibrotic tissue reaction, as shown in this axial contrast-enhanced computed tomography image (*asterisks*)	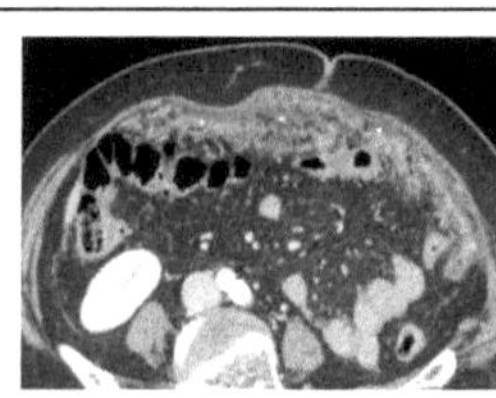

Plaque like	Confluence of multiple nodular implants forms irregular soft-tissue thickenings of inconstant extension that coat abdominal viscera and peritoneal walls, usually scalloping liver (*asterisks*) and splenic surfaces and presenting a lower attenuation than the parenchyma on contrast-enhanced scans. It is typically found in subdiaphragmatic spaces and better depicted on coronal reformatted images	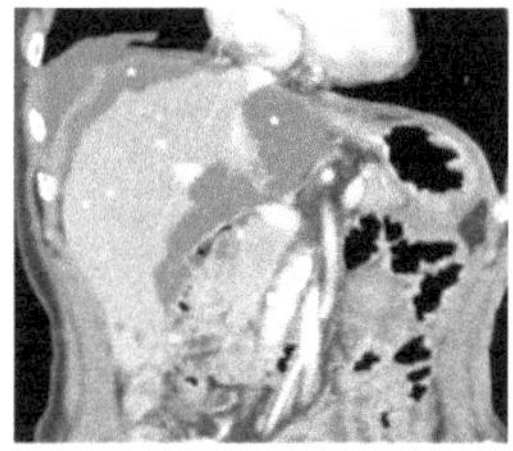
Mass like	Confluence of multiple nodular implants, usually in the pelvis, leads to formation of tissue mass that can reach sizes of several centimeters. When a single mass is ~ 10 cm in diameter or larger, it is called a bulky tumor (axial contrast-enhanced computed tomography, *asterisks*)	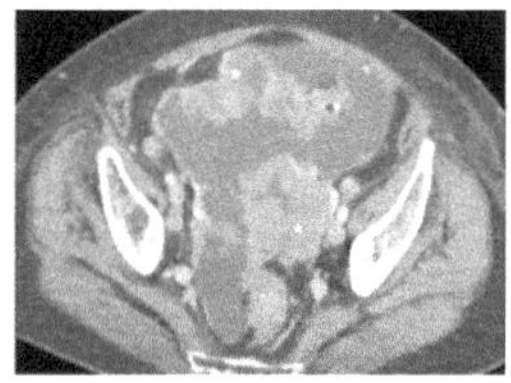
Teca aspect and ileal freezing	Small-bowel loops appear completely enveloped by a thickened layer of visceral peritoneum that covers the bowel loops as a sleeve, a condition called Teca aspect: **a** axial contrast-enhanced computed tomography (*arrow*). **b** Sometimes, neoplastic tissue that completely coated the small-bowel loops causes small-bowel obstruction with consequent dilatation of proximal loops (*asterisk*), a condition called ileal freezing	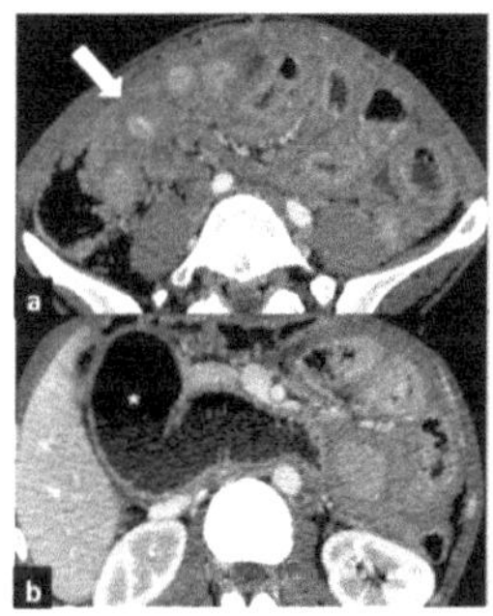
Ascites	The presence of ascites within the peritoneal cavity is usually one of the first indications of peritoneal carcinomatosis (PC) (*asterisks*). In patients with PC, increased peritoneal fluid, or ascites, is usually seen. In some cases, ascites is little or absent. The mechanism of fluid formation includes increased capillary permeability, fluid production, and obstructed lymphatic vessels with decreased absorption. At computed tomography (CT) and magnetic resonance imaging (MRI), respectively, scans are acquired with the patient in the supine position during and after inspiration. That is why fluid accumulates especially in subdiaphragmatic spaces, paracolic gutters, and epiploon retro-cavity	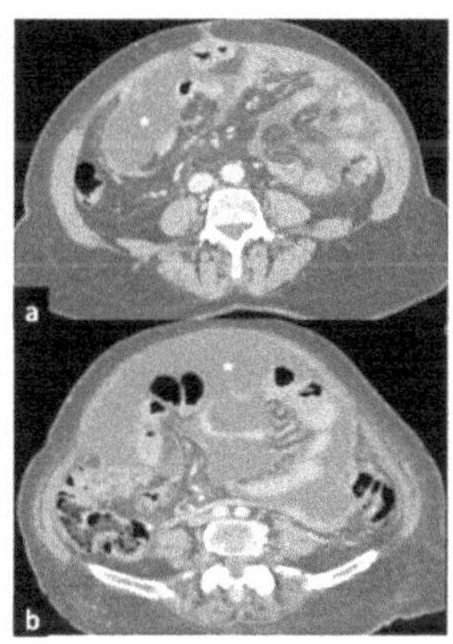

References

1. Patel CM, Sahdev A, Reznek RH (2011) CT, MRI and PET imaging in peritoneal malignancy Cancer Imaging 11:123-139
2. Iafrate F, Ciolina M, Laghi A et al (2012) Peritoneal carcinomatosis: imaging with 64-MDCT and 3T MRI with diffusion-weighted imaging. Abdom Imaging 37:616-627
3. Koh JL, Yan TD, Glenn D, Morris DL (2009) Evaluation of preoperative computed tomography in estimating peritoneal cancer index in colorectal peritoneal carcinomatosis. Ann Surg Oncol 16:327-333
4. Verwaal VJ, Bruin S, Boot H et al (2008) 8-Year follow-up of randomized trial: cytoreduction and hyperthermic intraperitoneal chemotherapy versus systemic chemotherapy in patients with peritoneal carcinomatosis of colorectal cancer. Ann Surg Oncol 15:2633–2635
5. Esquivel J, Sticca R, Sugarbaker P et al (2007) Cytoreductive surgery and hyperthermic intraperitoneal chemotherapy in the management of peritoneal surface malignancies of colonic origin: a consensus statement. Society of Surgical Oncology. Ann Surg Oncol 14:128–133
6. Kim SJ, Kim HH, Kim YH et al (2009) Peritoneal metastasis: detection with 16- or 64-detector row CT in patients undergoing surgery for gastric cancer. Radiology 253:407-415
7. Marin D, Catalano C, Baski M et al (2010) 64-Section multi- detector row CT in the preoperative diagnosis of peritoneal carci- nomatosis: correlation with histopathological findings. Abdom Imaging 35:694–700
8. Pannu HK, Bristow r, Montz F, Fishman EK (2003) Multidetector CT of peritoneal cersinomatosis from ovarian cancer. Radiographics 23:687-701
9. Jacquet P, Jelinek JS, Steves MA, Sugarbaker PH (1993) Evaluation of computed tomography in patients with peritoneal carcinomatosis. Cancer 72:1631–1636
10. Amendola MA (1985) The role of CT in the evaluation of ovarian malignancy. CRC Crit Rev Diagn Imaging 24:329–368
11. Coakley FV, Hricak H (1999) Imaging of peritoneal and mesenteric disease: key concepts for the clinical radiologist. Clin Radiol 54:563-574
12. Bristow RE, Duska LR, Lambrou NC et al (2000) A model for predicting surgical outcome in patients with advanced ovarian carcinoma using computed tomography. Cancer 89:1532–1540
13. Jang YJ, Kim JK, Park SB, Cho KS (2007) Variable CT findings of epithelial origin ovarian carcinoma according to the degree of histologic differentiation. Korean J Radiol 8:120-126
14. Tempany CM, Zou KH, Silverman SG et al (2000) Staging of advanced ovarian cancer: comparison of imaging modalities—report from the Radiological Diagnostic Oncology Group.Radiology 215:761–767
15. De Bree E, Koops W, Kröger R et al (2004) Peritoneal carcinomatosis from colorectal or appendiceal origin: correlation of pre-operative CT with intraoperative findings and evaluation of interobserver agreement. J Surg Oncol 86:64–73
16. Coakley FV, Choi P, Poturi B et al (2002) Peritoneal metastases detection with spiral CT in patient with ovarian cancer. Radiology 223:495-499
17. Patel CM, Sahdev A, Reznek RH (2011) CT, MRI and PET imaging in peritoneal malignancy. Cancer Imaging 11:123-139
18. Woodward PJ, Hosseinzadeh K, Saenger JS (2004) From the archives of the AFIP: radio- logic staging of ovarian carcinoma with pathologic correlation. RadioGraphics 24:225–246
19. Low RN, Barone RM, Lacey C et al (1997) Peritoneal tumor: MR imaging with dilute oral barium and intravenous gadolinium-containing contrast agents compared with unenhanced MR imaging and CT. Radiology 204:513–520
20. Fujii S, Matsusue E, Kanasaki Y et al (2008) Detection of peritoneal dissemination in gynecological malignancy: evaluation by diffusion-weighted MR imaging. Eur Radiol 18:18-23
21. Low RN1, Barone RM (2012) Combined diffusion-weighted and gadolinium-enhanced MRI can accurately predict the peritoneal cancer index preoperatively in patients being considered for cytoreductive surgical procedures. Ann Surg Oncol 19:1394-1401

22. Low RN (2007) MR imaging of the peritoneal spread of malignancy. Abdom Imaging 32:26783
23. Kyriazi S, Collins DJ, Morgan VA et al (2010) Diffusion-weighted imaging of peritoneal disease for noninvasive staging of advanced ovarian cancer. Radiographics 30:1269-1285
24. Low RN (2007) MR imaging of the peritoneal spread of malignancy. Abdom Imaging 32:267–283
25. Low RN, Sebrechts CP, Barone RM, Muller W (2009) Diffusion-weighted MRI of peritoneal tumors: comparison with conventional MRI and surgical and histopathologic findings—a feasibility study. AJR Am J Roentgenol 193:461–470
26. Koh DM, Collins DJ (2007) Diffusion-weighted MRI in the body: applications and challenges in oncology. AJR Am J Roentgenol 188:1622–1635
27. Kitajima K, Murakami K et al (2011) Present and future of FDG-PET/CT in ovarian cancer. Ann Nucl Med 25:155-164
28. Fanti S, Nanni C et al (2006) Supra-clavicular lymph node metastatic spread in patients with ovarian cancer disclosed a 18F-FDG-PET/CT: an unusual finding. Cancer Imaging 23:20-23
29. Nishiyama Y, Yamamoto Y et al (2008) Monitoring the neoadjuvant therapy response in gynecological cancer patients using FDG PET. Eur J Nucl Med Mol Imaging 35:287-295
30. Yuan Y, Gu ZX et al (2012) Computer tomography, magnetic resonance imaging, and positron emission tomography or positron emission tomography/computer tomography for detection of metastatic lymphnodes in patients with ovarian cancer: a meta-analysis. Eur J Radiol 81:1002-1006
31. Esquivel J, Sticca R, Sugarbaker P, Levine E, Yan TD, Alexander R, Baratti D, Bartlett D, Barone R, Barrios P, Bieligk S, Bretcha-Boix P, Chang CK, Chu F, Chu Q, Daniel S, de Bree E, Deraco M, Dominguez-Parra L, Elias D, Flynn R, Foster J, Garofalo A, Gilly FN, Glehen O, Gomez-Portilla A, Gonzalez-Bayon L,Gonzalez-Moreno S, Goodman M, Gushchin V, Hanna N, Hartmann J, Harrison L, Hoefer R, Kane J, Kecmanovic D, Kelley S, Kuhn J, Lamont J, Lange J, Li B,Loggie B, Mahteme H, Mann G, Martin R, Misih RA, Moran B, Morris D, Onate-Ocana L, Petrelli N, Philippe G, Pingpank J, Pitroff A, Piso P, Quinones M, Riley L,Rutstein L, Saha S, Alrawi S, Sardi A, Schneebaum S, Shen P, Shibata D, Spellman J, Stojadinovic A, Stewart J, Torres-Melero J, Tuttle T, Verwaal V, Villar J,Wilkinson N, Younan R, Zeh H, Zoetmulder F, Sebbag G; Society of Surgical Oncology Annual Meeting (2007) Cytoreductive surgery and hyperthermic intraperitoneal chemotherapy in the management of peritoneal surface malignancies of colonic origin: a consensus statement. Ann Surg Oncol 14:128–133
32. Nougaret S, Addley HC, Colombo PE et al (2012) Ovarian carcinomatosis: how the radiologist can help plan the surgical approach. Radiographics 32:1775-800
33. Sugarbaker PH, Ronnett BM, Archer A et al (1997) Pseudomyxoma peritonei syndrome. Adv Surg 30:233–80
34. Sugarbaker PH (1999) Results of treatment of 385 patients with peri- toneal surface spread of appendiceal malignancy. Ann Surg Oncol 6:727–31
35. Vaira M, Cioppa T, D'Amico S et al (2010) Peritoneal colorectal car- cinomatosis treated with surgery and perioperative intraperitoneal chemotherapy: retrospective analysis of 523 patients from a multicentric French study. J Clin Oncol 28:63–68
36. Glehen O, Kwiatkowski F, Sugarbaker PH et al (2005) Cytoreductive surgery combined with perioperative intraperitoneal chemother- apy for the management of peritoneal carcinomatosis from colo- rectal cancer: a multi-institutional study. J Clin Oncol 22:3284–3292
37. Klumpp BD1, Schwenzer N, Aschoff P et al (2013) Preoperative assessment of peritoneal carcinomatosis: intraindividual comparison of 18F-FDG PET/CT and MRI. Abdom Imaging 38:64-71
38. Chang MC, Chen JH, Liang JA et al (2013) PET or PET/CT for detection of peritoneal carcinomatosis: a meta-analysis. Clin Nucl Med 38:623-629
39. Glehen O, Kwiatkowski F, Sugarbaker PH et al (2004) Cytoreductive surgery combined with perioperative intraperitoneal chemotherapy for the management of peritoneal carcinomatosis from colorectal cancer: a multi-institutional study. J Clin Oncol 22:3284-3292

40. Yan TD, Sim J, Morris DL (2007) Selection of patients with colorectal peritoneal carcinomatosis for cytoreductive surgery and perioperative intraperitoneal chemotherapy. Ann Surg Oncol 14:1807-1817
41. Bakrin N, Bereder JM, Decullier E et al (2013) Peritoneal carcinomatosis treated with cytoreductive surgery and Hyperthermic Intraperitoneal Chemotherapy (HIPEC) for advanced ovarian carcinoma: a French multicentre retrospective cohort study of 566 patients. Eur J Surg Oncol 39:1435-1443
42. Glehen O, Gilly FN, Boutitie F et al (2010) Toward curative treatment of peritoneal carcinomatosis from nonovarian origin by cytoreductive surgery combined with perioperative intraperitoneal chemotherapy: a multi-institutional study of 1,290 patients. Cancer 116:5608–5618
43. Yan TD, Morris DL, Shigeki K et al (2008). Preoperative investigations in the management of peritoneal surface malignancy with cytoreductive surgery and perioperative intraperitoneal chemotherapy: Expert consensus statement. J Surg Oncol 98:224-227
44. Rutten MJ, Leeflang MM, Kenter GG et al (2014) Laparoscopy for diagnosing resectability of disease in patients with advanced ovarian cancer. Cochrane Database Syst Rev 21;2:CD009786
45. Pomel C, Appleyard TL, Gouy S et al (2005). The role of laparoscopy to evaluate candidates for complete cytoreduction of peritoneal carcinomatosis and hyperthermic intraperitoneal chemotherapy. Eur J Surg Oncol 31:540–543
46. Garofalo A, Valle M (2009) Laparoscopy in the management of peritoneal carcinomatosis. Cancer J 15:190–195
47. Laterza B, Kusamura S, Baratti D et al (2009) Role of explorative laparoscopy to evaluate optimal candidates for cytoreductive surgery and hyperthermic intraperitoneal chemotherapy (HIPEC) in patients with peritoneal mesothelioma. In Vivo 23:187–190
48. Fagotti A, Ferrandina G, Fanfani F et al (2006) A laparoscopy-based score to predict surgical outcome in patients with advanced ovarian carcinoma: a pilot study. Ann Surg Oncol 13:1156-1161
49. Fagotti A, Ferrandina G, Fanfani F et al (2008) Prospective validation of a laparoscopic predictive model for optimal cytoreduction in advanced ovarian carcinoma. Am J Obstet Gynecol 199:642.e1-6
50. Zivanovic O, Sonoda Y, Diaz JP et al (2008) The rate of port-site metastases after 2251 laparoscopic procedures in women with underlying malignant disease. Gynecol Oncol 111:431-437
51. Wang PH, Yuan CC, Lin G et al (1999) Risk factors contributing to early occurrence of port site metastases of laparoscopic surgery for malignancy. Gynecol Oncol 72:38-44
52. van Dam PA, DeCloedt J, Tjalma WA et al (1999) Trocar implantation metastasis after laparoscopy in patients with advanced ovarian cancer: can the risk be reduced? Am J Obstet Gynecol 181:536-541
53. Nagarsheth NP, Rahaman J, Cohen CJ et al (2004) The incidence of port-site metastases in gynecologic cancers. JSLS 8:133-139
54. Iversen LH, Rasmussen PC, Laurberg S (2013) Value of laparoscopy before cytoreductive surgery and hyperthermic intraperitoneal chemotherapy for peritoneal carcinomatosis. Br J Surg 100:285-292
55. Sugarbaker PH (Editor), van der Speeten K, Stuart OA et al (2012) Cytoreductive Surgery & Perioperative Chemotherapy for Peritoneal Surface Malignancy. Textbook and Video Atlas. Cine-Med Publishing: Woodbury, CT, pp. 84-85

Part II

Treatment

Prevention and Management of Peritoneal Metastases from Gastrointestinal Cancer: A Short History of a Paradigm for Peritoneal Surface Malignancies

7

Paul H. Sugarbaker

7.1 Introduction

Until the 1980s, carcinomatosis from gastrointestinal malignancy was a lethal condition. The treatments directed at peritoneal dissemination were best supportive care, palliative systemic chemotherapy, and palliative surgery when necessary. None of these treatments were in any way satisfactory. Treatment strategies that afforded prolonged survival or a chance for cure did not exist. Over the last three decades, progress with two treatment innovations continued. As a result of cytoreductive surgery (CRS) combined with hyperthermic perioperative chemotherapy (HIPEC), long-term survival has been demonstrated by institutions widely distributed around the globe. The term carcinomatosis has been abandoned because it implies this terminal condition with no substantial benefit from treatments. Rather, this dissemination of cancer into the peritoneal space is now referred to as peritoneal metastases. This is now a treatable condition in properly selected patients with gastrointestinal cancer, and a goal in selected patients is a curative approach. In this chapter, we explore the innovations that have resulted in this profound change in treatment options of peritoneal metastases from gastrointestinal cancer. Also reported are promising directions that require immediate exploration in order to continue the optimization of CRS plus HIPEC for peritoneal metastases from gastrointestinal cancer.

P. H. Sugarbaker (✉)
Center for Gastrointestinal Malignancies, Washington Cancer Institute, Washington, DC, USA
e-mail: Paul.Sugarbaker@medstar.net

A. Di Giorgio, E. Pinto (Eds), *Treatment of Peritoneal Surface Malignancies*,
Updates in Surgery
DOI: 10.1007/978-88-470-5711-1_7,

7.2 Cytoreductive Surgery and Hyperthermic Perioperative Chemotherapy as Current Standard of Care

A question of profound importance emerged as the development of treatments for peritoneal metastases progressed: Is its current acceptance by the oncologic community as a standard of care appropriate? Recent reviews from prominent centers of excellence in oncology would answer this question with a profound yes. Elias and colleagues advocated that combining complete CRS plus HIPEC can be expected to achieve cure in selected patients. They use CRS plus HIPEC for treating pseudomyxoma peritonei (PMP), malignant peritoneal mesothelioma (MPM), and colorectal peritoneal metastases with limited extent of disease on peritoneal surfaces. Also, in a limited setting, this combined treatment is of value for gastric cancer (GC) and neuroendocrine cancer to prevent or treat limited disease on peritoneal surfaces. The authors also indicate that certain rare tumors with a propensity for peritoneal dissemination but a small likelihood of systemic metastases should be considered for CRS plus HIPEC. Finally, prophylactic CRS plus HIPEC for patients with primary disease and a high risk of peritoneal metastases can be considered of value. Results of second-look surgery in selected patients must be considered an important treatment option. The authors conclude that complete CRS plus HIPEC is an "indispensible tool in the oncologist's armamentarium" [1].

A second prestigious center for cancer treatment, Memorial Sloan-Kettering Cancer Center in the USA, described their current practice. Kelly and Nash reviewed the literature and summarized the expected results for appendiceal mucinous neoplasms (AMN), colorectal cancer (CRC), GC, and diffuse MPM. They concluded that long-term survival is achieved for patients with AMN and justifies the perioperative morbidity and possible mortality of this aggressive approach. Cytoreduction with perioperative chemotherapy is "currently the standard of care for this disease." They conclude that CRC has the likelihood for systemic metastases, so that CRS plus HIPEC should be routinely combined with systemic chemotherapy. Also, patients with extensive peritoneal disease burden should be treated cautiously. However, CRS plus HIPEC can achieve long-term survival in patients with peritoneal metastases from CRC. The authors cite eight randomized trials evaluating patients with GC treated with CRS plus HIPEC or early postoperative intraperitoneal chemotherapy (EPIC) to prevent progression of peritoneal metastases. Also, they indicated promising results in managing limited peritoneal metastases in patients who can undergo gastrectomy. Finally, although the authors could not report on randomized prospective trials of CRS plus HIPEC for MPM, observational studies show superior median patient survival rates compared with historical controls, with acceptable morbidity and mortality. Currently, an aggressive regional approach to this disease is indicated. Treatment should be limited to patients with epithelioid histology, nuclear grades 1–3, and an absence of gross lymph node metastases [2].

Some institutions still do not recognize the great benefits that knowledgeable

Table 7.1 Nations approving treatment guidelines for cytoreductive surgery (CRS) and hyperthermic perioperative chemotherapy (HIPEC) as a standard of care for selected patients at experienced institutions. Approval is for appendiceal neoplasms, epithelial peritoneal mesothelioma, and colorectal cancer with limited peritoneal metastases

Nation	Year approved	Reference
France	2003	[3]
Holland	2003	[4]
Germany	2010	[5]
Spain	2012	[6]
United Kingdom	2013	[7]

and skillful application of CRS plus HIPEC have for managing peritoneal metastases. For the most part, these institutions do not have significant experience with these treatment modalities, have not seen the benefits that can be achieved in this group of patients with otherwise poor prognosis, and have been unwilling to invest in the requirements necessary to embark on this management strategy. Table 7.1 lists national guidelines of several nations around the world that now include CRS plus HIPEC as a standard of care for patients with AMN with peritoneal dissemination, epithelioid MPM, and CRC with limited peritoneal surface metastases. As shown in Table 7.1, these national guidelines occurred first in France [3], then in Holland [4], Germany [5], Spain [6], and the United Kingdom [7].

In the United States, the National Comprehensive Cancer Network guidelines have not as yet been changed to include CRS plus HIPEC for treating these three diseases. However, nearly all insurance companies in the United States authorize these treatments for their insured patients. Clearly, CRS plus HIPEC must be considered a treatment option in nations where modern cancer treatments are available.

7.3 Conceptual Changes that Contributed to the Progress of Cytoreductive Surgery and Perioperative Chemotherapy

Over the last three decades, oncologic, physiologic, and pharmacologic advances have contributed to the progress of CRS plus HIPEC treatment. No doubt, the initial success treating PMP was a "proof of principle," in which the combination of complete CRS along with a perioperative chemotherapy lavage of peritoneal surfaces could, in a select group of patients, result in long-term survival, and even a cancer cure. Two observations in patients with AMN were crucial: First, these patients rarely developed metastases to lymph nodes or liver [8]. Second, even though there was a large volume of mucinous malignancy infiltrating diaphragm undersurfaces, the omentum, pelvic peritoneum, and small bowel was uninvolved or uninvolved to the extent that CRS combined with the perioperative chemotherapy lavage could maintain the small bowel in a disease-free state [9].

A second conceptual change in the surgical approach was the development of five different peritonectomy procedures [10]. The loose attachment of the parietal peritoneum allowed complete stripping of the peritoneum from the anterior abdominal wall, the right and left subphrenic spaces, the pelvis, and the omental bursa. Because the visceral peritoneum was more intimately attached to underlying structures such as stomach, small bowel, and large bowel, these peritonectomy procedures were of necessity combined with visceral resections in order to achieve complete CRS. As time went on, methodological refinements whereby cancer nodules were removed from the small bowel were published by Bijelic and Sugarbaker [11].

A third conceptual change involves the use of intraperitoneally administered chemotherapy. Pharmacologically, a new concept regarding a peritoneal-space-to-plasma barrier was described and provided the rationale for intraperitoneal chemotherapy. The original pharmacologic principles regarding the movement of large molecules placed directly into the peritoneal space in a large volume of physiologic fluid were developed for the most part at the National Institutes of Health, Bethesda, MD, USA. Early publications by Flessner et al. in the experimental laboratory, and Myers and Collins and Speyer et al. in the clinic, suggested clinical utility of this new route of administration for cancer chemotherapy [12–14]. The importance of drug selection and proper dosimetry of intraperitoneal chemotherapy for vesicant drugs such as doxorubicin and for liver-metabolized drugs such as 5-fluorouracil (5-FU) was described by Sugarbaker et al. [15, 16]. The role of molecular size in maintaining this peritoneal-space-to-plasma barrier was clarified early on by Myers and colleagues [13].

Although little has changed over the course of the last three decades in the pharmacologic principles established by these early investigators, some clarifications of the use of chemotherapy within the peritoneal space have occurred [17]. First, it was made clear that the extent of peritonectomy had little to do with the continued presence of the peritoneal-space-to-plasma barrier. De Lima Vazquez et al. established that the percentage of parietal peritoneum removed had little or no impact on the pharmacology of intraperitoneal chemotherapy with 5-FU [18]. Second, the volume of intraperitoneal fluid used to dilute the chemotherapy solution and thereby fill the peritoneal space had an impact on the pharmacology of intraperitoneal drug instillation. Both Elias and Sideris and Sugarbaker et al. showed that a volume of intraperitoneal fluid had an impact on chemotherapy clearance into the body [19, 20]. If both volume and dose of chemotherapy were controlled, systemic exposure could be predicted, and intraperitoneal and systemic effects remained constant from patient to patient.

Perhaps the most clearly demonstrated clinical finding for successful treatment of peritoneal metastases is the absolute requirement for complete visible clearing of malignant disease from the peritoneal space for intraperitoneal chemotherapy to affect long-term survival [21].

The peritonectomy procedures were described initially by Sugarbaker in 1995 [10]. Yonemura and colleagues published similar procedures especially adapted for managing peritoneal metastases from GC [22]. Extensive visceral resections, including total gastrectomy, allowed surgical technology extension and the resulting optimal cytoreduction to a larger number of cancer patients [23].

Surgical technical advances associated with complete cytoreduction with peritonectomy involved the use of self-retaining retractors and ball-tip, high-voltage electrosurgery. A recent advance, results of which have not yet been completely realized, is the resurfacing of these extensive raw tissue surfaces with antisclerotic agents. Also needed are instructions at treatment centers in the advanced surgical technology required for complete CRS.

7.4 Early Postoperative Intraperitoneal Chemotherapy

The earliest reports of large numbers of patients with CRC and appendiceal malignancy showing long-term benefit from CRS combined with intraperitoneal chemotherapy were for treatment regimens using early postoperative intraperitoneal chemotherapy (EPIC) [21]. The most profound changes in the natural history of a peritoneal surface malignancy as a result of combined treatment seem to be in the minimally aggressive peritoneal surface malignancies, such as appendiceal cancer [24]. Elias and Pocard showed benefits from CRS with EPIC in CRC patients [25].

At the time of writing this chapter, EPIC remained the favored treatment plan for several chemotherapy agents when the intraperitoneal route of administration was favored. Drugs with a high rate of hepatic chemotherapeutic-agent extraction—so that a large proportion of the drug is detoxified with a single pass through the liver—are appropriate. These agents include 5-FU and doxorubicin [15, 26]. Also, taxanes, especially paclitaxel, are appropriate for EPIC. This drug is not significantly augmented by heat, works as a cell-cycle-specific drug that should be used over the long term, and is much better tolerated from the perspective of nausea and vomiting postadministration if given in divided doses over the first 5 days postoperatively. This drug has an area under the curve ratio of 1,000 and prolonged retention within the peritoneal space [27]. Clinical investigators are testing combinations of HIPEC and EPIC as a perioperative multidrug treatment plan, which may determine the optimal combination of these treatment strategies [28].

7.5 Heated Intraoperative Intraperitoneal Chemotherapy

The initial innovative efforts with heated intraoperative intraperitoneal chemotherapy (HIPEC) were by the efforts of Spratt et al. in 1980 [29]. Shortly thereafter, in 1988, Koga and colleagues at Tottori University, Japan, applied these treatments to patients with GC and peritoneal seeding [30]. Reports by Fujimoto et al. from Chiba University, Japan, and Yonemura et al. from Kanazawa University, Japan, should also be mentioned [31–34]. Studies from Japan involved GC patients with demonstrated peritoneal seeding or GC with adjuvant HIPEC.

Combining CRS with HIPEC was shown in a phase III trial to improve the survival of patients with CRC peritoneal seeding [35]. Also, a large retrospective multi-institutional study documented that in ~ 25% of patients with CRC treated with this combined therapy will be alive and disease free at 5 years [36]. All natural history studies suggest that these patients have a median survival limited to ≤ 6 months [37–39].

7.6 Evolution of Prognostic Indicators Useful for Patient Selection

In the early efforts to manage carcinomatosis, patients were scored as carcinomatosis present versus carcinomatosis absent. In a group of patients with peritoneal seeding, no survival at 3 years was expected in patients with gastrointestinal cancer [37–39]. It became apparent that all patients with peritoneal metastases were not the same. Four different scoring systems by which to quantitate peritoneal metastases were described. Perhaps the original one was the "P factor," utilized in the Japanese classification of GC: P1 (cancer seedlings limited to the stomach itself), P2 (cancer seedlings limited to the space above the transverse colon), and P3 (cancer seeding located throughout the peritoneal space) stood the test of time as a useful quantitation of gastric carcinomatosis [40]. For more precise quantitation of the distribution and extent of peritoneal metastases, the Peritoneal Cancer Index (PCI) was developed. This scoring system combines the distribution of peritoneal metastases and lesion size of nodules present throughout the abdomen and especially emphasizes cancerous involvement of the small bowel and its mesentery. The PCI can be scored preoperatively with a computed tomography (CT), at the time of abdominal and pelvic exploration, and after maximal efforts at cytoreduction have occurred [41]. Other methodologies for quantitating peritoneal cancer dissemination are the simplified PCI used at The Netherlands Cancer Institute and the Gilly Staging System from Lyon, France [35, 42].

As more publications on peritoneal metastases appeared, an assessment of the completeness of cytoreduction was necessary. It was suggested that the Completeness of Cytoreduction (CC) score will vary as the invasive character of the malignancy and its response to neoadjuvant chemotherapy vary. A CC scoring system is reported [41].

It is obvious to those working long term in this field that early interventions in patients who have not had extensive prior surgery provides the best results in terms of survival and the lowest incidence of morbidity and mortality. Some means of assessing the extent of prior surgery was found to be necessary; thus, the Prior Surgical Score (PSS) was presented by Jacquet and colleagues and shown to have a major impact in determining survival of patients with appendiceal malignancy or ovarian cancer [24, 41, 43].

An essential adjunct to assessing prognosis in these patients is renewed interest in the histomorphology of peritoneal surface malignancy. The work of Ronnett and colleagues clearly shows that the invasive character of a malignant process, as estimated by histology, has a profound effect upon the success of combined treatment [44]. Similar emphasis on histomorphology in the outcome of combined treatment in patients with MPM was demonstrated by Cerruto et al. and Deraco et al. [45, 46].

7.7 Hyperthermia

Perioperative chemotherapy treatments over the last two decades have applied hyperthermia along with IP-CHT, with a presumed benefit. Hyperthermia in animal models increases drug cytotoxicity [47] and depth of chemotherapy penetration [48]; perhaps, if used long enough and at high enough temperatures, causes apoptosis from the heat itself. A single report, by Yonemura and colleagues, suggests that IP-CHT with heat is more effective than IP-CHT at body temperature [49]. Other studies confirming the benefits of hyperthermia have not been forthcoming. Also, studies show that EPIC is equivalent to HIPEC in maintaining a complete surgical response and improving long-term survival [50]. Certainly, in a patient who has undergone many hours of surgery with the abdomen and pelvis widely exposed often has moderate to profound hypothermia. The 90-min of hyperthermic lavage of the peritoneal space returns these patients to an optimal physiologic condition. In this regard, hyperthermia is an essential part of perioperative cancer treatment.

7.8 Peritoneal Surface Malignancy Treatment Centers

To the credit of Heald and Moran [7], the importance of a treatment center in the UK for patients with PMP was made clear and 1998 became a reality. Moran and colleagues [7] added greatly to the quality of care of patients with appendiceal malignancy in the UK. In 2002, a second center was established under the direction of O'Dwyer [7] and colleagues in Manchester, UK. Other designated treatment centers throughout Europe have since developed.

New efforts to further develop and improve outcomes of patients with peritoneal surface malignancy are underway. It is now clear that early treatment of minimal residual disease is optimal for these patients. Certainly, a watch-and-wait policy with referral of symptomatic patients to a peritoneal surface oncology center is no longer acceptable. Second, perioperative treatments are now many and varied. A bidirectional approach is becoming standard of care. As reviewed by van der Speeten and colleagues, some chemotherapy agents are most appropriate for intravenous use with heat targeting to the peritoneal cavity. Others are more valuable because of their large molecular size, and heat augmentation is used as part of the HIPEC regimen [51, 52].

Long-term intraperitoneal taxanes are now being explored, especially in Japan, for GC. The high response rate of combined systemic and intravenous application of chemotherapy reported by Yonemura et al. presents an exciting new treatment direction for patients with a very poor prognosis [53]. Kitayama et al. also continued applying adjuvant therapies for patients with peritoneal seeding using a combination of chemotherapy via an intraperitoneal port and systemic agents, which remains to be fully explored [54]. A summary of treatment evolution for patients with peritoneal metastases is shown in Table 7.2.

Finally, to allow treatments to be extended beyond the operating theater, a new interest in the use of antisclerotic agents to diminish adhesions postoperatively has occurred. Numerous agents are now available, including methylcellulose, polylactide sheets, polyethylene glycol spray, and 5-FU early postoperative irrigations. Continued studies to maintain the integrity of the peritoneal cavity are needed.

Table 7.2 Evolution of treatments for peritoneal carcinomatosis from gastrointestinal cancer (modified from [51])

Authors	Year	Event	Reference
Spratt et al.	1980	Suggested a hyperthermic peritoneal perfusion system with the administration of intraperitoneal chemotherapy. University of Louisville, KY, USA	[29]
Speyer et al.	1981	Pharmacology of intraperitoneal 5-fluorouracil in humans. National Institutes of Health, Bethesda, MD, USA	[14]
Koga et al.	1984	Experimental study with prophylactic continuous hyperthermic peritoneal perfusion with mitomycin C. A significant prolongation of survival was obtained when 41.5°C hyperthermia was combined with mitomycin C. Tottori University, Japan	[55]
Flessner et al.	1985	Pharmacokinetic studies established the peritoneal plasma barrier. National Institutes of Health, Bethesda, MD, USA	[12]
Sugarbaker et al.	1985	Randomized controlled study of intravenous versus intraperitoneal 5-fluorouracil documented a diminished incidence of peritoneal carcinomatosis in patients with colon cancer. National Institutes of Health, Bethesda, MD, USA	[56]
Koga et al.	1988	First study of adjuvant intraoperative hyperthermic peritoneal perfusion with mitomycin C in gastric cancer. Tottori University, Japan	[30]

(cont.) →

Table 7.2 (*continued*)

Fujimoto et al.	1988	Use of intraoperative hyperthermic peritoneal perfusion with mitomycin C combined with extended surgery in patients with gastric cancer and established peritoneal carcinomatosis. After treatment, 12.8% survived 1 year compared with 0% after surgery alone. Chiba University, Japan	[31]
Sugarbaker	1995	Trial of early postoperative intraperitoneal mitomycin C and 5-fluorouracil in the management of carcinomatosis. Washington Hospital Center, Washington, DC, USA	[21]
Sugarbaker	1995	Peritonectomy procedures. Washington Hospital Center, Washington, DC, USA	[10]
Yonemura et al.	1996	Suggested peritoneal cavity expander for optimizing intraoperative intraperitoneal hyperthermic chemotherapy delivery in patients with gastric cancer. Kanazawa University, Japan	[57]
Sugarbaker and Jacquet	1996	Published methodologies by which to quantitate peritoneal metastases and their management	[41]
Yu et al.	2001	Positive results of randomized study on adjuvant early postoperative intraperitoneal chemotherapy for gastric cancer. Kyungpook National University, Taegu, Korea	[58]
Moran and Cecil	2003	Pseudomyxoma peritonei treatment center designated for the UK. North Hampshire Hospital, Basingstoke, England	[59]
Urano et al.	1999	In vivo chemohyperthermia parameters defined. Memorial Sloan- Kettering, New York, NY, USA	[47]
Pestieau and Sugarbaker	2000	Benefit of cytoreductive surgery and perioperative chemotherapy in the management of primary colorectal cancer with synchronous peritoneal metastases. Medstar Washington Hospital Center, Washington, DC, USA	[60]
Verwaal et al.	2003	Prospective randomized trial showing superiority of comprehensive CRS plus HIPEC for carcinomatosis from colon cancer. The Netherlands Cancer Institute, Amsterdam.	[35]
Glehen et al.	2004	Multi-institutional study from 28 institutions describing benefit of CRS and perioperative chemotherapy utilizing prognostic indicators. Centre Hospitalo Universitaire Lyon Sud, Pierre Benite cedex, France	[36]
Elias et al.	2008	Systematic second-look for patients at high risk for recurrence. Institut Gustav Roussy, Villejuif, France	[61]
Elias et al.	2008	Association of French Surgeons Monograph describing results of CRS and perioperative chemotherapy for gastrointestinal and ovarian cancer plus peritoneal mesothelioma. French guidelines declare CRS and perioperative chemotherapy as standard of care for appendiceal cancer, colorectal cancer, and peritoneal mesothelioma." Institut Gustav Roussy, Villejuif, France	[62]

References

1. Elias D, Goere D, Dumont F et al (2014) Role of hyperthermic intraoperative peritoneal chemotherapy in the management of peritoneal metastases. Eur J Cancer 50:332-340
2. Kelly KJ, Nash GM (2014) Peritoneal debulking/intraperitoneal chemotherapy – non-sarcoma. J Surg Oncol 109:14-22
3. Glehen O, Mithieux F, Osinsky D et al (2003) Surgery combined with peritonectomy procedures and intraperitoneal chemohyperthermia in abdominal cancers with peritoneal carcinomatosis: a phase II study. J Clin Oncol 21:799-806
4. Verwaal VJ, van Ruth S, de Bree E et al (2003) Randomized trial of cytoreduction and hyperthermic intraperitoneal chemotherapy versus systemic chemotherapy and palliative surgery in patients with peritoneal carcinomatosis of colorectal cancer. J Clin Oncol 21:3737-3743
5. Hypertherme intraperitoneale Chemotherapie (HIPEC) in Kombination mit Peritonektomie und ggf. mit Multiviszeralresektion, ZE2007-4, Institut für das Entgeltsystem im Krankenhaus gGmbH, 2013
6. Losa F, Barrios P, Salazar R et al (2014) Cytoreductive surgery and intraperitoneal chemotherapy for treatment of peritoneal carcinomatosis from colorectal origin. Clin Transl Oncol 16:128-140
7. NHS Commissioning Board. Clinical Commissioning Policy for Cytoreductive Surgery with Hyperthermic Intraperitoneal Chemotherapy for Peritoneal Carcinomatosis. April 2013 http://www.england.nhs.uk/wp-content/uploads/2013/09/a08-p-a.pdf
8. Gonzalez-Moreno S, Brun E, Sugarbaker PH (2005) Lymph node metastases in epithelial malignancies of the appendix with peritoneal dissemination does not reduce survival in patients treated by cytoreductive surgery and perioperative intraperitoneal chemotherapy. Ann Surg Oncol 12:72-80
9. Carmignani P, Sugarbaker TA, Bromley CM, Sugarbaker PH (2003) Intraperitoneal cancer dissemination: Mechanisms of the patterns of spread. Cancer Metastasis Rev 22:465-472
10. Sugarbaker PH (1995) Peritonectomy procedures. Ann Surg 221:29-42
11. Bijelic L, Sugarbaker PH (2008) Cytoreduction of the small bowel surfaces. J Surg Oncol 97:176-179
12. Flessner MF, Dedrick RL, Schultz JS (1985) Exchange of macromolecules between peritoneal cavity and plasma. Am J Physiol 248:H15-25
13. Myers CE, Collins JM (1983) Pharmacology of intraperitoneal chemotherapy. Cancer Invest 1:395-407
14. Speyer JL, Sugarbaker PH, Collins JM et al (1981) Portal levels and hepatic clearance of 5 fluorouracil after intraperitoneal administration in humans. Cancer Res 41:1916-1922
15. Sugarbaker PH, Graves T, DeBruijn EA et al (1990) Rationale for early postoperative intraperitoneal chemotherapy (EPIC) in patients with advanced gastrointestinal cancer. Cancer Res 50:5790-5794
16. Sugarbaker PH (1991) Early postoperative intraperitoneal adriamycin as an adjuvant treatment for advanced gastric cancer with lymph node or serosal invasion. (In) Sugarbaker PH (ed); Management of Gastric Cancer. Kluwer: Boston pp. 277-284
17. Sugarbaker PH, Mora JT, Carmignani P et al (2005) Update on chemotherapeutic agents utilized for perioperative intraperitoneal chemotherapy. Oncologist 10:112-122
18. De Lima Vazquez V, Stuart OA, Sugarbaker PH (2003) Extent of a parietal peritonectomy does not change intraperitoneal chemotherapy pharmacokinetics. Cancer Chemother Pharmacol 52:108-112
19. Elias DM, Sideris L (2003) Pharmacokinetics of heated intraoperative intraperitoneal oxaliplatin after complete resection of peritoneal carcinomatosis. Surg Oncol Clin N Am 12:755-769
20. Sugarbaker PH, Stuart OA, Carmignani CP (2006) Pharmacokinetic changes induced by the volume of chemotherapy solution in patients treated with hyperthermic intraperitoneal mitomycin C. Cancer Chemother Pharmacol 57:703-708

21. Sugarbaker PH, Jablonski KA (1995) Prognostic features of 51 colorectal and 130 appendiceal cancer patients with peritoneal carcinomatosis treated by cytoreductive surgery and intraperitoneal chemotherapy. Ann Surg 221:124-132
22. Yonemura Y, Fujimura T, Fushida S et al (1999) Peritonectomy as a treatment modality for patients with peritoneal dissemination from gastric cancer. In: Nakajima T, Yamaguchi T (Eds). Multimodality Therapy for Gastric Cancer. Springer-Verlag, Tokyo
23. Sugarbaker PH (2002) Cytoreduction including total gastrectomy for pseudomyxoma peritonei. Br J Surg 89:208-212
24. Sugarbaker PH (1999) Results of treatment of 385 patients with peritoneal surface spread of appendiceal malignancy. Ann Surg Oncol 6:727-731
25. Elias DM, Pocard M (2003) Treatment and prevention of peritoneal carcinomatosis from colorectal cancer. Surg Oncol Clin N Am 12:543-559
26. Sugarbaker PH (2014) Intraperitoneal doxorubicin: Rationale, pharmacokinetic studies and clinical results. In: Pache M (ed); Doxorubicin: Biosynthesis, Clinical Uses and Clinical Results. Nova Science Publishers: New York, pp 1-20
27. Mohamed F, Sugarbaker PH (2003) Intraperitoneal taxanes. Surg Oncol Clin N Am 12:825-833
28. Yonemura Y, Bandou E, Sawa T et al (2006) Neoadjuvant treatment of gastric cancer with peritoneal dissemination. Eur J Surg Oncol 32:661-665
29. Spratt JS, Adcock RA, Muskovin M et al (1980) Clinical delivery system for intraperitoneal hyperthermic chemotherapy. Cancer Res 40:256-260
30. Koga S, Hamazoe R, Maeta M et al (1988) Prophylactic therapy for peritoneal recurrence of gastric cancer by continuous hyperthermic peritoneal perfusion with mitomycin C. Cancer 61:232-237
31. Fujimoto S, Shrestha RD, Kokubun M et al (1988) Intraperitoneal hyperthermic perfusion combined with surgery effective for gastric cancer patients with peritoneal seeding. Ann Surg 208:36-41
32. Fujimoto S, Takahashi M, Mutou T et al (1999) Successful intraperitoneal hyperthermic chemoperfusion for the prevention of postoperative peritoneal recurrence in patients with advanced gastric carcinoma. Cancer 85:529-534
33. Yonemura Y, Fujimura T, Fushida S et al (1991) Hyperthermo-chemotherapy combined with cytoreductive surgery for the treatment of gastric cancer with peritoneal dissemination. World J Surg 15:530-535
34. Fujimura T, Yonemura Y, Muraoka K et al (1994) Continuous hyperthermic peritoneal perfusion for the prevention of peritoneal recurrence of gastric cancer: randomized controlled study. World J Surg 18:150-155
35. Verwaal VJ, van Ruth S, de Bree E et al (2003) Randomized trial of cytoreduction and hyperthermic intraperitoneal chemotherapy versus systemic chemotherapy and palliative surgery in patients with peritoneal carcinomatosis of colorectal cancer. J Clin Oncol 21:3737-3743
36. Glehen O, Kwiatkowski F, Sugarbaker PH et al (2004) Cytoreductive surgery combined with perioperative intraperitoneal chemotherapy for the management of peritoneal carcinomatosis from colorectal cancer: A multi-institutional study. J Clin Oncol 22:3284-3292
37. Chu DZ, Lang NP, Thompson C et al (1989) Peritoneal carcinomatosis in nongynecologic malignancy. A prospective study of prognostic factors. Cancer 63:364-367
38. Sadeghi B, Arvieux C, Glehen O et al (2000) Peritoneal carcinomatosis from non-gynecologic malignancies: results of the EVOCAPE 1 multicentric prospective study. Cancer 88:358-363
39. Jayne DG, Fook S, Loi C, Seow-Choen F (2002) Peritoneal carcinomatosis from colorectal cancer. Br J Surg 89:1545-1550
40. Japanese Research Society for Gastric Cancer. Japanese Classification of Gastric Carcinoma. First Edition. Tokyo: Kanehara & Co., Ltd., 1995
41. Jacquet P, Sugarbaker PH (1996) Current methodologies for clinical assessment of patients with peritoneal carcinomatosis. J Exp Clin Cancer Res 15:49-58
42. Glehen O, Gilly FN (2003) Quantitative prognostic indicators of peritoneal surface malignan-

cy: carcinomatosis, sarcomatosis, and peritoneal mesothelioma. Surg Oncol Clin N Am 12:649-671
43. Look M, Chang D, Sugarbaker PH (2004) Long-term results of cytoreductive surgery for advanced and recurrent epithelial ovarian cancers and papillary serous carcinoma of the peritoneum. Int J Gynecol Cancer 14:35-41
44. Ronnett BM, Shmookler BM, Sugarbaker PH, Kurman RJ (1997) Pseudomyxoma peritonei: New concepts in diagnosis, origin, nomenclature, relationship to mucinous borderline (low malignant potential) tumors of the ovary. In: Fechner RE, Rosen PP, eds. Anatomic Pathology. ASCP Press:Chicago pp 197-226
45. Cerruto CA, Brun EA, Chang D, Sugarbaker PH (2006) Prognostic significance of histomorphologic parameters in diffuse malignant peritoneal mesothelioma. Arch Pathol Lab Med 130:1654-1661
46. Deraco M, Nonaka D, Baratti D et al (2006) Prognostic analysis of clinicopathologic factors in 49 patients with diffuse malignant peritoneal mesothelioma treated with cytoreductive surgery and intraperitoneal hyperthermic perfusion. Ann Surg Oncol 13:229-237
47. Urano M, Kuroda M, Nishimura Y (1999) For the clinical application of thermochemotherapy given at mild temperatures. Int J Hyperthermia 15:79-107
48. Jacquet P, Averbach A, Stuart OA et al (1998) Hyperthermic intraperitoneal doxorubicin: pharmacokinetics, metabolism, and tissue distribution in a rat model. Cancer Chemother Pharmacol 41:147-154
49. Yonemura Y, de Aretxabala X, Fujimura T et al (2001) Intraoperative chemohyperthermic peritoneal perfusion as an adjuvant to gastric cancer: final results of a randomized controlled study. Hepatogastroenterology 48:1776-1782
50. Sørensen O, Flatmark K, Reed W et al (2012) Evaluation of complete cytoreductive surgery and two intraperitoneal chemotherapy techniques in Pseudomyxoma peritonei. Eur J Surg Oncol 38:969-976
51. Sugarbaker PH (2007) Management of peritoneal surface malignancy: A short history. Recent Results Cancer Res 169:1-9
52. Van der Speeten K, Stuart OA, Sugarbaker PH (2012) Pharmacology of perioperative cancer chemotherapy. (In) Sugarbaker PH (Ed). Cytoreductive Surgery & Perioperative Chemotherapy for Peritoneal Surface Malignancy. Textbook and Video Atlas. Cine-Med Publishing: Woodbury, CT, pp 159-182
53. Yonemura Y, Bandou E, Sawa et al (2006) Neoadjuvant treatment of gastric cancer with peritoneal dissemination. Eur J Surg Oncol 32:661-665
54. Kitayama J, Ishigami H, Yamaguchi H et al (2014) Salvage gastrectomy after intravenous and intraperitoneal paclitaxel (PTX) administration with oral S-1 for peritoneal dissemination of advanced gastric cancer with malignant ascites. Ann Surg Oncol 21:539-546
55. Koga S, Hamazoe R, Maeta M et al (1984) Treatment of implanted peritoneal cancer in rats by continuous hyperthermic peritoneal perfusion in combination with an anticancer drug. Cancer Res 44:1840-1842
56. Sugarbaker PH, Gianola FJ, Speyer JL et al (1985) Prospective randomized trial of intravenous versus intraperitoneal 5 fluorouracil in patients with advanced primary colon or rectal cancer. Surgery 98:414 421
57. Yonemura Y, Fujimura T, Nishimura G et al (1996) Effects of intraoperative chemohyperthermia in patients with gastric cancer with peritoneal dissemination. Surgery 119:437-444
58. Yu W, Whang I, Chung HY, Averbach A, Sugarbaker PH (2001) Indications for early postoperative intraperitoneal chemotherapy of advanced gastric cancer: Results of a prospective randomized trial. World J Surg 25:985-990
59. Moran BJ, Cecil TD (2003) The etiology, clinical presentation, and management of pseudomyxoma peritonei. Surg Oncol Clin N Am 12:585-603
60. Pestieau SR, Sugarbaker PH (2000) Treatment of primary colon cancer with peritoneal carcinomatosis: A comparison of concomitant versus delayed management. Dis Colon Rectum 43:1341-1348

61. Elias D, Goéré D, Di Pietrantonio D (2008) Results of systematic second-look surgery in patients at high risk of developing colorectal peritoneal carcinomatosis. Ann Surg 247:445-450
62. Elias D, Gilly F, Glehen O (2008) Carcinoses peritoneales d'origine digestive et primitive. Monographies de L'association Francaise de Chirurgie. Walters Kluwer, France

Rationale for Integrated Procedures: Cytoreduction and Hyperthermic Intraperitoneal Chemotherapy (HIPEC) Combined

8

Paolo Sammartino, Fabio Accarpio, Tommaso Cornali, Daniele Biacchi, Maurizio Cardi, and Giammaria Fiorentini

8.1 Introduction

Diffuse peritoneal malignancy raises major therapeutic problems and puts the patient's life at high risk. In the past, systemic chemotherapy regimens functioned as a purely palliative approach, and palliative surgery aimed merely at reducing the symptoms, being unable to alter the natural course of the disease [1]. At the beginning of the 1990s, thanks to Sugarbaker's pioneering efforts, research began to develop integrated procedures for treating peritoneal surface malignancies based on a therapeutic approach. This approach involved cytoreductive surgery (CRS) (peritonectomy procedures) combined with perioperative intraperitoneally administered chemotherapy (IP-CHT)—eventually integrated with hyperthermia—done immediately after surgical cytoreduction ended [hyperthermic intraperitoneal chemotherapy (HIPEC)], or during the early postoperative course [early postoperative intraperitoneal chemotherapy (EPIC)] [2]. The therapeutic rationale underlying integrated treatment originates from advances in systemic chemotherapy and improved knowledge about the pharmacological mechanisms underlying endoperitoneal drug delivery. The rationale for cancer chemotherapy hinges upon several well-known theoretical hypotheses. According to the Gompertzian cellular kinetic model (the tumor-growth profile can be depicted as an S-shaped curve), a tumor initially grows slowly and then rapidly becomes fast growing [3]. As the tumor enlarges, its blood supply and growth slows down, and a larger tumor cell percentage gradually enters a nonproliferative cell-cycle stage (Fig. 8.1). At the same time as the growth fraction slows down, tumor heterogeneity increases and drug sensi-

P. Sammartino (✉)
Department of Surgery "Pietro Valdoni", Sapienza University of Rome, Rome, Italy
e-mail: paolo.sammartino@uniroma1.it

A. Di Giorgio, E. Pinto (Eds), *Treatment of Peritoneal Surface Malignancies*, Updates in Surgery
DOI: 10.1007/978-88-470-5711-1_8, © Springer-Verlag Italia 2015

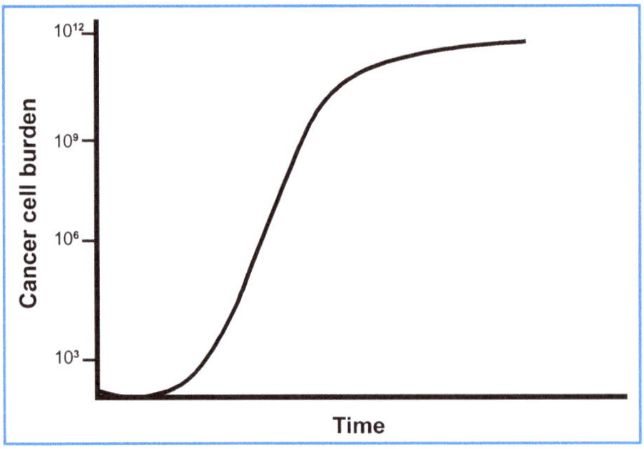

Fig. 8.1 Gompertzian growth kinetics

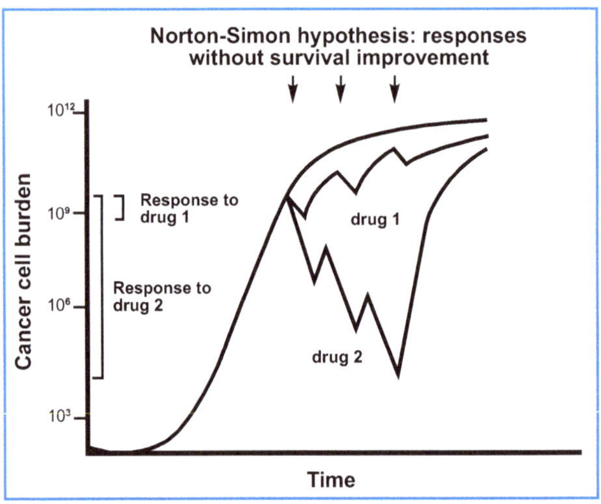

Fig. 8.2 Norton–Simon hypothesis: progressive improvements in drug response do not change actual cancer survival

tivity decreases. Advances in the Gompertzian model led to the Norton–Simon hypothesis [4, 5]. According to this model, chemotherapy results in tumor regression volume rates proportional to the growth rate expected for a tumor of that size. Smaller tumors grow more rapidly and undergo greater log kill (cell kill on a logarithmic scale) when chemotherapy is applied. If rapid regrowth makes it impossible to eradicate all tumor cells (an essential requirement in the Gompertzian model) cancer-killing efficacy is no longer reflected in cancer survival (Fig. 8.2). The Goldie–Coldman hypothesis is a mathematic model predicting that tumor cells mutate to a drug-resistant phenotype at a time-dependent rate related also to the tumor's intrinsic genetic instability [6]. Drug resistance is a selection process, and with each new cellular division, new subclones arise, some becoming drug resistant. Even the smallest detectable cancers would contain at least one drug-resistant clone. Expanding the Norton–Simon hypothesis and focusing on the heterogeneous cancer population, Norton proposed a therapeutic strategy intended to treat first the cell population in a growth phase and then the other (slow-growing and chemotherapy-resistant) cell population. This strategy entailed several cycles repeating an effective regimen A, followed by several cycles repeating regimen B (AAA plus BBB), acquiring the dose intensity for each regimen [7]. Even this approach failed to eradicate the disease, and recurrent disease developed. These observations emphasized the need to drastically reduce tumor cell numbers before applying chemotherapy, thus opening the way to integrated maximal cytoreduction plus systemic and locoregional chemotherapy. Extensive debulking surgery to reduce the tumor mass decreases the likelihood that resistance develops, thereby making it less likely that new resistant subclones will appear. Equally important, cytoreduction stimulates the remaining cells to enter into a proliferative phase that is potentially more responsive to chemotherapy. Hence, the rationale underlying cytoreduction is that the fewer tumor cells left after cytoreduction, the better they respond to chemotherapy [8–10]. For various reasons, CRS and IP-CHT must be done at the same time. First, because surgery alone could lead to fibrin entrapment of microscopic intra-abdominal residual disease (tumor cell entrapment), thus causing peritoneal surface malignancies to recur rapidly and progress. Second, because if patients undergo IP-CHT after surgery, adhesions create multiple barriers to the free access of fluid, with nonuniform drug distribution that may lead to treatment failure. Third, undertaking IP-CHT weeks or months after surgery raises difficulties and dangers related to long-term peritoneal access [2].

8.2 Intraperitoneal Chemotherapy: Physical and Biological Principles

The pharmacological rationale behind endoperitoneal chemotherapy consists of dose intensification determined by the peritoneal plasma barrier. The two compartments (peritoneal cavity and blood) are separated by a semipermeable membrane that allows a high peritoneal drug concentration, thus optimizing its effect on the endoperitoneal target and at the same time limiting drug passage into the plasma stream, which causes treatment toxicity. From experience gained in peritoneal dialysis, Dedrick et al. stated that peritoneal permeability to a certain drug is notably lower than the same drug's plasma clearance. Peritoneal drug clearance is inversely proportional to the square root of its molecular weight [11]. Figure 8.3 shows the equation that describes the pharmacokinetic advantages gained by giving a drug by the endoperitoneal route rather than the intravenous route and the traditional two-compartment model of peritoneal transport with the equation showing the rate of mass transfer. Drugs pass in a parallel fashion from the peritoneal cavity into the various surrounding tissues, and multiplying tissue permeability by the area exposed to peritoneal fluid shows how much a given tissue type contributes to overall transport (Fig. 8.4).

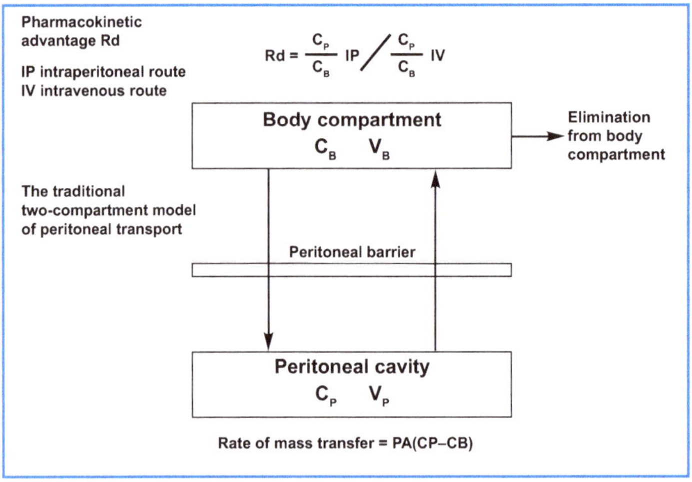

Fig. 8.3 Mass transfer coefficient for a specific drug has conventionally been considered a single parameter. The permeability *P* could be considered a property of the membrane with units of cm/min; when *P* is multiplied by the effective area *A* of the membrane (expressed in cm^2), a clearance term, cm^3/min, results. It has enabled prediction of peritoneal and plasma concentration and the resulting regional advantage in a clinical setting if the systemic pharmacokinetics are known. *PA*, permeability area (effective contact area *A* × permeability of a specific drug *P*); *CP*, free drug concentration in peritoneal fluid; *CB*, free drug concentration in blood; *VP*, volume of peritoneal cavity; *VB*, volume of drug distribution in the body

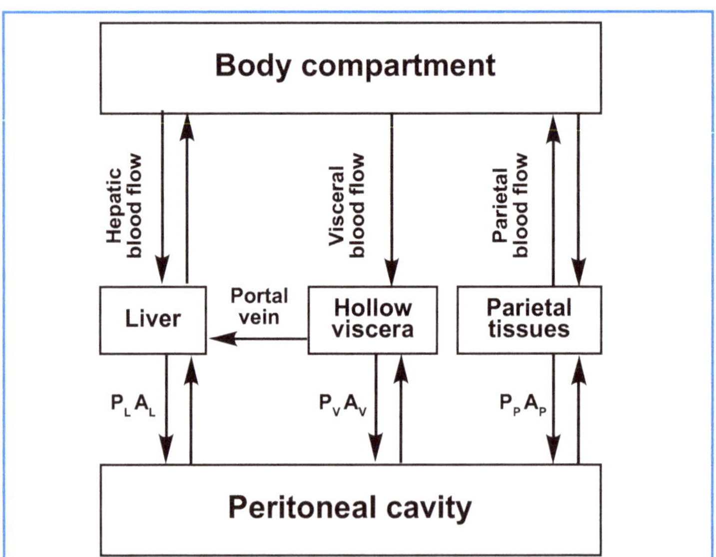

Fig. 8.4. How drug transfer from the peritoneal cavity into surrounding tissue-specific permeabilities *P* and area *A* where the subscript can be *L* for liver, *V* for hollow viscera, and *P* for parietal tissue. Low-molecular-weight drugs move from the peritoneal tissues into the rest of the body primarily via blood flow. (Reproduced from [28], with permission)

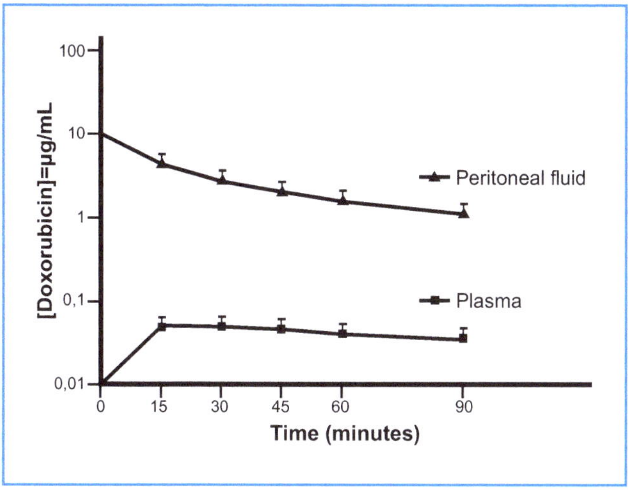

Fig. 8.5 Concentration-time graph of doxorubicin in peritoneal fluid and plasma in 145 patients. Area under the curve (AUC) ratio of peritoneal fluid to plasma was 78.6 (+ 27.7). (Reproduced from [12], with permission)

8.3 Pharmacokinetic and Pharmacodynamic Variables Related to Intraperitoneal Chemotherapy

One reason for delivering chemotherapeutic agents into the peritoneum is that this route allows relatively lengthy contact between the drug and its therapeutic target. The pharmacokinetic advantage of dose intensification arises from the higher drug concentration achieved in the peritoneum than in the plasma, as expressed by the area-under-the curve (AUC) ratio. The simplest way to illustrate the pharmacokinetic advantage is to construct a concentration-time curve. The endoperitoneal AUC reflects therapeutic effectiveness, whereas the intravenous AUC expresses drug toxicity (Fig. 8.5) [12]. A high peritoneal drug concentration does not itself, however, guarantee therapeutic effectiveness insofar as the real pharmacological aim is for the drug to penetrate into the target tumor. An approximate measure of the result obtained is therefore provided by inserting into the preceding graph the chemotherapeutic drug concentration achieved within the malignant nodule (Fig. 8.6) [13]. Hence whereas pharmacokinetic variables (dose, volume of the chemotherapy solution, duration, carrier solution, and pressure) influence peritoneal drug bioavailability; a series of pharmacodynamic variables (size of the malignant nodule, vascularization, interstitial pressure, and temperature) reflect how much drug reaches the oncologic target.

8.3.1 Pharmacokinetic Variables

A major controversial problem is the wide variability in the chemotherapeutic drug doses used for endoperitoneal chemotherapy. Most groups base the doses delivered, as happens for systemic chemotherapy, on body surface area (BSA)

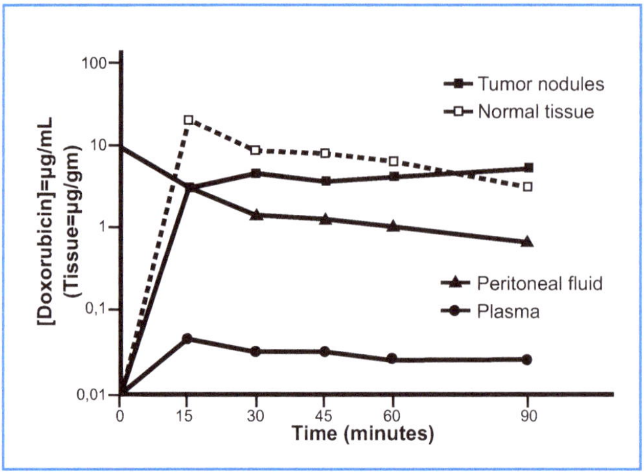

Fig. 8.6 Doxorubicin concentration in plasma, peritoneal fluid, tumor nodules, and normal adjacent tissues. Data obtained from a single patient. (Reproduced from [13], with permission)

(mg/m^2), considering BSA as a peritoneal surface area (PSA). Despite the substantial difference between BSA and PSA [14], BSA is a reasonably reliable method for assessing predictable toxicity. Other groups use a concentration-based method that calculates the pharmacological dose in mg/m^2 per liter perfusate and usually increase this dose up to 6 l [15–17]. According to the aforementioned Dedrick formula for transport through the peritoneal membrane, the volume of IP-CHT will increase the solution contact area (A) and will improve mass transfer from the peritoneal cavity to the plasma. The great advantage of a concentration-based system is that the residual tumor nodules after cytoreduction are exposed to increased cytotoxicity, but this advantage pays the price of highly unpredictable systemic side effects. Reported IP-CHT protocols vary in duration from 30 to 120 min. According to a mathematical model proposed by Gardner [18], the dose–response curves and their dependency on exposure time reach a cell-kill plateau, after which prolonging exposure time offers no further cytotoxic advantage. The most advantageous exposure time for cytotoxic effects in peritoneal carcinomatosis (PC) should be weighed against systemic toxicity. Other pharmacokinetic variables include perfusate osmolality (most perfusates are isotonic saline or dextrose solutions) [19] and pressure as a determinant variable reflecting drug penetration into tissues [20]. Hydrostatic pressure, especially for HIPEC, depends partly on the two principal technologies (open vs closed) used, and despite debate over recent years on their advantages and disadvantages, no definitive conclusions have been reached [21]. Two studies conducted by Ortega-Deballon et al. and Facey et al. show in animal experiments (pigs) an increased drug tissue penetration after HIPEC given with the open technique. The investigators obtained the highest tissue concentrations by combining open HIPEC with increased hydrostatic pressure obtained with a special device fixed to the skin margins, and to a Thompson retractor equipped with a vertical latex expander able to increase hydrostatic pressure to 25 cm of water [22, 23].

Table 8.1 Multivariate modeling analysis to evaluate the association between clinicopathologic factors and the area under the curve (AUC) ratio. (Reproduced from [12], with permission)

Clinicopathologic factors	Analysis	*P* value
Age	Not significant	0.153
Gender	Men have a significantly higher AUC ratio than women	0.025
Completeness of cytoreduction	Not significant	0.572
Peritoneal space	Patients with a restricted peritoneal space have a significantly higher AUC ratio	0.002
Number of peritonectomies	The number of peritonectomies has a significant negative correlation with the AUC ratio (a higher number of peritonectomies tends to have a lower AUC ratio)	0.003
Number of visceral resections	The number of visceral resections has a significant positive correlation with the AUC ratio (a higher number of visceral resections tends to have a higher AUC ratio)	0.001

Pharmacokinetic variables also vary according to the surgical procedure used, and surgical and clinical factors may require changes in chemotherapy administration. In a study conducted on 145 patients with appendiceal cancer and colorectal carcinomatosis who underwent CRS plus HIPEC with doxorubicin as part of a multidrug regimen, Sugarbaker et al. observed that the number of surgical procedures (number of peritonectomy procedures or entity of visceral resections or both) can influence the AUC ratio. Doxorubicin peritoneal clearance differs as the number of peritonectomy procedures or the entity of visceral resections done (gastrectomies or total colectomies) progressively increases (Table 8.1) [12]. The number of peritonectomy procedures increases peritoneal drug clearance, whereas the entity of visceral resections increases the AUC ratio. This observation depends solely on the different rates at which doxorubicin penetrates through the peritoneal–plasma diffusion pathways into the various organs and structures [24].

8.3.2 Pharmacodynamic Variables

Pharmacodynamic variables, expressing what the drug does to the body, focus on the tumor nodule, rightly considering it the pharmacological endpoint for endoperitoneal therapies. The equations in Fig. 8.3 allow us to calculate the pharmacological advantages of endoperitoneal chemotherapy and illustrate drug-transfer mechanisms between the two compartments. However, they provide no information on the real mechanisms that regulate drug penetration into tumor nodules. In vitro experiments with multicellular models show that most

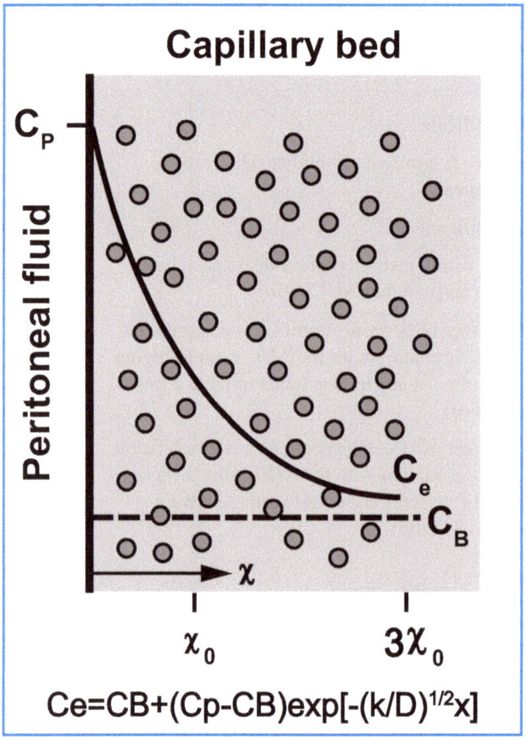

Fig. 8.7 Exponential decrease (*solid line*) in the free tissue interstitial concentration, *Ce*, as the drug diffuses down the concentration gradient and is removed by loss to blood perfusing the tissue. Also shown are the characteristics diffusion length, *x0*, at which the concentration difference between tissue and blood has decreased to 37 % of its maximum value, and *3x0*, at which the difference has decreased to 5 % of its maximum value. *Cp*, free drug concentration in peritoneal fluid; *CB,* free drug concentration in blood (or plasma). (Reproduced from [28], with permission)

cytotoxic agents penetrate poorly into tumor tissue (< 1 mm) [25]. After intraperitoneal cisplatinum administration in an animal model, Los et al., reported a 1- to 2-cm penetration [26, 27]. As the model proposed by Dedrick et al. [28] and the related equation show (Fig. 8.7), low-molecular-weight drugs (up to 6,000 Daltons) present at a given concentration in the peritoneal cavity (Cp) diffuse through the tissues (Ce) according to a concentration that diminishes exponentially until it reaches the concentration in blood (Cb). Drug movement through the tissues is measured by the drug's diffusion constant (D) (cm^2/min) and the rate constant k (min $^{-1}$), a variable that measures the amount that can be removed from the tissue by blood capillary diffusion. The k constant takes into account capillary permeability, the capillary surface per unit tissue, and capillary blood flow per unit tissue volume. Last, *x* indicates the distance in centimeters from the serosal surface, assuming that *x0* is the distance from the serosal surface at which the concentration difference between tissue and blood has decreased to 37% of its maximum value. The distance from the serosa surface, *3x0*, is a reference value at which the concentration difference decreases to 5% of the maximum value. Obtaining increased tissue penetration for low-molecular-weight drugs is no easy task, because it requires an increased D value (diffusion coefficient) or a reduced k value, or both. Drug diffusion into tissue depends on tissue structure and drug properties. In locoregional therapy, because the drug has to pass from the periphery to reach the tumor center, a major influential factor is the interstitium and interstitial fluid pressure. Interstitial pressure in tumors is usually increased. Because lymph flows from the tumor center toward the periphery, it flows in the opposite direction to peritoneally administered drugs [29]. Interstitium, or the so-called microenvironment, consists of collagen fibers linked through adhesion molecules, such as beta-1 integrins to fibroblast, parenchymal cells, and other interstitial cells. Emerging evidence suggests that giving drugs such as bortezomib, a proteasome inhibitor, can disrupt cell–cell adhesion, lower interstitial fluid pressure, and thus enhance drug diffusion into tumor tissue [30]. Some researchers tried to reduce the k constant with vasoactive agents able to regulate peritoneal-tissue blood flow, thus delaying drug clearance from the peritoneal cavity. Because these studies using vasoactive agents yielded conflicting data, mainly owing to the various experimental systems used, further studies are needed before vasoactive agents can be recommended [31].

Another pharmacodynamic variable is hyperthermia. Hyperthermia unites the pharmacokinetic advantages inherent to intraperitoneal perfusion of cytotoxic drugs (regional dose intensification) with the direct cytotoxic effect induced by heat. Combining hyperthermia with intraperitoneally perfused chemotherapy agents increases tumor response through numerous mechanisms. Hyperthermia > 41°C inhibits DNA repair mechanisms in neoplastic cells, denatures proteins, induces lysosomal activation, and increases cell death [32, 33]. Hyperthermia also potentiates chemotherapy drug activity inhibiting intracellular drug-detoxification pathways and drug-induced DNA adduct repair mechanisms [34]. Last, hyperthermia helps drugs penetrate more deeply into tumor tissue. In a study investigating this hypothesis, Leunig et al. reported that heat induced a dose-dependent reduction in interstitial pressure, thereby increasing drug penetration into tissues [35]. Pichè et al., using a murine model, showed that increasing the temperature for oxaliplatin HIPEC delivery increases tissue penetration without changing the pharmacokinetic advantages of the administration route and even reduces systemic toxicity [36]. Hyperthermia both induces and reverses certain forms of drug resistance, although the clinical importance of these interactions is still poorly understood. From a clinical point of view, the chance of reversing drug resistance using hyperthermia outweighs the dangers of inducing thermotolerance [37].

8.4 Bidirectional (Intraperitoneal plus Intravenous) Intraoperative Chemotherapy

Some have proposed bidirectional chemotherapy (intravenous plus endoperitoneal) drug infusion to obtain a bidirectional diffusion gradient in peritoneal neoplastic tissues. The first to propose this strategy was Elias et al., who sug-

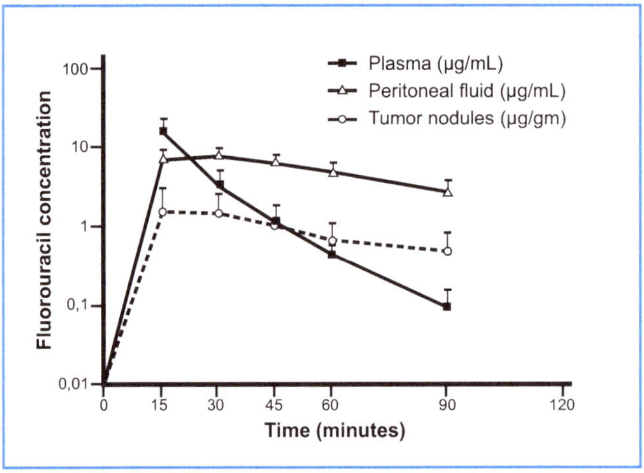

Fig. 8.8 Concentrations of 5-fluorouracil in plasma, peritoneal fluid, and tumor nodules after intravenous administration during hyperthermic intraperitoneal chemotherapy (HIPEC) procedure. (Reproduced from [41], with permission)

gested perioperative intravenous 5-fluorouracil (5-FU) and leucovorin in conjunction with oxaliplatin-based HIPEC [38], thus extending information from earlier studies suggesting that the two drugs induced a synergic effect [39, 40]. 5-FU is a thymidylate synthase inhibitor, enters the cell directly, and is then intracellularly metabolized to its active metabolite. Mild hyperthermia only slightly increases the 5-FU-induced effect, and the drug is not chemically compatible with other drugs in mixed solution. A study investigating the pharmacological rationale for perioperative 5-FU intravenous infusion during HIPEC in patients with PC from appendiceal cancer showed a definite pharmacologic locoregional advantage [41] (Fig. 8.8). The 5-FU concentration in peritoneal fluid is high 15 min after infusion, and this high drug level persists over 90 min. Single heated tumor nodules harvested at 15-min intervals showed 5-FU penetration. The study shows that perioperative bidirectional chemotherapy is pharmacokinetically, useful given that intravenous 5-FU application reaches a high concentration in the peritoneal fluid. By acting synergistically, bidirectional chemotherapy provides a high drug concentration in the tumor nodule. The bidirectional therapeutic approach is widely used by French and German centers for treating colorectal carcinomatosis [42, 43]. Similar results have been obtained after intravenous administration of ifosfamide (1,300 mg/m^2 per liter continuous saline solution for 90 min) during HIPEC containing cisplatin and doxorubicin in a series of patients who underwent peritonectomy procedures for PC or mesothelioma [44]. This therapeutic strategy has enjoyed widespread use for various cancers at different time points (neoadjuvant or adjuvant) before or after surgical resection. Japanese investigators have obtained promising results by associating systemic and normothermic IP-CHT in a neoadjuvant setting in patients with advanced gastric cancers (GC) and neoadjuvant intraperitoneal and systemic (NIPS) therapy [45, 46]. Sugarbaker and Bijelic proposed using bidirectional (systemic and normothermic intraperitoneal) chemotherapy in an adjuvant setting to reduce locoregional recurrence after peritonectomy procedures plus HIPEC [47].

8.5 Overview of Drugs Commonly Used in Protocols for Perioperative Intraperitoneal Cancer Chemotherapy

8.5.1 Mitomycin C

Mitomycin C is an alkylating antibiotic (extracted from *Streptomyces* species) that acts mainly through DNA cross-linking. Mitomycin C has been extensively used in IP-CHT treatment protocols in appendiceal and colorectal carcinomatosis [48–50]. Although mitomycin is not regarded as a prodrug, it is not active against cancerous tissue as is the unchanged molecule. The drug changes into its active state as it enters the cell [51], and in vitro data suggest heat enhances mitomycin's antitumoral activity [52]. Extending these findings, Jacquet et al. reported that intraperitoneally infused mitomycin C had a clear pharmacokinetic advantage over intravenous infusion, with an AUC IP/IV ratio of 23.5, findings confirmed by Van der Speeten [53, 54]. Drug dosimetry differs notably between the various research groups. Some institutions use mitomycin in a single dose, others a double dose, and still others a triple dose infused over 90 mins [55, 56]. A study from the Dutch Cancer Institute suggests that mitomycin at a dose of 35 mg/m^2 yields the highest AUC IP/IV ratio with acceptable toxicity [55]. To maintain the concentration throughout the 90-min perfusion time, the dose was divided into three fractions: 50 % at the start, 25 % after 30 mins, and 25 % at 60 mins. Ample evidence describes the toxicity profile for mitomycin C, including anastomotic dehiscence and impaired wound healing [57, 58].

8.5.2 Cisplatin

Cisplatin is a well-known chemotherapy drug. It was the first member in the platinum family drug class, which now includes oxaliplatin and carboplatin. These platinum complexes react in vivo, binding to DNA and causing DNA crosslinking. Cisplatin induces cell death by causing DNA adducts to form [59]. The drug has been well studied for adjuvant IP-CHT in residual small-volume ovarian cancers (OC) after CRS. Three randomized trials showed a significant survival benefit [60–62]. For CRS plus HIPEC, cisplatin has been used for intracavitary therapy in patients with OC, GC, and malignant peritoneal mesothelioma (MPM). In their study, Urano and coworkers showed that cisplatin provided excellent in vitro and in vivo thermal augmentation [63]. Several groups have studied cisplatin penetration into tumor nodules. For example, Los et al. described intratumoral cisplatin distribution after intraperitoneal infusion and suggested that intraperitoneal cisplatin distribution reached its maximal advantage versus the intravenous route in the first 1.5 mm [64]. In a similar study, van der Vaart et al. investigated cisplatin-induced DNA-adduct formation and measured this drug-induced change 3–5 mm into the tumor tissue [65]. In an experimental model, Esquis et al. reported enhanced cisplatin penetration when they infused cisplatin at increased pressure [20].

8.5.3 Oxaliplatin

Oxaliplatin is a third-generation platinum compound that possesses a wide antitumor effect in vitro and in vivo, a better safety profile than cisplatin, and no cross-resistance with cisplatin or carboplatin. Oxaliplatin has a nonhydrolysable diaminocyclohexane (DACH) carrier ligand, which the final cytotoxic drug metabolites maintain. The bulky DACH ring retained by activated oxaliplatin is thought to cause formation of platinum–DNA adducts. These platinum–DNA adducts seem more effective than cisplatin adducts at blocking DNA replication and are more cytotoxic [66, 67]. The clinical use of oxaliplatin during bidirectional intraoperative chemotherapy in patients with PC was pioneered by Elias et al. [38, 68]. In a dose-escalation and pharmacokinetic study, they showed that 460 mg/m^2 in 2 L/m^2 of chemotherapy solution infused over 30 mins is well tolerated. The low AUC ratio is compensated by the rapid drug absorption into the tissue. In contrast to cisplatin and mitomycin, oxaliplatin is unstable in chloride-containing solutions and can only be given in 5 % dextrose, a solution that may result in severe electrolyte disturbances and hyperglycemia during intracavitary therapy [69, 70]. A recent study using oxaliplatin in a murine model confirmed that heat increased its antitumoral activity [36]. In clinical practice, oxaliplatin given during HIPEC has proven activity in colorectal and appendiceal malignancies and has been used in patients with recurrent OC [71, 72].

8.5.4 Carboplatin

Carboplatin was introduced in the late 1980s and has since gained popularity in clinical treatment, inducing far fewer adverse effects than its parent compound, cisplatin. Carboplatin is a platinum compound with a higher molecular weight than cisplatin. Carboplatin is mostly used in intraperitoneal normothermic and, rarely, in hyperthermic chemotherapy protocols in patients with advanced OC [73, 74]. In a clinical study, investigators reported that normothermic carboplatin achieves acceptable bioavailability (calculated as AUC values), remaining at least six times higher in the intraperitoneal fluid than in the serum for 48 h [75]. Continuing research into bioavailability, Los et al compared the ability of carboplatin and cisplatin to penetrate into peritoneal cancer nodules in a rat model, and even though intraperitoneally administered carboplatin had a clear pharmacokinetic advantage over cisplatin, it proved far less able than cisplatin to penetrate into tumor cells [27]. A report showing opposite results has now revived clinical interest in intraperitoneally administered carboplatin [76].

8.5.5 Doxorubicin

Doxorubicin, or hydroxyl daunorubicin, is an antibiotic belonging to the anthracycline family. Although categorized as a DNA-intercalating drug, its true mechanism of action involves its critical interaction with the cell-surface membrane [77], and this interaction is influenced by temperature [78]. Given its wide in vitro and in vivo activity against a broad range of malignancies, its slow clearance from the peritoneal compartment due to the high molecular weight of the hydrochloride salt (579, 99 Dalton), its favorable AUC ratio of intraperitoneal to intravenous concentration times of 230, and the absence of risk for dose-limiting cardiotoxicity in intraperitoneal infusion, made doxorubicin a potential beneficial agent for perioperative intraperitoneal delivery. This advantage received support from experimental and clinical pharmacokinetic data [12, 13, 79]. Based on ex vivo studies, Pilati et al. suggested that during hyperthermia, doxorubicin uptake increases, and tumor cells become more sensitive to the drug [80]. Pegylated liposomal doxorubicin has generated interest for HIPEC because of its favorable pharmacokinetics [81]. Doxorubicin-based HIPEC has been used in peritoneal surface malignancy from appendiceal, GC, OC, and colon cancer, and MPM.

8.5.6 Gemcitabine

Gemcitabine is a nucleoside analog in which the hydrogen atoms on the 2' deoxycytidine carbon are replaced by fluorine atoms. As with pyrimidines, the triphosphate gemcitabine analog replaces one of the nucleic acid building blocks, in this case cytidine, during DNA replication. This process arrests tumor growth, because only one additional nucleoside can be attached to the "faulty" nucleoside, thus resulting in cell death. Another gemcitabine target is the enzyme ribonucleotide reductase. Gemcitabine exerts widely ranging in vitro and in vivo cytotoxic activity, particularly against pancreatic and lung cancer. To extend knowledge on its actions, Pestieau et al. investigated intraperitoneally delivered gemcitabine pharmacokinetics and tissue distribution in a rat model [82]. The AUC ratio (IP/IV) after intraperitoneal infusion was 26.8 ± 5.8 favoring intraperitoneal use. Several investigators explored the use of normothermic intraperitoneally delivered gemcitabine in advanced cancer outside the setting of CRS [83, 84]. Resected advanced pancreatic cancer at high risk of locoregional recurrence is a potential indication for intraoperative intraperitoneally delivered heated gemcitabine in an adjuvant setting [85–87].

8.5.7 Melphalan

Melphalan is an antineoplastic alkylating agent that causes interstrand DNA crosslinks to form and the activity of which increases with heat [88, 89]. Melphalan remains the principal agent used in isolated limb perfusion for the treatment of in-transit metastases from melanoma [90]. The first to investigate the pharmacokinetics of intraperitoneally delivered melphalan were Alberts et al., [91]. Later, Glehen et al. showed in an animal model that intraperitoneally delivered melphalan combined with heat is effective in delaying tumor growth and that the effect of hyperthermia on the pharmacokinetics and tissue distribution of intraperitoneally delivered melphalan indicated increased intra-abdominal tissue concentrations [92]. In a pharmacokinetic and phase II study of intraoperative intraperitoneally delivered melphalan, Sugarbaker et al. showed that 90 % of the cancer chemotherapy drug was absorbed during the 90-min procedure, with a 30-times higher exposure at the peritoneal surface than in the blood and concentrations in tumor nodules ten times higher than concentrations in blood [93]. In a later study, Bijelic et al., in a series of 34 patients treated with hyperthermic intraperitoneally administered melphalan, showed an average peritoneal fluid-to-plasma AUC ratio of 35 and recommended a dosage of 60 mg/m^2 for 60 mins, with a favorable pharmacologic and safety profile. These findings warrant including melphalan in future studies, especially for patients with peritoneal recurrence after initial cytoreduction plus HIPEC [94].

8.5.8 Paclitaxel and Docetaxel

Paclitaxel and docetaxel are taxanes used for IP-CHT. The taxanes stabilize the microtubule against depolymerization, thereby disrupting normal microtubule dynamics [95], and exert cytotoxic activity against a broad range of tumors. Owing to their high molecular weight, these agents have a remarkably high AUC ratio—paclitaxel 853 and docetaxel 861—which translates into a clear pharmacokinetic advantage for the intraperitoneal route [96]. Data regarding possible taxane-induced thermal augmentation are conflicting [97–99]. Taxanes have been used in a neoadjuvant intraperitoneal setting as well as intraoperatively and postoperatively. Their cell-cycle-specific mechanism of action makes them a particularly good candidate for repeat application; for example, in EPIC, NIPS, or normothermic adjuvant postoperative IP-CHT [45, 61, 62]. Research efforts now focus on developing novel taxane formulations to increase bioavailability [100].

8.5.9 Irinotecan

Irinotecan is a topoisomerase-I inhibitor that has little if any cytotoxic activity and exerts its anticancer activity only through its metabolite SN-38. Irinotecan has a high molecular weight (677 Daltons) and was considered a pharmacokinetically advantageous molecule for intraperitoneal infusion. In their pharmacokinetic study, Guichard et al. reported high CPT-11 and SN-38 AUCs and low clearance rates from the peritoneal cavity after intracavitary infusion in mice [101]. Conflicting human pharmacokinetic data were reported by Maruyama et al., who showed in patients with malignant ascites from gastric and colon cancer that little or no CPT-11 was converted intraperitoneally to SN-38 after intraperitoneal administration [102, 103]. In a phase I study, Elias et al. combined intraperitoneally delivered oxaliplatin with escalating irinotecan doses during HIPEC, and at 400 mg/m^2 reported a tissue concentration 16–23 times higher than that in unbathed tissues despite grades 3–4 hematological toxicity [104]. Heated combined intraperitoneal perfusion of oxaliplatin plus irinotecan after cytoreduction has achieved disappointing results in recurrent ovarian granulosa-cell tumor [105].

8.5.10 Pemetrexed

Pemetrexed is a multitargeted antifolate that is a folinic acid analog and is in the class of chemotherapy drugs called antimetabolites. It acts by inhibiting three enzymes used in pyrimidine and purine synthesis. By inhibiting the formation of precursor purine and pyrimidine nucleotides, pemetrexed prevents the formation of RNA and DNA, the molecules required for normal cells and cancer cells to grow and survive. Pemetrexed possesses cytotoxic activity against various malignancies, especially mesothelioma, OC, and colon cancer. It acts mainly as a thymidylate synthase inhibitor. Significantly improved survival rates after intravenous infusion in patients with peritoneal and pleural mesothelioma, and the drug's favorable pharmacokinetics, generated interest in its intraperitoneal use [106–108]. Pemetrexed is under investigation for intraperitoneal treatment of MPM and OC [109].

8.6 Conclusions

The past two decades have witnessed advances in perioperative cancer chemotherapy protocols for treating patients with PC. These efforts, combined with improved surgical techniques and better postoperative care, have already led to extremely satisfactory clinical results. Now that technical expertise in high-volume tertiary referral centers has reached a plateau that is hard to overcome, the time has come to concentrate our efforts on pharmacological advances and seek further knowledge on tumor biology.

References

1. Sadeghi B, Arvieux C, Glehen O et al (2000) Peritoneal carcinomatosis from non-gynecologic malignancies: results of the EVOCAPE 1 multicentric prospective study. Cancer 88:358-363
2. Sugarbaker P (1996) Peritoneal carcinomatosis: principle of management. Kluwer Academic Publisher
3. Norton L, Simon R, Brereton HD, Bogden AE (1976) Predicting the course of Gompertzian growth. Nature 264:542-545
4. Norton L, Simon R (1977) Tumor size, sensitivity to therapy, and design of treatment schedules. Cancer treatment reports 61:1307-1317
5. Norton L, Simon R (1986) The Norton-Simon hypothesis revisited. Cancer treatment reports 70:163-169
6. Goldie JH, Coldman AJ (1979) A mathematic model for relating the drug sensitivity of tumors to their spontaneous mutation rate. Cancer treatment reports 63:1727-1733
7. Norton L (1985)Implications of kinetic heterogeneity in clinical oncology. Seminars in oncology 12:231-249
8. Simpson-Herren L, Sanford AH, Holmquist JP (1976) Effects of surgery on the cell kinetics of residual tumor. Cancer treatment reports 60:1749-1760
9. Gunduz N, Fisher B, Saffer EA (1979) Effect of surgical removal on the growth and kinetics of residual tumor. Cancer research 39:3861-3865
10. Tanaka K, Inoue Y, Toiyama J (2010)The role of cytoreduction for metastatic and recurrent colorectal cancer in the era of multidisciplinary treatments J Clin Oncol 28:14091
11. Dedrick RL, Myers CE, Bungay PM, DeVita VT Jr (1978) Pharmacokinetic rationale for peritoneal drug administration in the treatment of ovarian cancer. Cancer treatment reports 62:1-11
12. Sugarbaker PH, Van der Speeten K, Anthony Stuart O, Chang D (2011) Impact of surgical and clinical factors on the pharmacology of intraperitoneal doxorubicin in 145 patients with peritoneal carcinomatosis. European journal of surgical oncology 37:719-726
13. Van der Speeten K, Stuart OA, Mahteme H, Sugarbaker PH (2009) A pharmacologic analysis of intraoperative intracavitary cancer chemotherapy with doxorubicin. Cancer chemotherapy and pharmacology 263:799-805
14. Rubin J, Clawson M, Planch A, Jones Q (1988) Measurements of peritoneal surface area in man and rat. The American journal of the medical sciences 295:453-458
15. Rossi CR, Deraco M, De Simone M et al (2004) Hyperthermic intraperitoneal intraoperative chemotherapy after cytoreductive surgery for the treatment of abdominal sarcomatosis: clinical outcome and prognostic factors in 60 consecutive patients. Cancer 100:1943-1950
16. Baratti D, Kusamura S, Martinetti A et al (2007) Prognostic value of circulating tumor markers in patients with pseudomyxoma peritonei treated with cytoreductive surgery and hyperthermic intraperitoneal chemotherapy. Annals of surgical oncology 14:2300-2308
17. Glehen O, Schreiber V, Cotte E et al (2004) Cytoreductive surgery and intraperitoneal chemohyperthermia for peritoneal carcinomatosis arising from gastric cancer. Archives of surgery 139:20-26
18. Gardner SN (2000) A mechanistic, predictive model of dose-response curves for cell cycle phase-specific and -nonspecific drugs. Cancer research 60:1417-1425
19. Kusamura S, Elias D, Baratti D et al (2008) Drugs, carrier solutions and temperature in hyperthermic intraperitoneal chemotherapy. Journal of surgical oncology 98:247-252
20. Esquis P, Consolo D, Magnin G et al (2006) High intra-abdominal pressure enhances the penetration and antitumor effect of intraperitoneal cisplatin on experimental peritoneal carcinomatosis. Annals of surgery 244:106-112
21. Gonzalez-Moreno S, Gonzalez-Bayon L, Ortega-Perez G (2012) Hyperthermic intraperitoneal chemotherapy: methodology and safety considerations. Surgical oncology clinics of North America 21:543-557

22. Ortega-Deballon P, Facy O, Jambet S et al (2010) Which method to deliver hyperthermic intraperitoneal chemotherapy with oxaliplatin? An experimental comparison of open and closed techniques. Annals of surgical oncology 17:1957-1963
23. Facy O, Al Samman S, Magnin G et al (2012) High pressure enhances the effect of hyperthermia in intraperitoneal chemotherapy with oxaliplatin: an experimental study. Annals of surgery 256:1084-1088
24. Katz MH, Barone RM (2003) The rationale of perioperative intraperitoneal chemotherapy in the treatment of peritoneal surface malignancies. Surgical oncology clinics of North America 12:673-688
25. Tannock IF, Lee CM, Tunggal JK et al (2002) Limited penetration of anticancer drugs through tumor tissue: a potential cause of resistance of solid tumors to chemotherapy. Clinical cancer research 8:878-884
26. Los G, Mutsaers PH, Lenglet WJ et al (1990) Platinum distribution in intraperitoneal tumors after intraperitoneal cisplatin treatment. Cancer chemotherapy and pharmacology 25:389-394
27. Los G, Verdegaal EM, Mutsaers PH, McVie JG (1991) Penetration of carboplatin and cisplatin into rat peritoneal tumor nodules after intraperitoneal chemotherapy. Cancer chemotherapy and pharmacology 28:159-165
28. Dedrick RL, Flessner MF (1997) Pharmacokinetic problems in peritoneal drug administration: tissue penetration and surface exposure. Journal of the National Cancer Institute 89:480-487
29. Flessner MF, Choi J, Credit K et al (2005) Resistance of tumor interstitial pressure to the penetration of intraperitoneally delivered antibodies into metastatic ovarian tumors. Clinical cancer research 11:3117-3125
30. Grantab RH, Tannock IF (2012) Penetration of anticancer drugs through tumour tissue as a function of cellular packing density and interstitial fluid pressure and its modification by bortezomib. BMC cancer12:214
31. Molucon-Chabrot C, Isambert N, Benoit L et al (2006) Feasibility of using intraperitoneal epinephrine and cisplatin in patients with advanced peritoneal carcinomatosis. Anti-cancer drugs 17:1211-1217
32. Sticca RP, Dach BW (2003) Rationale for hyperthermia with intraoperative intraperitoneal chemotherapy agents. Surgical oncology clinics of North America 12:689-701
33. Dahl O, Dalene R, Schem BC, Mella O (1999) Status of clinical hyperthermia. Acta oncologica (Stockholm, Sweden) 38:863-873
34. Kampinga HH (2006) Cell biological effects of hyperthermia alone or combined with radiation or drugs: a short introduction to newcomers in the field. International journal of hyperthermia 22:191-196
35. Leunig M, Goetz AE, Dellian M et al (1992) Interstitial fluid pressure in solid tumors following hyperthermia: possible correlation with therapeutic response. Cancer research 52:487-490
36. Piche N, Leblond FA, Sideris L et al (2001) Rationale for heating oxaliplatin for the intraperitoneal treatment of peritoneal carcinomatosis: a study of the effect of heat on intraperitoneal oxaliplatin using a murine model. Annals of surgery 254:138-144
37. Souslova T, Averill-Bates DA (2004) Multidrug-resistant hela cells overexpressing MRP1 exhibit sensitivity to cell killing by hyperthermia: interactions with etoposide. International journal of radiation oncology, biology, physics 60:1538-1551
38. Elias D, Bonnay M, Puizillou JM et al (2002) Heated intra-operative intraperitoneal oxaliplatin after complete resection of peritoneal carcinomatosis: pharmacokinetics and tissue distribution. Annals of oncology 13:267-272
39. Mathe G, Kidani Y, Segiguchi M et al (1989) Oxalato-platinum or 1-OHP, a third-generation platinum complex: an experimental and clinical appraisal and preliminary comparison with cis-platinum and carboplatinum. Biomedicine & pharmacotherapy 43:237-250
40. de Gramont A, Tournigand C, Louvet C et al (1997) Oxaliplatin, folinic acid and 5-fluorouracil (FOLFOX) in pretreated patients with metastatic advanced cancer. The GERCOD. La Revue de medecine interne / fondee par la Societe nationale francaise de medecine interne 18:769-775

41. Van der Speeten K, Stuart OA, Mahteme H, Sugarbaker PH (2010) Pharmacology of perioperative 5-fluorouracil. Journal of surgical oncology 102:730-735
42. Elias D, Goere D, Dumont F et al (2014) Role of hyperthermic intraoperative peritoneal chemotherapy in the management of peritoneal metastases. European journal of cancer 50:332-340
43. Glockzin G, Rochon J, Arnold D et al (2013) A prospective multicenter phase II study evaluating multimodality treatment of patients with peritoneal carcinomatosis arising from appendiceal and colorectal cancer: the COMBATAC trial. BMC cancer 13:67
44. Van der Speeten K, Stuart OA, Mahteme H, Sugarbaker PH (2011) Pharmacokinetic study of perioperative intravenous Ifosfamide. International journal of surgical oncology 2011:185092
45. Fujiwara Y, Takiguchi S, Nakajima K et al (2012) Intraperitoneal docetaxel combined with S-1 for advanced gastric cancer with peritoneal dissemination. Journal of surgical oncology 105:38-42
46. Canbay E, Mizumoto A, Ichinose M et al (2014) Outcome data of patients with peritoneal carcinomatosis from gastric origin treated by a strategy of bidirectional chemotherapy prior to cytoreductive surgery and hyperthermic intraperitoneal chemotherapy in a single specialized center in Japan. Annals of surgical oncology 21:1147-1152
47. Sugarbaker PH, Bijelic L (2012) Adjuvant bidirectional chemotherapy using an intraperitoneal port. Gastroenterology research and practice 2012:752643
48. Verwaal VJ, van Ruth S, de Bree E et al (2003) Randomized trial of cytoreduction and hyperthermic intraperitoneal chemotherapy versus systemic chemotherapy and palliative surgery in patients with peritoneal carcinomatosis of colorectal cancer. Journal of clinical oncology 21:3737-3743
49. Sugarbaker PH (2009) Epithelial appendiceal neoplasms. Cancer journal (Sudbury, Mass)15:225-235
50. Weber T, Roitman M, Link KH (2012) Current status of cytoreductive surgery with hyperthermic intraperitoneal chemotherapy in patients with peritoneal carcinomatosis from colorectal cancer. Clinical colorectal cancer 11:167-176
51. Bachur NR, Gordon SL, Gee MV, Kon H (1979) NADPH cytochrome P-450 reductase activation of quinone anticancer agents to free radicals. Proceedings of the National Academy of Sciences of the United States of America 76:954-957
52. Barlogie B, Corry PM, Drewinko B (1980) In vitro thermochemotherapy of human colon cancer cells with cis-dichlorodiammineplatinum(II) and mitomycin C. Cancer research 40:1165-1168
53. Jacquet P, Averbach A, Stephens AD et al (1998) Heated intraoperative intraperitoneal mitomycin C and early postoperative intraperitoneal 5-fluorouracil: pharmacokinetic studies. Oncology 55:130-138
54. Van der Speeten K, Stuart OA, Chang D et al (2011) Changes induced by surgical and clinical factors in the pharmacology of intraperitoneal mitomycin C in 145 patients with peritoneal carcinomatosis. Cancer chemotherapy and pharmacology 68:147-156
55. van Ruth S, Verwaal VJ, Zoetmulder FA (2003) Pharmacokinetics of intraperitoneal mitomycin C. Surgical oncology clinics of North America 12:771-780
56. Esquivel J (2009) Technology of hyperthermic intraperitoneal chemotherapy in the United States, Europe, China, Japan, and Korea. Cancer journal (Sudbury, Mass) 15:249-254
57. Smeenk RM, Verwaal VJ, Zoetmulder FA (2006) Toxicity and mortality of cytoreduction and intraoperative hyperthermic intraperitoneal chemotherapy in pseudomyxoma peritonei—a report of 103 procedures. European journal of surgical oncology 32:186-190
58. Sugarbaker PH, Alderman R, Edwards G et al (2006) Prospective morbidity and mortality assessment of cytoreductive surgery plus perioperative intraperitoneal chemotherapy to treat peritoneal dissemination of appendiceal mucinous malignancy. Annals of surgical oncology 13:635-644
59. Cepeda V, Fuertes MA, Castilla J et al (2007) Biochemical mechanisms of cisplatin cytotoxicity. Anti-cancer agents in medicinal chemistry 7:3-18

60. Alberts DS, Liu PY, Hannigan EV et al (1996) Intraperitoneal cisplatin plus intravenous cyclophosphamide versus intravenous cisplatin plus intravenous cyclophosphamide for stage III ovarian cancer. The New England journal of medicine 335:1950-1955
61. Markman M, Bundy BN, Alberts DS et al (2001) Phase III trial of standard-dose intravenous cisplatin plus paclitaxel versus moderately high-dose carboplatin followed by intravenous paclitaxel and intraperitoneal cisplatin in small-volume stage III ovarian carcinoma: an intergroup study of the Gynecologic Oncology Group, Southwestern Oncology Group, and Eastern Cooperative Oncology Group. Journal of clinical oncology 19:1001-1007
62. Armstrong DK, Bundy B, Wenzel L et al (2006) Intraperitoneal cisplatin and paclitaxel in ovarian cancer. The New England journal of medicine 354:34-43
63. Urano M, Kuroda M, Nishimura Y (1999) For the clinical application of thermochemotherapy given at mild temperatures. International journal of hyperthermia 15:79-107
64. Los G, Mutsaers PH, van der Vijgh WJ et al (1989) Direct diffusion of cis-diamminedichloroplatinum(II) in intraperitoneal rat tumors after intraperitoneal chemotherapy: a comparison with systemic chemotherapy. Cancer research 49:3380-3384
65. van de Vaart PJ, van der Vange N, Zoetmulder FA et al (1998) Intraperitoneal cisplatin with regional hyperthermia in advanced ovarian cancer: pharmacokinetics and cisplatin-DNA adduct formation in patients and ovarian cancer cell lines. European journal of cancer 34:148-154
66. Raymond E, Faivre S, Woynarowski JM, Chaney SG (1998) Oxaliplatin: mechanism of action and antineoplastic activity. Seminars in oncology 25:4-12
67. Di Francesco AM, Ruggiero A, Riccardi R (2002) Cellular and molecular aspects of drugs of the future: oxaliplatin. Cellular and molecular life sciences 59:1914-1927
68. Elias DM, Sideris L (2003) Pharmacokinetics of heated intraoperative intraperitoneal oxaliplatin after complete resection of peritoneal carcinomatosis. Surgical oncology clinics of North America 12:755-769
69. Jerremalm E, Hedeland M, Wallin I et al (2004) Oxaliplatin degradation in the presence of chloride: identification and cytotoxicity of the monochloro monooxalato complex. Pharmaceutical research 21:891-894
70. De Somer F, Ceelen W, Delanghe J et al (2008) Severe hyponatremia, hyperglycemia, and hyperlactatemia are associated with intraoperative hyperthermic intraperitoneal chemoperfusion with oxaliplatin. Peritoneal dialysis international 28:61-66
71. Stewart JHt, Shen P, Russell G et al (2008) A phase I trial of oxaliplatin for intraperitoneal hyperthermic chemoperfusion for the treatment of peritoneal surface dissemination from colorectal and appendiceal cancers. Annals of surgical oncology 15:2137-2145
72. Fagotti A, Costantini B, Petrillo M et al (2012) Cytoreductive surgery plus HIPEC in platinum-sensitive recurrent ovarian cancer patients: a case-control study on survival in patients with two year follow-up. Gynecologic oncology 127:502-505
73. Esselen KM, Rodriguez N, Growdon W (2012) Patterns of recurrence in advanced epithelial ovarian, fallopian tube and peritoneal cancers treated with intraperitoneal chemotherapy. Gynecologic oncology 127:51-54
74. Argenta PA, Sueblinvong T, Geller MA et al (2013) Hyperthermic intraperitoneal chemotherapy with carboplatin for optimally-cytoreduced, recurrent, platinum-sensitive ovarian carcinoma: a pilot study. Gynecologic oncology 129:81-85
75. Czejka M, Jager W, Schuller J, Teherani D (1991) [Pharmacokinetics of carboplatin after intraperitoneal administration]. Archiv der Pharmazie 324:183-184
76. Jandial DD, Messer K, Farshchi-Heydari S (2009) Tumor platinum concentration following intraperitoneal administration of cisplatin versus carboplatin in an ovarian cancer model. Gynecologic oncology 115:362-366
77. Tritton TR (1991) Cell surface actions of adriamycin. Pharmacology & therapeutics 49:293-309
78. Lane P, Vichi P, Bain DL, Tritton TR (1987) Temperature dependence studies of adriamycin uptake and cytotoxicity. Cancer research 47:4038-4042

79. Jacquet P, Averbach A, Stuart OA et al (1998) Hyperthermic intraperitoneal doxorubicin: pharmacokinetics, metabolism, and tissue distribution in a rat model. Cancer chemotherapy and pharmacology 41:147-154
80. Pilati P, Mocellin S, Rossi CR et al (2003) Doxorubicin activity is enhanced by hyperthermia in a model of ex vivo vascular perfusion of human colon carcinoma. World journal of surgery 27:640-646
81. Harrison LE, Bryan M, Pliner L, Saunders T. Phase I trial of pegylated liposomal doxorubicin with hyperthermic intraperitoneal chemotherapy in patients undergoing cytoreduction for advanced intra-abdominal malignancy. Annals of surgical oncology. 2008;15(5):1407-13.
82. Pestieau SR, Stuart OA, Chang D et al (1998) Pharmacokinetics of intraperitoneal gemcitabine in a rat model. Tumori 84:706-711
83. Sabbatini P, Aghajanian C, Leitao M et al (2004) Intraperitoneal cisplatin with intraperitoneal gemcitabine in patients with epithelial ovarian cancer: results of a phase I/II Trial. Clinical cancer research 10:2962-2967
84. Morgan RJ, Jr, Synold TW, Xi B et al (2007) Phase I trial of intraperitoneal gemcitabine in the treatment of advanced malignancies primarily confined to the peritoneal cavity. Clinical cancer research 13:1232-1237
85. Gamblin TC, Egorin MJ, Zuhowski EG et al (2008) Intraperitoneal gemcitabine pharmacokinetics: a pilot and pharmacokinetic study in patients with advanced adenocarcinoma of the pancreas. Cancer chemotherapy and pharmacology 62:647-653
86. Sugarbaker PH, Stuart OA, Bijelic L (2011) Intraperitoneal gemcitabine chemotherapy treatment for patients with resected pancreatic cancer: rationale and report of early data. International journal of surgical oncology 2011:161862
87. Tentes AA, Kyziridis D, Kakolyris S et al (2012) Preliminary results of hyperthermic intraperitoneal intraoperative chemotherapy as an adjuvant in resectable pancreatic cancer. Gastroenterology research and practice 2012:506571
88. Sarosy G, Leyland-Jones B, Soochan P, Cheson BD (1988) The systemic administration of intravenous melphalan. Journal of clinical oncology 6:1768-1782
89. Urano M, Ling CC (2002) Thermal enhancement of melphalan and oxaliplatin cytotoxicity in vitro. International journal of hyperthermia 18:307-315
90. Testori A, Verhoef C, Kroon HM et al (2011) Treatment of melanoma metastases in a limb by isolated limb perfusion and isolated limb infusion. Journal of surgical oncology 104:397-404
91. Alberts DS, Chen HS, Chang SY, Peng YM (1980) The disposition of intraperitoneal bleomycin, melphalan, and vinblastine in cancer patients. Recent results in cancer 74:293-299
92. Glehen O, Stuart OA, Mohamed F, Sugarbaker PH (2004) Hyperthermia modifies pharmacokinetics and tissue distribution of intraperitoneal melphalan in a rat model. Cancer chemotherapy and pharmacology. 54:79-84
93. Sugarbaker PH, Stuart OA (2007) Pharmacokinetic and phase II study of heated intraoperative intraperitoneal melphalan. Cancer chemotherapy and pharmacology 59:151-155
94. Bijelic L, Sugarbaker PH, Stuart OA (2012) Hyperthermic intraperitoneal chemotherapy with melphalan: a summary of clinical and pharmacological data in 34 patients. Gastroenterology research and practice 2012:827534
95. Ceelen WP, Pahlman L, Mahteme H (2007) Pharmacodynamic aspects of intraperitoneal cytotoxic therapy. Cancer treatment and research 134:195-214
96. Mohamed F, Sugarbaker PH (2003) Intraperitoneal taxanes. Surgical oncology clinics of North America 12:825-833
97. Rietbroek RC, Katschinski DM, Reijers MH et al (1997) Lack of thermal enhancement for taxanes in vitro. International journal of hyperthermia 13:525-533
98. Schrump DS, Zhai S, Nguyen DM et al (2002) Pharmacokinetics of paclitaxel administered by hyperthermic retrograde isolated lung perfusion techniques. The Journal of thoracic and cardiovascular surgery 123:686-694
99. Mohamed F, Stuart OA, Glehen O et al (2004) Docetaxel and hyperthermia: factors that modify thermal enhancement. Journal of surgical oncology 88:14-20

100. Bouquet W, Ceelen W, Adriaens E et al (2010) In vivo toxicity and bioavailability of Taxol and a paclitaxel/beta-cyclodextrin formulation in a rat model during HIPEC. Annals of surgical oncology 17:2510-2517
101. Guichard S, Chatelut E, Lochon I et al (1998) Comparison of the pharmacokinetics and efficacy of irinotecan after administration by the intravenous versus intraperitoneal route in mice. Cancer chemotherapy and pharmacology 42:165-170
102. Maruyama M, Toukairin Y, Baba H et al (2000) Experimental study on CPT-11 intraperitoneal chemotherapy—metabolism of CPT-11 in malignant ascites. Gan to kagaku ryoho Cancer & chemotherapy 27:1858-1860
103. Maruyama M, Toukairin Y, Baba H et al (2001) Pharmacokinetic study of the intraperitoneal administration of CPT-11 for patients with peritoneal seedings of gastric and colonic cancers. Gan to kagaku ryoho Cancer & chemotherapy 28:1505-1507
104. Elias D, Matsuhisa T, Sideris L et al (2004) Heated intra-operative intraperitoneal oxaliplatin plus irinotecan after complete resection of peritoneal carcinomatosis: pharmacokinetics, tissue distribution and tolerance. Annals of oncology 15:1558-1565
105. Gouy S, Uzan C, Pautier P et al (2013) Results of oxaliplatin-based hyperthermic intraperitoneal chemotherapy in recurrent ovarian granulosa cell tumors. European journal of obstetrics, gynecology, and reproductive biology 170:464-467
106. Pestieau SR, Stuart OA, Sugarbaker PH et al (2000) Multi-targeted antifolate (MTA): pharmacokinetics of intraperitoneal administration in a rat model. European journal of surgical oncology 26:696-700
107. Vogelzang NJ, Rusthoven JJ, Symanowski J et al (2003) Phase III study of pemetrexed in combination with cisplatin versus cisplatin alone in patients with malignant pleural mesothelioma. Journal of clinical oncology 21:2636-2644
108. Janne PA, Wozniak AJ, Belani CP et al (2005) Open-label study of pemetrexed alone or in combination with cisplatin for the treatment of patients with peritoneal mesothelioma: outcomes of an expanded access program. Clinical lung cancer 7:40-46
109. Chambers SK, Chow HH, Janicek MF et al (2012) Phase I trial of intraperitoneal pemetrexed, cisplatin, and paclitaxel in optimally debulked ovarian cancer. Clinical cancer research 18:2668-2678

Peritonectomy Techniques

9

Angelo Di Giorgio

9.1 Introduction

The treatment of peritoneal carcinomatosis (PC) and of primary tumors of the peritoneum with peritoneal diffusion—two conditions known as peritoneal surface malignancies (PSM)—currently includes peritonectomy combined with hyperthermic intraperitoneal chemotherapy (PRT plus HIPEC). PRT plus HIPEC consists of two phases: in the first phase, which lasts about 8 h, peritoneal disease is surgically removed; in the second phase, HIPEC is administered over 30–90 min, depending on drug regimen. This integrated procedure has a curative intent and aims to improve patient quality of life (QoL) and increase survival rates.

9.2 Principles of Management

Surgical procedures aimed at maximal cytoreduction of PSM are known as PRT, according to the definition given by Paul Sugarbaker [1]. This term identifies the actual aim of such cytoreductive surgery (CRS): excision of parietal and visceral peritoneal areas in which the tumor is present. The rationale of those procedures is complete removal of macroscopically evident disease. Residual cancer cells or minimal implants, if present after cytoreduction, are exposed to the action of HIPEC. A marked cytoreduction plays a crucial role in maximizing the efficacy of HIPEC: indeed, during HIPEC, drugs penetrate tissues for ~4 mm, allowing highest efficacy on microscopic or minimal cancer residuals. In addi-

A. Di Giorgio (✉)
Department of Surgery "Pietro Valdoni", Sapienza University of Rome,
Rome, Italy
e-mail: angelo.digiorgio@uniroma1.it

A. Di Giorgio, E. Pinto (Eds), *Treatment of Peritoneal Surface Malignancies*,
Updates in Surgery
DOI: 10.1007/978-88-470-5711-1_9,

tion, surgical procedures include complete lysis of bowel adhesions and opening of all intra-abdominal recesses: these actions permit adequate circulation of chemotherapeutic agents during HIPEC and optimal exposure of the peritoneal cavity and its contents to the drugs. Maximal cytoreduction represents the fundamental factor for the success of integrated treatment. Its prognostic value has been confirmed for all forms of PSM, both in primary and recurrent settings. PRT consists of a number of techniques, which can be used according to anatomical districts and to dimensions and quality of carcinosis. Carcinomatosis can be removed with wide resection of parietal peritoneum, visceral and parenchymal exeresis, local excision, or in situ destruction of implants. It requires adequate surgical instrumentation, which should include high-quality electrosurgery with a full set of tips of various shapes and dimensions, argon-beam laser, UltraCision, radiofrequency, and all tools useful for removing malignant implants of different shapes and to control bleeding. Particular attention must be paid to hemostasis, vein ligation, and anastomosis, as sutures and ligations are potentially susceptible to HIPEC aggression, particularly when administered via a closed-abdomen technique (closed HIPEC). Vein ligations should always be doubled. The use of metal clips should be reserved exclusively for treating small vessels and should be avoided for medium and large vessels because of the long duration of procedure, during which manipulation of anatomical structures is particularly intense and may involve the risk of clip dislocation. In addition, UltraCision for vascular sectioning and sealing should be used with care. Anastomosis, even when performed with mechanical staplers, should be reinforced with continuous suture or single stitches, especially when closed HIPEC will be performed. During PRT, large excisions require careful hemostasis. An electrosurgical handpiece with ball tip, argon-beam laser, and adhesive products (paste, foam, sheets) are especially useful. Radiofrequency tools help achieve hemostasis in narrow and difficult-to-access areas.

Patients eligible for PRT plus HIPEC are enrolled into specific protocols for each neoplastic form. The evaluation of eligibility to surgery is based on morphological [computed tomography (CT), positron emission tomography (PET), magnetic resonance imaging (MRI), ultrasound (US)] and clinical assessment. In particular, criteria for absolute contraindications for surgery should be identified. These include massive involvement of the radix mesenterii or small bowel, first intestinal loop, duodenum or pancreas (head, body), liver, diaphragmatic pillars, large vessels (vena cava), bladder, diffuse hepatic metastases, or metastatic lymphadenopathy above renal vessels. For specific forms of carcinosis, the extension of endoperitoneal diffusion as assessed by specific protocols can be indicative of ineligibility for surgery.

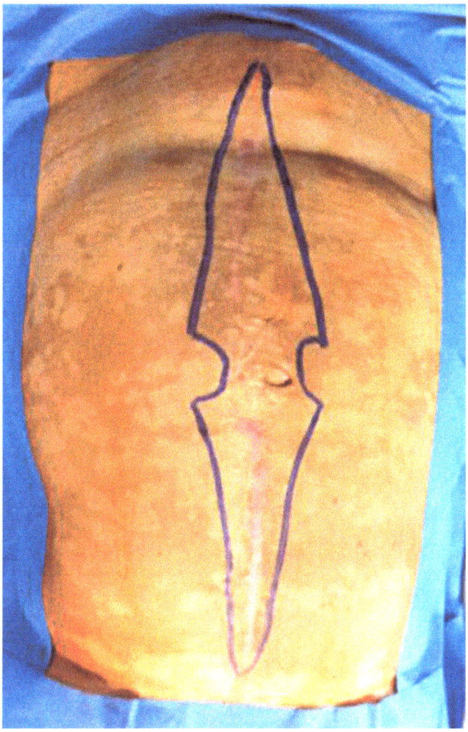

Fig. 9.1 Skin resection in repeat laparotomy includes umbilicus. Incision drawing is aimed at cosmetic umbilical reconstruction

9.3 Surgical Procedure

9.3.1 Incision

The patient is placed in a modified lithotomy position with legs extended. Access is always performed by a complete midline incision from xiphoid to pubis. In secondary cytoreduction, the scar should be completely removed, including umbilicus, skin, musculoaponeurotic, and peritoneal margins, which are common sites of disease diffusion in patients with recurrences (Fig. 9.1). In patients with previous laparoscopy for treatment of the primary tumor or those with a previous diagnostic laparoscopy, particular attention should be given to trocar sites, which can be potentially contaminated by neoplastic implants.

9.3.2 Examination of the Abdominal Cavity

A complete abdominal lysis of adhesions is performed to evaluate the possibility of surgical exeresis and carcinosis extension. The latter can be classified according to different criteria, the most frequently used being the Peritoneal

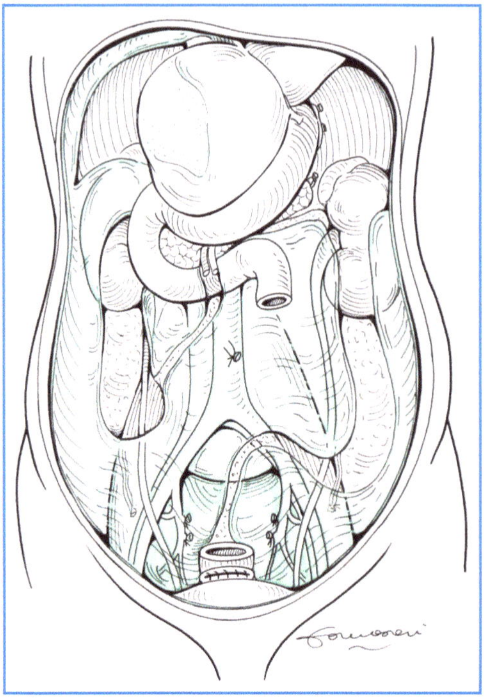

Fig. 9.2 Parietal peritoneum

Cancer Index (PCI) [2]. Exeresis of parietal and visceral peritoneum represents the fundamental step of PRT. This goal is achieved by evaluating localization, type, extension, and number of carcinomatosis implants. Proper assessment of these parameters allows correct planning of the extent of visceral exeresis and parietal PRT and identifies the most suitable techniques for implant removal and/or destruction.

9.3.3 Peritonectomy

PRT comprises:

- Removal of parietal peritoneum
- Removal of visceral peritoneum (visceral and parenchymal resections)
- Removal/in situ destruction of implants
- Resection of abdominal wall, muscle implants, and trocar sites
- Lymphadenectomy

9.3.3.1 Removal of Parietal Peritoneum

The peritoneum entirely covers the abdominal wall, pelvic cavities (Fig. 9.2) and endoabdominal organs (visceral peritoneum). Several thickenings, such as liga-

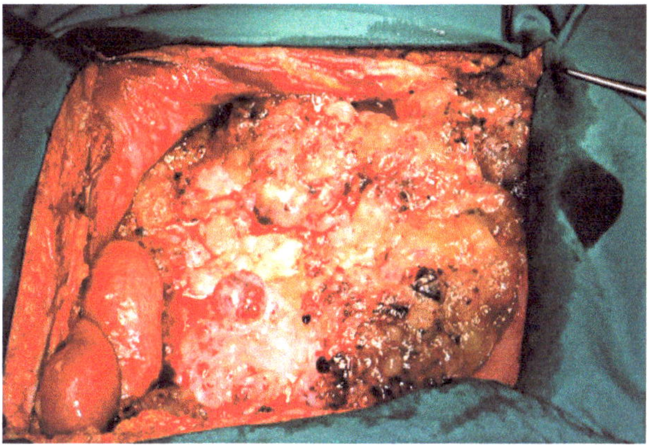

Fig. 9.3 Massive carcinomatous infiltration of the greater omentum: "omental cake"

ments, connect visceral and parenchymal organs to each other and to the abdominal wall, thus forming anatomical recesses, including omental bursa. Carcinosis can affect all those areas and is promoted by the peculiar circulation of endoabdominal fluids and ascites, ligamentous obstacles to fluid circulation, and the possibility of ascites trapped in natural or newly formed (e.g., due to previous surgical interventions) cavities. Specific anatomical structure and function of some abdominal districts can promote the development of carcinomatosis implants. In particular, the high number of milky spots in the pelvic peritoneum and epiploon—organs for ascites reabsorption—promotes implant formation and penetration of neoplastic cells into the peritoneal lamina and underlying tissues (Fig. 9.3).

The peritoneum is the substratum for carcinomatosis; however, it also represents an effective barrier, helping to maintain disease in the peritoneal cavity. During PRT, cutting the ligaments and complete visceral adhesiolysis represents a preliminary step necessary to evaluate disease extend and to perform HIPEC. In fact, only complete cutting of ligaments and extended removal of adherence allow adequate diffusion of HIPEC agents.

At a parietal level, exeresis comprises complete or partial removal of the peritoneum, which covers the abdominal wall, the diaphragm, and the pelvis, according to disease extension (Fig. 9.4). In the presence of carcinosis involving the parietal peritoneum, there is general consensus on the need to remove only the parietal peritoneum that presents implants, without removing unaffected areas. When the abdominal wall presents extensive and deeply penetrating disease, removal of some tracts of the musculoaponeurotic layer may be necessary (Fig. 9.5a, b). Wide peritoneal resection should be reserved to areas with extensive disease, whereas *à la demande* resection is suggested when implants are isolates with large areas of healthy tissue in between. If the healthy areas are limited, large peritonectomies—which can include entire anatomical sectors or even complete PRT—should be performed.

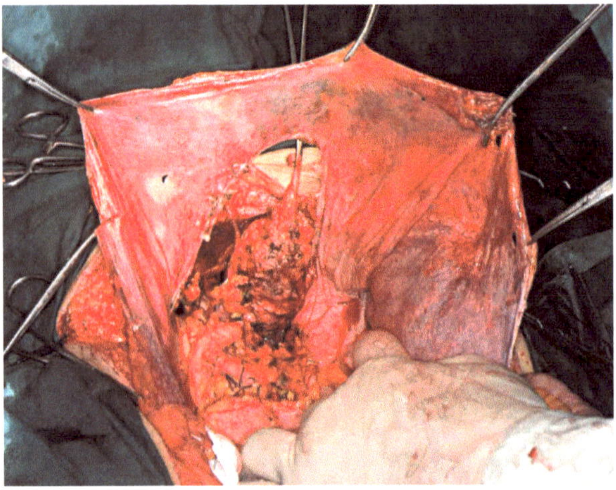

Fig. 9.4 Pelvic parietal peritonectomy

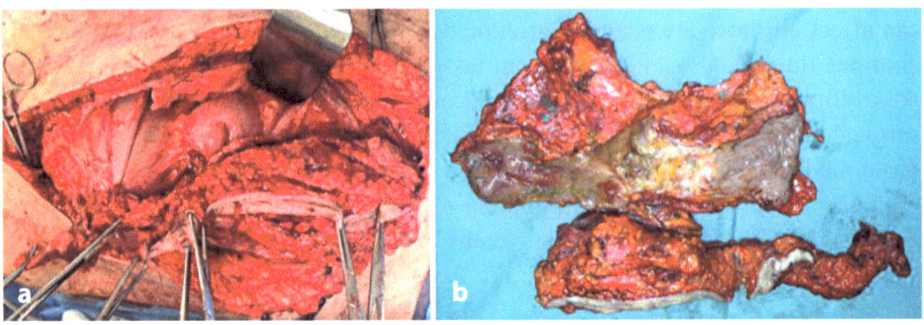

Fig. 9.5a, b En bloc resection of abdominal wall and ileum for carcinomatous involvement

When carcinomatosis involves pelvis and diaphragm, large excisions are required: they should comprise pelvic PRT and PRT of iliac fossae below the umbilical transverse line when the pelvis is involved, and diaphragm PRT associated with resection of the falciform and round ligament when the diaphragm is involved. Falciform and round ligament resection, in association with left hepatic triangular ligament resection, should be performed in all PRT procedures, with the aim of allowing correct placement of HIPEC catheters and optimal diffusion of chemotherapy solution.

Diaphragmatic PRT is technically complex. The diaphragmatic peritoneum adheres strongly to the diaphragm and tendinous center. Therefore—especially when implants are deeply infiltrating—there is a high risk of opening the pleural cavity and it subsequently becoming contaminated by neoplastic cells. In these cases, fluid penetration into the pleural cavity should be avoided by constant use of the aspirator and by sealing the opening. When action is taken immediately and the opening is sutured, the precautionary placement of pleural

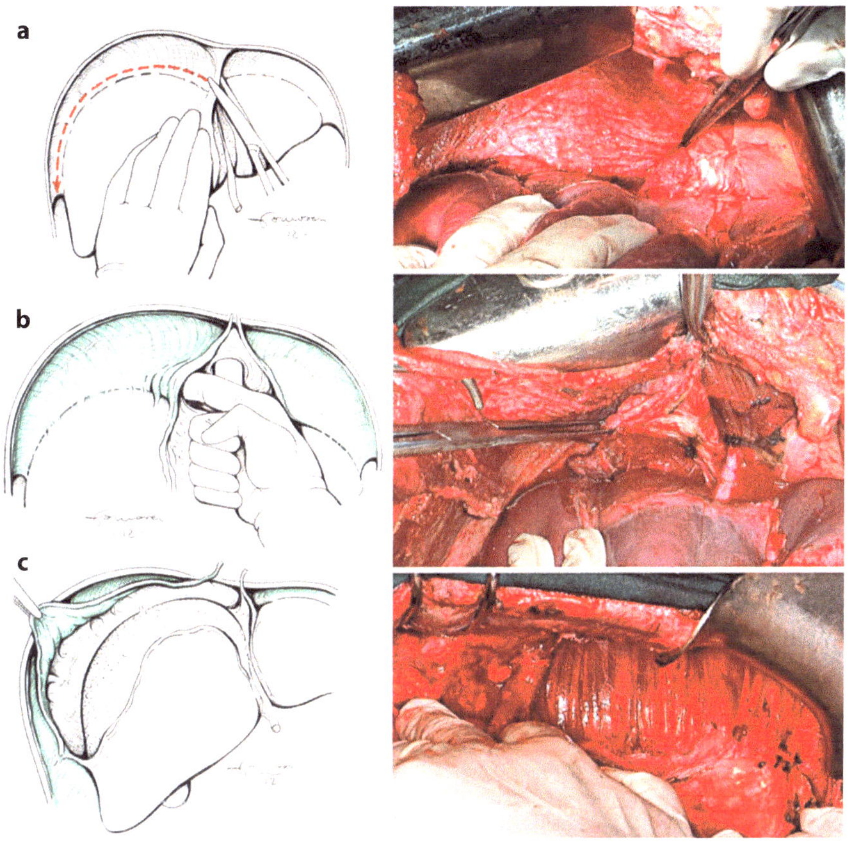

Fig. 9.6 Right-diaphragm peritonectomy: hepatic mobilization (**a**); exposition of vena cava and right suprahepatic vein (**b**); stripping of the diaphragmatic perinoneum (**c**)

drainages is not necessary. If a PRT of both diaphragms is necessary, the right and left resections should be performed separately. PRT of the right diaphragm is the more complex of the two (Fig. 9.6a–c). It begins with the sectioning of the falciform, umbilical, coronary, and triangular ligaments to allow complete liver mobilization. Sectioning of the falciform ligament up to the coronary ligament allows exposure of the precaval space and vena caval estrangement. Excision of the diaphragmatic peritoneum should begin at the margin of the laparotomy incision and continued by detaching the serous membrane from muscles and tendons, paying particular attention to preserving diaphragmatic and muscle vessels. Removing the right diaphragmatic peritoneum is completed by traction on the falciform and coronary ligaments. Glisson's capsule is often involved: in these cases, either removing the tracts of Glisson's capsule or in situ destruction of implants can be performed (see later chapters). The gall bladder is also frequently involved and should be removed as necessary.

PRT of the left diaphragm is based—as for the right diaphragm—on falciform, umbilical, coronary, and left triangular ligament section. Detaching the peritoneum is begun at the left margin of the middle abdominal incision and progresses backward. Contemporary ligament traction helps in complete removal of the left peritoneum. The spleen is often involved, and in such cases, it should be removed.

The parietal PRT comprises stripping the omental bursa peritoneum and resecting the greater and lesser omentum. Removing the greater omentum should be performed in all surgical procedures for PC. In fact, the omentum is rich in milky spots and therefore attracts neoplastic cells. Moreover, removing the greater omentum is mandatory for treating different primary tumors associated with carcinosis, such as ovarian or stomach cancer. Removing the greater omentum should be always complete and includes skeletonization of the greater curvature of the stomach. Vessels of the omentum should be ligated and cut near the gastric wall; ligation is safer than UltraCision. The right gastroepiploic vein must be cut at the intersection with the middle colic vein. Involvement of the omentum between the greater curvature and the spleen is often associated with parenchymal spleen involvement or hilar lymph node metastases: in these cases, splenectomy is mandatory (Fig. 9.7a–c)

Lesser omentum resection should save the arteries of the lesser curvature to preserve stomach vascularization and innervation. Resection may be optionally associated with pylorotomy to control loss of tone of gastric wall. Greater omentum resection is always required and of the lesser omentum only when necessary to expose the omental bursa. Cleaning the omental bursa can also include resecting the upper sheath of the transverse mesocolon and prepancreatic peritoneum and should extend to Morrison's pouch and the gastrohepatic ligament peritoneum when infiltrated by carcinomatosis. Resecting the peritoneum of the paracolic gutters, iliac fossae, and anterior wall does not present a technical issue; however, caution must be taken to verify integrity of the epigastric vessels to avoid postoperative bleeding (Fig. 9.8).

The pelvic peritoneum, analogously with the greater omentum, is rich in milky spots that filter and reabsorb endoperitoneal liquid. Viable neoplastic cells are thus concentrated, producing pelvic carcinomatosis. The degree of peritoneal infiltration and volume of pelvic carcinomatosis influence the strategy of pelvic cytoreduction. Simple pouch stripping without rectal resection can be performed when carcinomatosis spread is superficial. More frequently, removing pelvic and iliac fossae is associated with en bloc resection of endopelvic organs, such as female genitals and rectosigmoid colon with mesorectum (Fig. 9.9). Urinary bladder and prevesical peritoneal resection is frequent, whereas total cystectomy is exceptional.

The parietal peritoneum is stripped off the posterior rectus sheath starting at the margins of the median laparotomy, round ligaments are cut (in women), and the bladder and iliac fossae peritoneum is then detached to expose the retroperitoneum. In women, ovarian vessels are ligated and cut.

Ureters are identified and underpassed with vessel loops. Iliac vessels are dissected; temporary clamping or ligation of the internal iliac artery below the

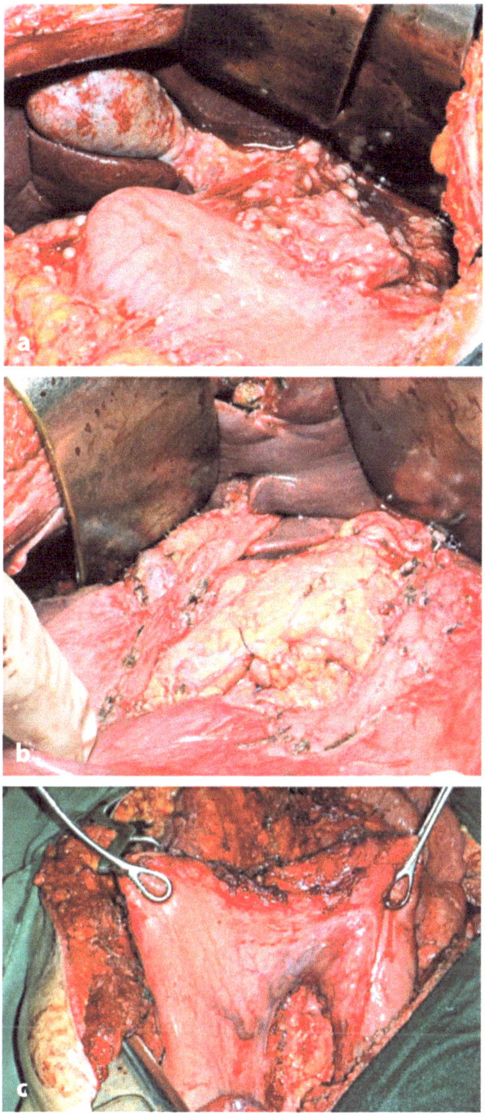

Fig. 9.7a–c **a** Peritoneal carcinomatosis of the lesser and greater omentum. **b** Lesser omentectomy and stripping of the peritoneum from hepatoduodenal ligament. **c** Lesser and greater omentectomy

origin of the superior gluteal artery may be performed to prevent major pelvic bleeding and is optionally associated with external iliac artery clamping.

Sigmoid colon and descending colon are mobilized. The inferior mesenteric artery is ligated and cut at the aortic origin, and the inferior mesenteric vein is ligated and cut at the ligament of Treitz; the descending colon is cut below the splenic flexure.

After capsizing the left colon and dissecting the rectum and mesorectum, uterine vessels are ligated where they cross the ureters. The bladder is dissected

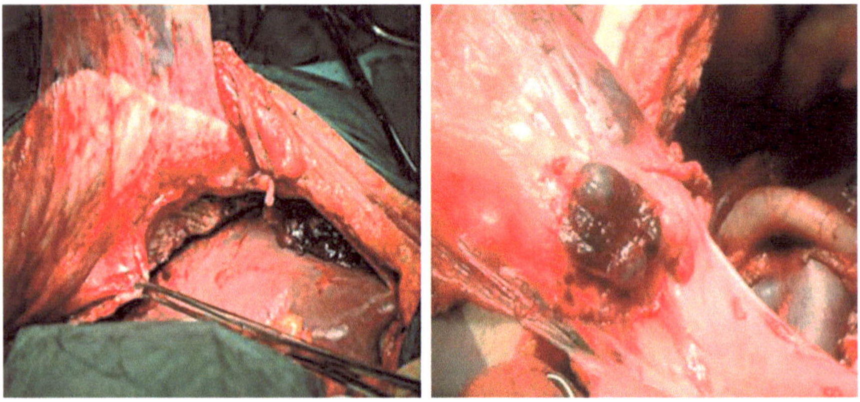

Fig. 9.8 Parietal peritonectomy

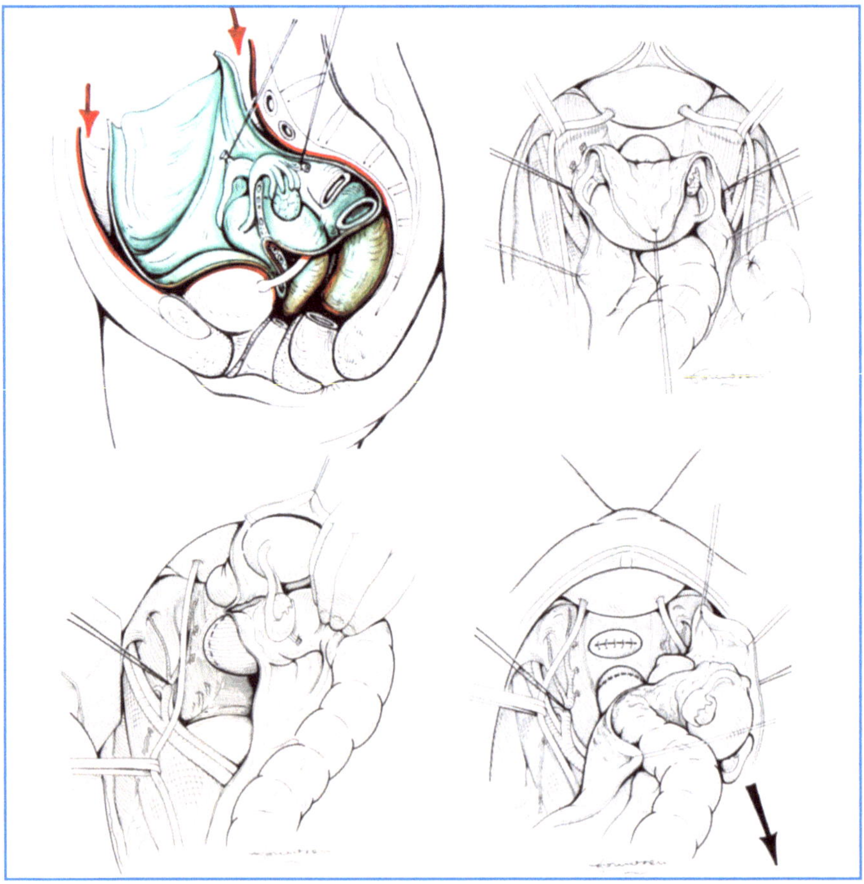

Fig. 9.9 Pelvic peritonectomy: en bloc resection of parietal peritoneum and endopelvic organs; temporary ligature of the internal iliac artery below the origin of the superior gluteal artery is optional

from the uterus neck, and the vagina is opened to allow complete detachment of the uterus neck. The vagina is then closed with interrupted sutures, and the anterior rectum wall is further prepared. The rectum and mesorectum are dissected up to the levator muscles; the rectum is stapled with a Roticulator, cut, and all structures are removed en bloc (Fig. 9.10).

In patients with primary ovarian carcinomatosis, iliac-obturator lymphadenectomy is performed. In rare cases, pelvic peritoneum and, in particular, the pouch of Douglas peritoneum, can be removed, saving endopelvic structures (Fig. 9.11). The pouch peritoneum can be resected (douglassectomy) when implants are superficial. In most female patients, douglassectomy is associated with hysteroadnexectomy. Dissection of the pouch peritoneum from the rectum–sigmoid colon anterior wall should be carefully performed, avoiding opening viscera and being sure to insert muscle sutures in case of parietal injury. Stripping the peritoneum from the bladder is aided by traction of the urachus and sometimes may require partial bladder resection, in relation to implant depth, whereas the need for total cystectomy is unlikely.

9.3.3.2 Removal of Visceral Peritoneum

The visceral peritoneum cannot be dissected from underlying layers and separately removed, which is different from parietal and diaphragmatic peritoneum. Thus, visceral PRT requires resecting viscera or organs in which peritoneal serous membrane is involved by carcinosis. Less frequently, stripping the visceral peritoneum only is an option; this occurs when carcinosis is restricted, does not deeply infiltrate the visceral wall, and is related to specific tumors (peritoneal pseudomyxoma and mesothelioma) (Fig. 9.12). Resection/destruction of single visceral implants in situ is mandatory for treating superficial carcinosis.

In primary cytoreduction, primary tumor exeresis is routinely performed with radical intent: therefore, viscera or organs with primary cancer are removed en bloc with regional lymph nodes. The initial phase of exeresis for the most frequent primary forms is represented by total gastrectomy, colorectal resection, hemicolectomy, total colectomy, and hysteroadnexectomy, all being associated in principle with total greater omentectomy, appendicectomy, and bilateral adnexectomy; resection of umbilical and falciform ligaments are routinely associated. Then, exeresis of further organs or other structures affected by carcinosis is performed: on principle all endoperitoneal organs can be removed if affected by carcinosis. Sacrificing an organ or viscus depends on carcinomatosis entity, implant size and location, and anatomic structure. Conservative treatments for bowel implants with in situ destruction are possible for small lesions and are mandatory when large resections could compromise intestinal function. When an organ or viscus is involved in massive carcinosis, its removal is recommended; splenectomy, cholecystectomy, hysterectomy, adnexectomy, and small- and large-bowel resection are the most common.

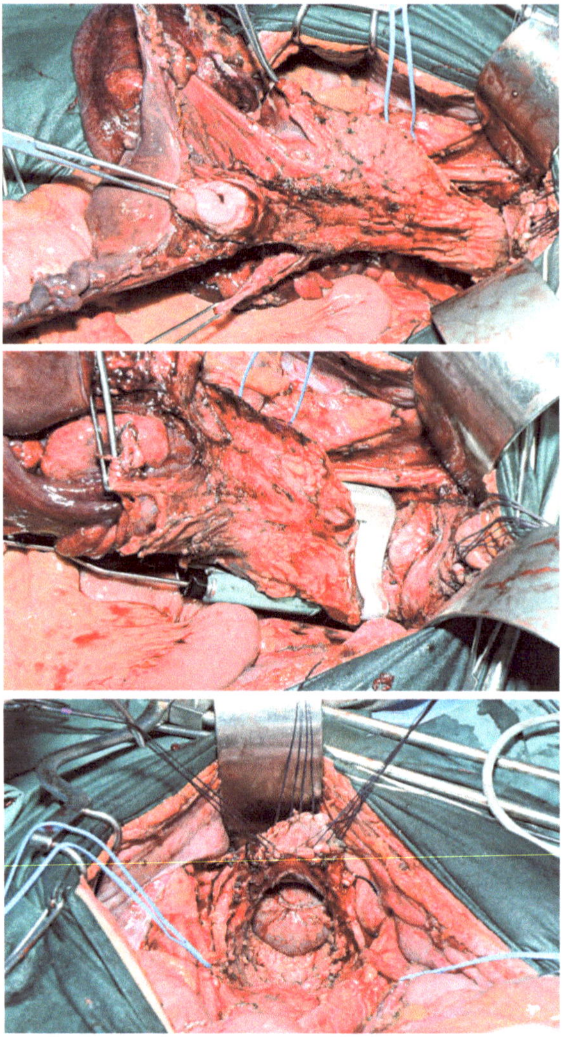

Fig. 9.10 Pelvic peritonectomy: en bloc resection of rectum, uterus, and adnexa comprising the pouch

Liver

Hepatic implants may involve Glisson's capsule only or infiltrate the underlying parenchyma less or more deeply. Removing hepatic Glisson's capsule or locally destroying implants are the most frequently used techniques, whereas atypical resections of peripheral parenchyma are rarely required to remove deeply infiltrating implants. In selected cases, hepatic resection is acceptable for hematogenous metastases, as long as the lesions are single, small, and easy to resect. In selected cases with multiple hepatic metastases that are small and few, intraoperative radiofrequency could be considered. However, treating hematogenous metastases is justified only when it is possible to achieve complete cytoreduc-

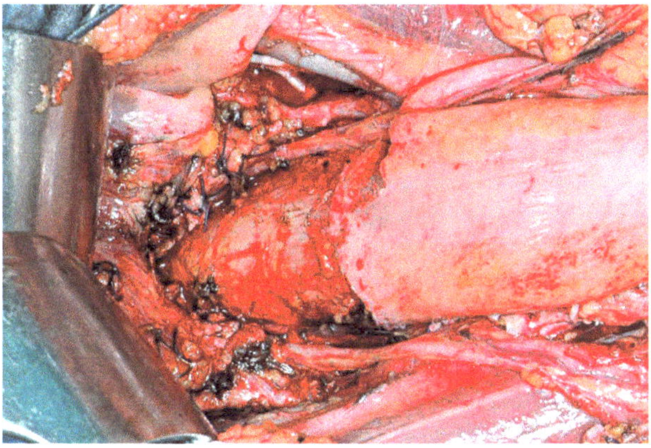

Fig. 9.11 Douglassectomy

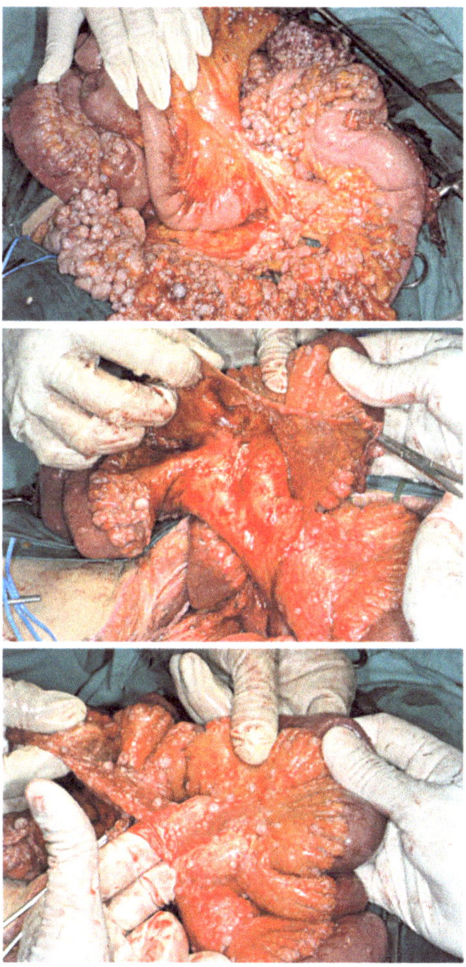

Fig. 9.12 Stripping of visceral peritoneum (peritoneal mesothelioma)

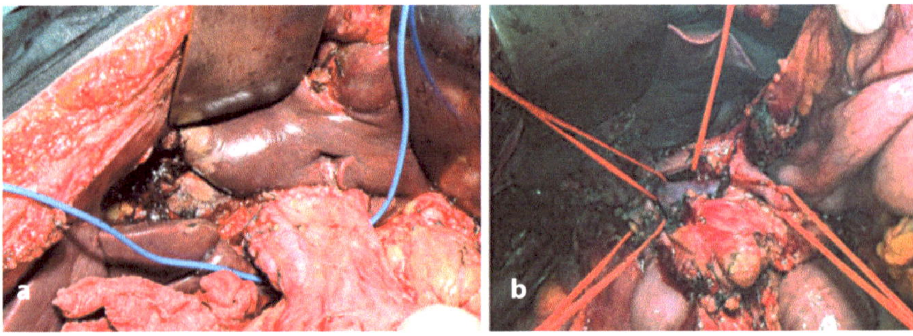

Fig. 9.13a, b **a** Stripping of anterior and posterior peritoneal sheath of hepatic pedicle; **b** exeresis of peritoneum and lymph nodes of hepatic pedicle

tion (CC-0). The carcinosis frequently involves the ligamentum teres in its intrahepatic pathway. Resecting round and falciform ligaments should be performed in all carcinosis forms to guarantee optimal flow of chemohyperthermic solution. When a parenchymal bridge is present at the level of third inferior of the round ligament, it should be sectioned to expose the umbilical fissure of the liver and treat implants if present [3].

Carcinosis may involve the serous membrane of the gallbladder or hepatoduodenal ligament: cholecystectomy is mandatory, and stripping the peritoneum requires complete dissection of pedicle elements from the porta hepatis to the head of the pancreas. Only in the case of superficial carcinosis in the anterior sheath of the ligament is it technically possible to remove the serous covering or destroy in situ the implants. Direct infiltration of the elements of the hepatoduodenal ligament does not allow complete removal of implants, and the cytoreductive approach should thus be re-evaluated. Lymphadenectomy in this area is essential during PRT for carcinomatosis from primary gastric cancer and is also useful in other forms of carcinosis when lymph node involvement is evident or suspected (Fig. 9.13a, b)

Spleen

The presence of carcinosis in the greater omentum, left hemidiaphragm, colonic splenic flexure, or in the omental bursa may involve the perisplenic peritoneum, spleen surface, or splenic hilum. In all these cases, splenectomy is mandatory and may be associated with pancreatic tail resection, left and transversal colectomy, and gastric-wall resection. Also, lymph node involvement of the splenic hilum is a condition determining spleen removal (Fig. 9.14).

Bladder and Ureter

Involvement of pelvic and prevesical peritoneums is frequent, and removal is usually associated with resection of other organs and endopelvic structures. Vesical resection is performed when implants deeply infiltrate the wall.

Cystectomy is rarely suggested and should be indicated only in the case of massive parietal and trigone infiltration. Cystectomy should be performed only

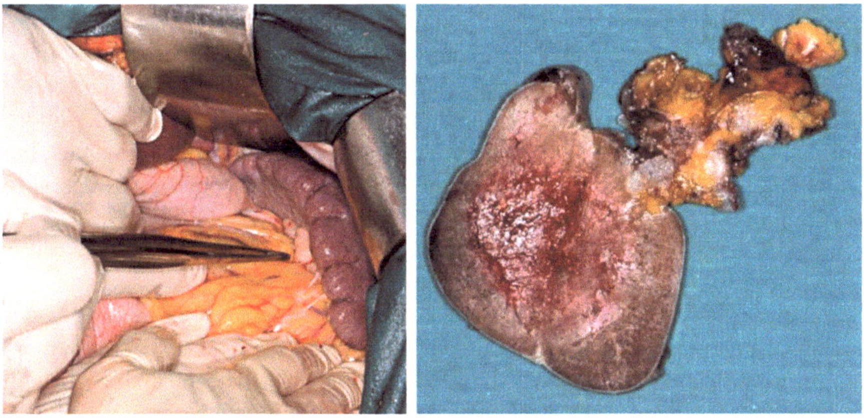

Fig. 9.14 Splenectomy for carcinomatosis involving splenic hilum

if this sacrifice achieves CC score 0 and if carcinosis has good prognosis. Pelvic PRT requires a mandatory and meticulous ureter preparation. In case of massive carcinosis, ureters can be usually isolated, and sacrificing them must be an exception. Isolating a long ureter tract as required during PRT does not generate any particular risk if accurately performed and if periureteric vascularization is preserved. Also, when the ureter seems to be totally encapsulated into the carcinomatous mass, correct preparation allows that structure to be preserved. Ureter size and absence of dilatation upstream of carcinomatous masses are essential to guarantee anatomical integrity and, therefore, stimulate maintenance. Only when infiltration massively involves the ureteric wall with stenosis and upstream dilatation is resection justified. In these cases, if a concomitant cystectomy is not required, the ureter is reimplanted on the bladder, with the introduction of a double-J catheter as support.

Uterus and Ovaries

Carcinomatosis from primary uterine or ovarian cancer requires bilateral hysteroadnexectomy in association with removal of other viscera or endopelvic structures if they are involved by primary tumor or concomitant carcinomatosis. In all other forms of extraovarian carcinomatosis, ovaries should be always removed, even if they appear macroscopically healthy, whereas the uterus should be removed only if directly involved in the tumoral mass or if the pouch or prevesical peritoneum are involved. In case of local and superficial involvement, the uterus may be spared and treated locally.

Stomach and Duodenum

In extragastric carcinomatosis, implants prevailingly involve the lower third of the stomach, the greater and lesser omentum, and the omental bursa. Generally, subtotal or total gastrectomy is unnecessary, as the relevant depth of the gastric wall allows partial-thickness resection or in situ destruction of implants. Major resections should be chosen only if complete CRS is possible. Distal gastrectomy is essential when antropyloric involvement causes stenosis.

Duodenal or duodenojejunal junction involvement rarely allows an effective local treatment without risk of fistulization and represents a strong limitation for optimal CRS. In selected cases, it is possible to destroy or remove nodules, but when this is not achievable and when the risk of stenosis is high, it is useful to perform a gastrojejunal bypass.

Small Intestine

Small intestine is one of the most involved structures in carcinosis. Correct evaluation of carcinosis quality and spread helps to determine the best treatment approaches. The extent of small-bowel resection must be well balanced with conservative treatments when other bowel resections or ostomy are needed; this is necessary to reduce surgical risk and preserve adequate digestive function. The percentage of expendable small intestine is < 50% of total intestinal length. A single comprehensive resection comprising major regions involved in carcinosis using a single anastomosis to restore continuity is preferred in order to reduce the risk of fistulization. When residual implants persist after optimal small-bowel resection, it is possible to destroy them in situ using argon-beam laser, ball-tipped electrosurgery, radiofrequency, (tissue link), or surgery to remove local implants. The same procedure is used when implants in the small intestine are few, small, and superficial and the distance between them is considerable. Conservative treatments are very difficult for implants that involve the small intestine at the bowel wall and mesentery junction. Partial exeresis or local destruction should be carefully performed, and suturing should be done whenever the intestinal wall is weak.

Colon and Rectum

In patients with diffuse carcinomatosis, colon involvement may require different types of large-bowel resection, and partial or total colectomy should be performed. Also, in extracolic carcinosis, all colorectal resections must be performed according to the same radical criteria applied to primary tumors of the large bowel. This approach allows resection of wide portions of mesocolon where implants are present and adequate lymphadenectomy to treat a high percentage of lymph node metastases detectable regardless primary origin, as previously reported by us and other authors [4–6].

Rectal involvement is usual, because pelvic carcinosis is one of the most frequent locations and often penetrates the pelvic–peritoneal barrier, thus involving the mesorectum and requiring low rectal resection. In the presence of massive involvement of colon and rectum, right hemicolectomy and Hartmann resection may be performed contemporaneously, sparing transverse colon and splenic colon flexure. In this way, colostomy is possible rather than total colectomy or ileostomy, neither of which is generally well tolerated by patients (Fig. 9.15).

Pelvic involvement with deep infiltration of the pouch and rectal wall

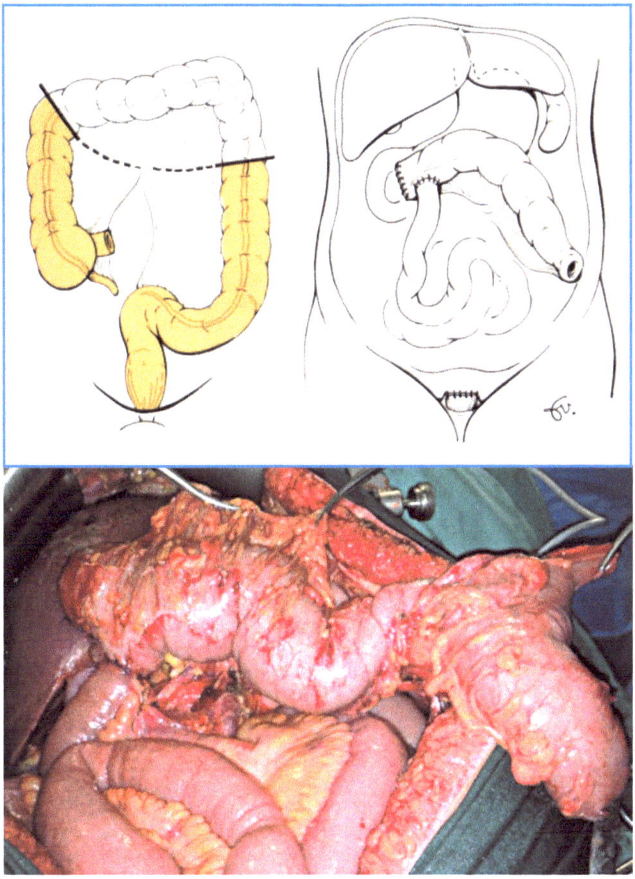

Fig. 9.15 Right and left hemicolectomy sparing transverse colon

requires colorectal resection, including mesorectum, with a residual rectal stump no longer than 5–6 cm.

In colorectal resection, it is preferable not to proceed to rectal anastomosis when other gastrointestinal resections with multiple anastomoses have already been performed. Indeed, the risk of fistulization is very high due to concomitant chemohyperthermia and when patients have been operated on under occlusion/subocclusion, without adequate colic cleaning. Rectal-stump anastomosis may also be avoided when patients have received treatment with bevacizumab. Furthermore, the pelvis has the highest risk of recurrence when wide pelvic carcinomatosis is present at first CRS. Thus, in these cases, restoring continuity can be postponed and performed at the end of adjuvant chemotherapeutic treatment and after a further follow-up of at least 6 months.

Local exeresis or in situ destruction of colonic implants is difficult to attain with safety because of the thin wall, especially at the level of the right colon, or because of concomitant diverticular disease. Full-thickness resection of a small

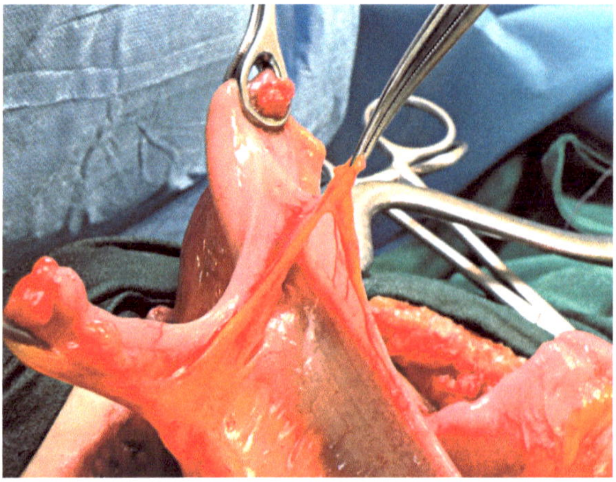

Fig. 9.16 Appendectomy and resection of periappendicular ligaments

portion of the colonic wall and excessive use of in situ destruction on long tracts are not recommended because of the risk of fistulization, especially in occluded patients. Epiploic appendices, if macroscopically involved or edematous and hypertrophic, must be removed. In the digestive tract, the colon can be sacrificed with minor functional impact and major advantages in terms of radicality, unlike in the small intestine; its resection with ostomy limits the risk of fistulization, which is strongly related to HIPEC in the closed-abdomen technique and to blood loss. Also, when the colon is macroscopically healthy, appendectomy is routinely performed, with contextual resection of the peritoneal plica, which defines the ileocecal fossa and peritoneal junction with the cecum (Fig. 9.16).

Removal/In Situ Implant Destruction

Treating peritoneal implants does not absolutely require exeresis of wide portions of the peritoneum or mandatory sacrifice of wide tracts of gut or other structures involved in the disease. In relation to quality, quantity, and macroscopic and microscopic (histology) characteristics of carcinomatous implants, exeresis should respond to general criteria to save structures and avoid useless tissue and visceral sacrifice when local removal or in situ destruction with an appropriate technology allow radical results. A conservative approach is achievable when implants are superficial, few infiltrate underlying structures, and are prevailingly mucinous. In these conditions, it is possible to save wide visceral resection, especially when the small or large intestine is involved. Exeresis or local treatment can be assured effectively with curved scissors, electric scalpels with various tips, radiofrequency (Tissue Link), and argon-beam laser (Fig. 9.17). It is even possible to remove accurately and effectively implants from anatomical sites difficult to reach.

The use of advanced technologies for in situ destruction of carcinomatous implants is highly useful when it is not possible to totally free nonexpendable structures from malignant nodules, e.g., ureter, large vessels, or hepatic pedicle.

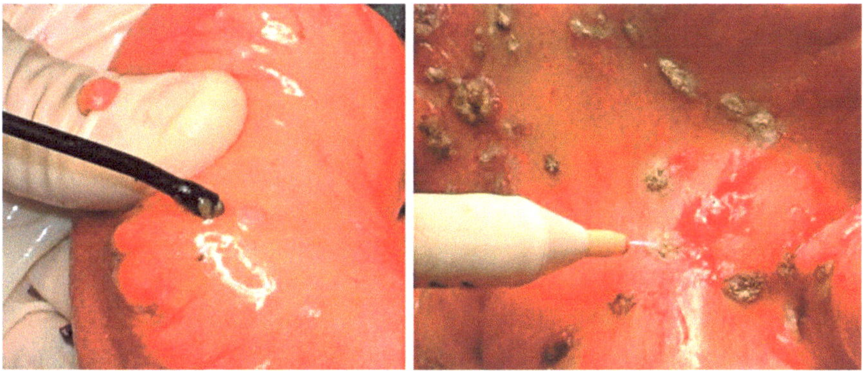

Fig. 9.17 In situ destruction of carcinomatous implants with radiofrequency technology or argon-beam laser

In these cases, cytoreduction with advanced technologies may allow significant debulking of masses and major HIPEC efficacy in involved regions. In patients have undergone neoadjuvant treatments, an additional contribution to HIPEC efficacy is achieved using argon-beam or electric scalpels in peritoneal areas where an apparent response to chemotherapy was achieved. These areas are identified by the presence of specific morphological changes, including opacification, thickening, fibrosis of serous peritoneal membrane, and presence of red spots (Fig. 9.18) Extensive treatment on such areas with argon-beam or ball-tip electrosurgery permits diffuse local damage and partial destruction of fibrosis. The loss of structural continuity will permit deeper tissue penetration of chemotherapeutics during HIPEC and better contact with eventual encapsulated microscopic residuals in postchemotherapy fibrosis.

9.3.3.4 Abdominal Wall, Muscle Implant, and Trocar-site Resection

When PC infiltrates the abdominal wall, it is necessary to perform parietal resection proportional to implant size. Trocar access sites previously used in diagnostic laparoscopy or in laparoscopic intervention for primary neoplasia should be carefully evaluated. In the presence of macroscopic involvement by tumor tissue or a suspected implant, full-thickness resections are performed. Parietal defects, if small, may be sutured or used to pass drains and catheters for perfusion. If trocars sites are massively involved, it is necessary to proceed with wide abdominal resection and then rebuild with dual mesh prosthesis and by sliding musculoaponeurotic sheaths (Fig. 9.19). The umbilicus may be a frequent location for carcinosis, regardless of previous laparoscopy, and its removal is justified especially in recurrent forms. A particular form of implant is represented by metastasis in the context of psoas muscle, which is frequent in recurrent forms. Such metastasis is generally endomuscular, and it is difficult to ascribe its presence to local recurrence or hematogenous metastasis. Its exeresis is easy and effective by opening or resecting muscle fibers.

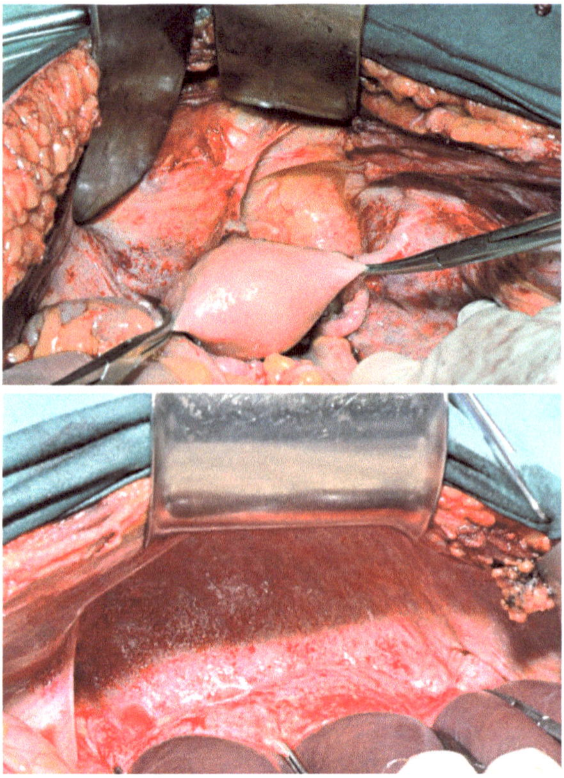

Fig. 9.18 Effects of carcinomatosis chemoreduction: red spots; fibrosis; peritoneal opacification

9.3.3.5 Lymphadenectomy

An important phase of PRT is represented by locoregional lymphadenectomy. In the primary setting, lymphadenectomy is performed in relation to the specific rules required for each primary tumor. In recurrences, locoregional lymphadenectomy is performed when it has not been performed in previous interventions or when lymph node recurrence in addition to peritoneal recurrence is present. Carcinomatous infiltration of serosa and underlying layers of the wall of the small and large intestine involves the subserosal lymphatic system in the early stages, thus producing locoregional lymph node metastases. The high rate of such metastases necessitates specific surgical approaches. Therefore in extracolic carcinosis, if the colon–rectum is involved by carcinomatosis, locoregional lymphadenectomy should be performed as in primary forms in these organs. In case of small-intestine involvement, enlarged mesenteric lymph nodes must be biopsied to evaluate metastatic spread and the advisability of continuing the procedure. Guidelines for surgical treatment of primary epithelial ovarian cancer (EOC) suggest pelvic and para-aortic lymphadenectomy (Fig. 9.20). When treating primary ovarian carcinomatosis, this procedure should be done routinely. When treating recurrent ovarian carcinomatosis, lymphadenectomy should be

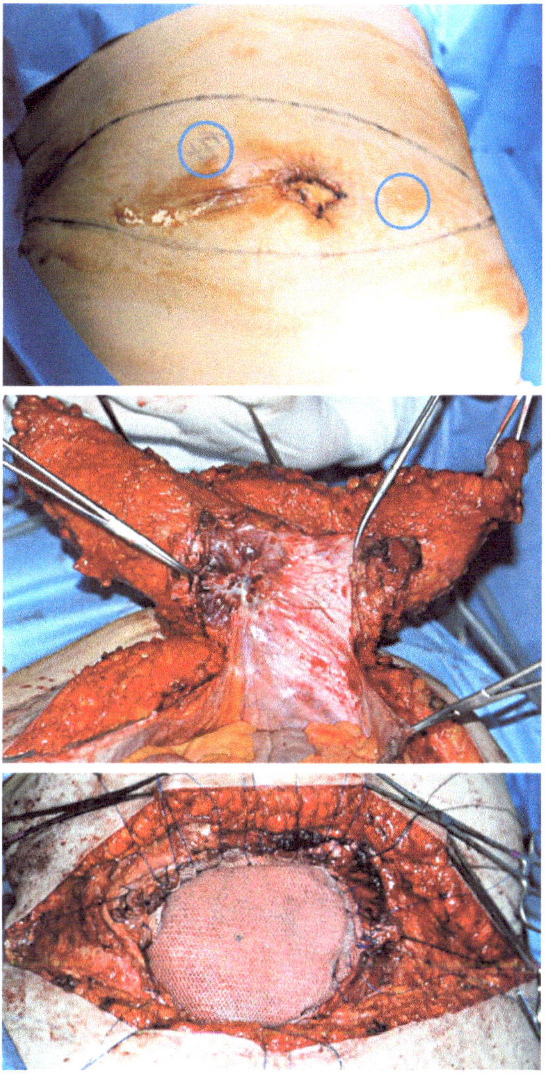

Fig. 9.19 Abdominal-wall resection, including port sites involved by tumor implants

done if not performed during the first CRS. The prognostic role of lymphadenectomy is relevant, improving overall and progression-free survival [7–11].

9.3.4 Closing Abdominal-wall Drainages and Catheter Positioning for HIPEC

After completing the surgical phase, it is important to clean meticulously the peritoneal cavity with a solution of hydrogen peroxide to remove cellular debris

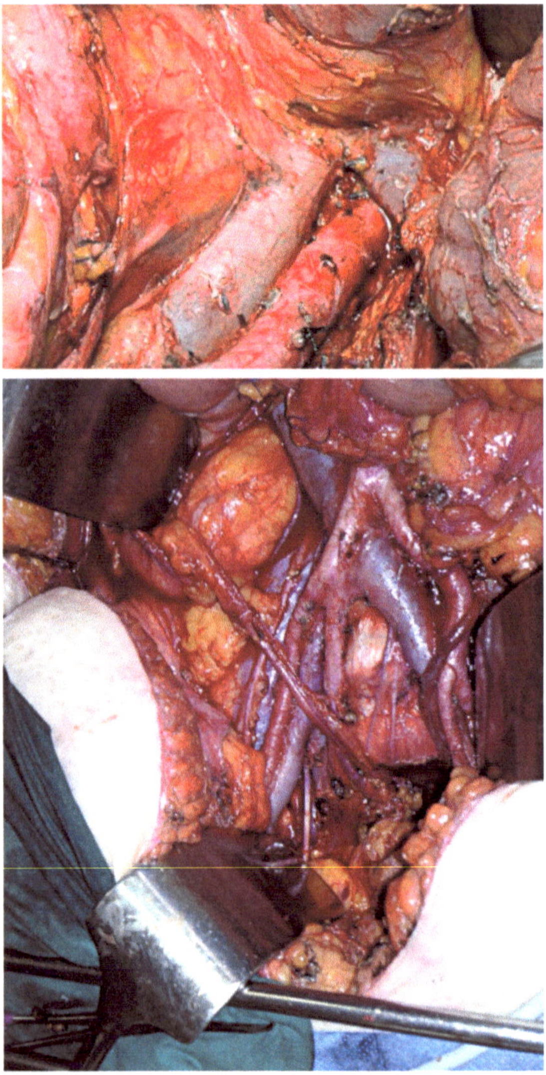

Fig. 9.20 Para-aortic, iliac, and obturator lymphadenectomy

and tissue fragments detached during cytoreduction procedures. It is crucial to verify complete adhesion lysis and viscerovisceral sectioning and visceroparietal ligaments in allow optimal flow of chemohyperthermic solution, regardless of the technique chosen for HIPEC: open or closed.

Before closing the abdominal wall or creating an abdominal tank (for open coliseum technique or open/closed technique), three or four catheters, or fenestrated or spiral drains are positioned for drug solution inflow and outflow. The catheters are placed as shown in Fig. 9.21:

- A catheter, introduced below the right costal arch, is placed under the diaphragm and over the superior edge of liver;

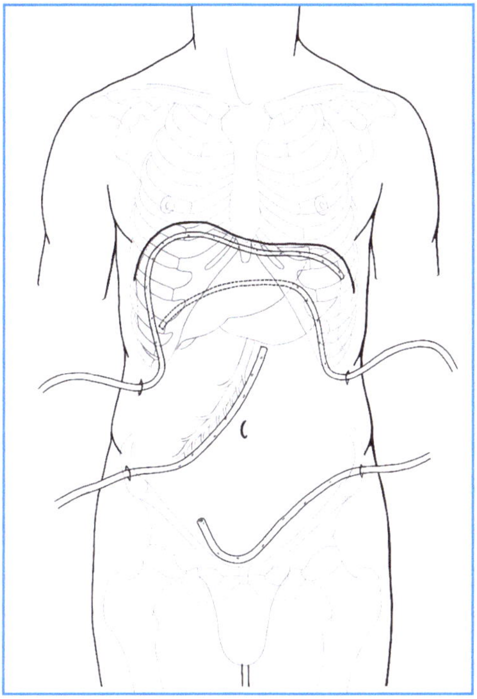

Fig. 9.21 Hyperthermic intraperitoneal chemotherapy (HIPEC) catheter positioning

- A catheter, introduced at the level of the right iliac fossa, is placed along the mesenteric root;
- A catheter, introduced under the left costal arch, is placed under the liver;
- A catheter, introduced from the left iliac fossa, is placed in the pelvis.

Catheters used for HIPEC are left in situ and will be useful as drains for post-operative procedures. In closed HIPEC, anastomoses and ostomy are generally performed before closing the laparotomy. In open HIPEC, anastomoses are performed after completing chemohyperthermia.

9.4 Discussion

PRT procedures were described by Sugarbaker in 1995 and then integrated with other publications [1, 2, 12, 13]. However, few technical contributions are described in the literature, even if the importance of maximal cytoreduction is recognized in all PSM as the most significant prognostic factor [14–20].

The main aim of CRS is to remove completely the evident disease or leave a residual disease < 2.5 mm and allow HIPEC to sterilize microscopic or millimetric residuals. To date, achieving this goal is the main indication for success when evaluating favorable prognostic scenarios after optimal integration of the procedure with neoadjuvant or adjuvant systemic chemotherapy. This approach is valid both for primary and recurrent or plurirecurrent carcinomatosis. For several types of PSM, some authors have indicated limits of PC spread determined by the PCI classification beyond which PRT should be avoided because of poor impact on survival, and an increased risk of morbidity and mortality [21–24]. To date, there is no evidence to confirm this hypothesis, and for several forms of PSM, maximal cytoreduction represents a therapeutic advantage irreplaceable with other therapies, even in the more advanced forms of the disease. Thus, the main factor pertaining to treating PSM, even when widely diffuse, is represented by the technical feasibility of cytoreduction rather than peritoneal extent of disease. Furthermore, maximal exeresis provides the only possible palliation for patients with bowel obstruction or chemoresistance after multiple chemotherapy lines.

PRT entails complex surgical procedures that require specialized knowledge and practice of oncologic abdominal surgery and a strong technical basis of gynecological, urological, and vascular surgery. The surgeon facing PRT must know the various forms of PSM in order to choose the better surgical approaches. If the main aim of PRT is maximal removal of peritoneal disease, a correct balance between wide exeresis and local conservative treatments should be respected when implant quality and site permits in situ implant destruction or local removal. This aspect must be especially considered when treating the small intestine and is determined by the need to maintain an acceptable digestive function. Alternately, when PC involves the colon–rectum, treatment must be aggressive, with left colon, rectum, mesorectum, female genitals, and pelvic peritoneum resection, according to studies that we and other authors have previously described [3–5]. Lymphadenectomy represents an essential element in the treatment of primary carcinosis from stomach, colon–rectum, and ovarian cancer. Indeed, it is inconceivable to perform extensive PRT without specific radical treatment of primary neoplasia, including the corresponding lymphadenectomy.

Some recent reports emphasize the opportunity to treat PC using laparoscopic techniques, but this approach is feasible only for minimal forms of peritoneal disease and involves significant risk of undertreatment for carcinosis substadiation [25, 26]. Indeed, for an exhaustive inspection and evaluation of all abdominal and pelvic cavities, both direct visual and manual contributions are crucial. Moreover, this technique—prevailingly, if not exclusively—is feasible in primary tumors and correlates with high risks of neoplastic contamination of trocar sites, as demonstrated in the literature [27–29].

References

1. Sugarbaker PH (2007) Peritonectomy procedures. Cancer treatment and research 134:247-264
2. Jacquet P, Sugarbaker PH (1996) Clinical research methodologies in diagnosis and staging of patients with peritoneal carcinomatosis. Cancer treatment and research 82:359-374

3. Sugarbaker PH (2010) Pont hepatique (hepatic bridge), an important anatomic structure in cytoreductive surgery. Journal of surgical oncology 101:251-252
4. Di Giorgio A, Cardi M, Biacchi D et al (2013) Depth of colorectal-wall invasion and lymph-node involvement as major outcome factors influencing surgical strategy in patients with advanced and recurrent ovarian cancer with diffuse peritoneal metastases. World journal of surgical oncology 11:64
5. O'Hanlan KA, Kargas S, Schreiber M et al (1995) Ovarian carcinoma metastases to gastrointestinal tract appear to spread like colon carcinoma: implications for surgical resection. Gynecologic oncology 59:200-206
6. Scarabelli C, Gallo A, Franceschi S et al (2000) Primary cytoreductive surgery with rectosigmoid colon resection for patients with advanced epithelial ovarian carcinoma. Cancer 88:389-397
7. du Bois A, Reuss A, Harter P, Ray-Coquard I, Pfisterer J, Arbeitsgemeinschaft Gynaekologische Onkologie Studiengruppe O, Groupe d'Investigateurs Nationaux pour l'Etude des Cancers O (2010) Potential role of lymphadenectomy in advanced ovarian cancer: a combined exploratory analysis of three prospectively randomized phase III multicenter trials. Journal of clinical oncology 28:1733-1739
8. Jaffre I, Bordes V, Dejode M et al (2010) Management of retroperitoneal lymphadenectomy in advanced epithelial ovarian cancer. Bulletin du cancer 97:65-71
9. Chan JK, Urban R, Hu JM et al (2007) The potential therapeutic role of lymph node resection in epithelial ovarian cancer: a study of 13918 patients. British journal of cancer 96:1817-1822
10. Chang SJ, Bristow RE, Ryu HS et al (2012) Prognostic significance of systematic lymphadenectomy as part of primary debulking surgery in patients with advanced ovarian cancer. Gynecologic oncology 126:381-386
11. Pereira A, Perez-Medina T, Magrina JF et al (2012) The role of lymphadenectomy in node-positive epithelial ovarian cancer. International journal of gynecological cancer 22:987-992
12. Kusamura S, O'Dwyer ST, Baratti D et al (2008)Technical aspects of cytoreductive surgery. Journal of surgical oncology 98:232-236
13. Bijelic L, Sugarbaker PH (2008) Cytoreduction of the small bowel surfaces. Journal of surgical oncology 97:176-179
14. Coccolini F, Gheza F, Lotti M et al (2013) Peritoneal carcinomatosis. World journal of gastroenterology 19:6979-6994
15. Weber T, Roitman M, Link KH (2012) Current status of cytoreductive surgery with hyperthermic intraperitoneal chemotherapy in patients with peritoneal carcinomatosis from colorectal cancer. Clinical colorectal cancer 11:167-176
16. Verwaal VJ, Bruin S, Boot H et al (2008) 8-year follow-up of randomized trial: cytoreduction and hyperthermic intraperitoneal chemotherapy versus systemic chemotherapy in patients with peritoneal carcinomatosis of colorectal cancer. Annals of surgical oncology 15:2426-2432
17. Shih KK, Chi DS (2010) Maximal cytoreductive effort in epithelial ovarian cancer surgery. Journal of gynecologic oncology 21:75-80
18. Schorge JO, McCann C, Del Carmen MG (2010) Surgical debulking of ovarian cancer: what difference does it make? Reviews in obstetrics and gynecology 3:111-117
19. Yonemura Y, Elnemr A, Endou Y et al (2010) Multidisciplinary therapy for treatment of patients with peritoneal carcinomatosis from gastric cancer. World journal of gastrointestinal oncology 2:85-97
20. Bristow RE, Puri I, Chi DS (2009) Cytoreductive surgery for recurrent ovarian cancer: a meta-analysis. Gynecologic oncology 112:265-274
21. Elias D, Dumont F, Honoré C, Goéré D (2013) Role of aggressive surgery for peritoneal metastases. European Journal of Cancer Supplements 11:268–269
22. Kulu Y, Muller-Stich B, Buchler MW, Ulrich A (2014) Surgical treatment of peritoneal carcinomatosis: current treatment modalities. Langenbeck's archives of surgery/Deutsche Gesellschaft fur Chirurgie 399:41-53
23. Bakrin N, Cotte E, Golfier F et al (2012) Cytoreductive surgery and hyperthermic intraperi-

toneal chemotherapy (HIPEC) for persistent and recurrent advanced ovarian carcinoma: a multicenter, prospective study of 246 patients. Annals of surgical oncology 19:4052-4058
24. Glehen O, Gilly FN, Arvieux C et al (2010) Peritoneal carcinomatosis from gastric cancer: a multi-institutional study of 159 patients treated by cytoreductive surgery combined with perioperative intraperitoneal chemotherapy. Annals of surgical oncology 17:2370-2377
25. Passot G, Bakrin N, Isaac S et al (2013) Postoperative outcomes of laparoscopic vs open cytoreductive surgery plus hyperthermic intraperitoneal chemotherapy for treatment of peritoneal surface malignancies. European journal of surgical oncology doi: 10.1016/j.ejso.2013.10.002 [Epub ahead of print]
26. Liu CS, Nagarsheth NP, Nezhat FR (2009) Laparoscopy and ovarian cancer: a paradigm change in the management of ovarian cancer? Journal of minimally invasive gynecology 16:250-262
27. Reymond MA, Schneider C, Hohenberger W, Kockerling F (1998) The pneumoperitoneum and its role in tumour seeding. Digestive surgery 15:105-109
28. Nagarsheth NP, Rahaman J, Cohen CJ et al (2004) The incidence of port-site metastases in gynecologic cancers. Journal of the Society of Laparoendoscopic Surgeons 8:133-139
29. Vergote I, Marquette S, Amant F et al (2005) Port-site metastases after open laparoscopy: a study in 173 patients with advanced ovarian carcinoma. International journal of gynecological cancer 15:776-779

Hyperthermic Intraperitoneal Chemotherapy (HIPEC) Techniques

10

Salvatore Virzì, Domenico Rosario Iusco, Serena Bonomi, and Antonio Grassi

10.1 Introduction

Peritoneal carcinomatosis has long been considered a terminal condition and constitutes a difficult therapeutic challenge given the dismal prognosis associated with this entity and the debilitating effect it exerts on affected patients. Over the past decade, novel therapeutic approaches to peritoneal surface malignancies have emerged. These new approaches are all based on a strong rationale: most frequently, peritoneal carcinosis is a locoregional condition that should be approached with locoregional treatments, such as cytoreductive surgery and peritonectomy procedures for macroscopic disease in combination with perioperative intraperitoneal chemotherapy for microscopic residual disease. In order to take advantage of this synergistic effect, different devices and techniques have been developed. Perioperative intraperitoneal chemotherapy is a milestone of the combined approach to peritoneal surface malignancy. Two main modalities for administering chemotherapeutic agents have been described: intraoperative hyperthermic intraperitoneal chemotherapy (HIPEC), and early postoperative normothermic; the former has gained greater acceptance among peritoneal surface malignancy centers.

10.2 Intraoperative Hyperthermic Intraperitoneal Chemotherapy

Intraoperative administration of intraperitoneal hyperthermic chemotherapy has been described using multiple names. The term HIPEC was adopted as the

S. Virzì (✉)
General Surgery Unit, Bentivoglio Hospital, Bentivoglio (BO), Italy
e-mail: st.virzi@gmail.com

A. Di Giorgio, E. Pinto (Eds), *Treatment of Peritoneal Surface Malignancies*, Updates in Surgery
DOI: 10.1007/978-88-470-5711-1_10, © Springer-Verlag Italia 2015

standardized acronym for this procedure during the fourth workshop on peritoneal surface malignancy held in Madrid in 2004 [1, 2]. HIPEC combines the pharmacokinetic advantage inherent to the intracavitary delivery of certain cytotoxic drugs, which results in regional dose intensification, with the direct cytotoxic effect of hyperthermia. Hyperthermia alone, in fact, has a selective cell-killing effect on malignant cells, potentiates the cytotoxic effect of certain chemotherapeutic agents, and enhances tissue penetration of the administered drug. In order to take advantage of this synergistic effect, different devices and techniques have been developed.

10.3 Perfusion Technology

Basically, all devices for administering certain chemotherapeutic agents are composed of a closed, continuous circuit, with a pump, a heater with a heat exchanger, and a real-time temperature monitor. Different temperature probes are positioned in different sites of the circuit and abdominal cavity to secure a constant temperature: heat generator, inflow and outflow drains, bladder, liver, and mesentery. A computerized, continuous recording of thermal data that may be displayed in situ for monitoring during the procedure and then exported or printed with different formats is usually included with the device. This adds security and comfort for the patient, avoids the need to create written records, and allows efficient data recording for clinical research [3].

Numerous compact HIPEC machines, approved by the US Food and Drug Administration or with a CE marking have been developed and commercialized since the late 1990s. The choice of a specific HIPEC device should be based upon certain characteristics, such as its ability to achieve adequate hyperthermia in a short period, adjustable flow rate, user-friendliness, ease of assembly, ease of reading, and continuous registration of temperatures, availability of technical support, and affordability of the machine itself and the disposable circuit tubing kits.

10.4 Perfusion Techniques

HIPEC can be conducted in various ways, without clear proven advantage of one method over the others. Four major perfusion techniques are described in the literature: open-abdomen technique(coliseum technique) closed-abdomen technique, peritoneal cavity expanders (PCE), and semiopen techniques . Procedure duration varies from 30 to 120 min according to the surgeon's discretion and drug used [4, 5].

10.4.1 Open-abdomen Technique

The open method, first described by Sugarbaker, is usually performed using the "coliseum technique" (Fig. 10.1) [6]. At the end of cytoreductive phase, a Tenckhoff catheter and closed suction drains are placed through the abdominal wall. Temperature probes, secured to the skin edge, are used for intraperitoneal temperature monitoring: one in the inflow line and another one at a distance from this point (pelvis). A silastic sheet is sutured over a Thompson retractor and to the patient's skin over the abdominal incision in order to prevent the chemotherapy solution from splashing. Abdominal-wall suspension, obtained with such a suture, will create a coliseum- or soup-bowl-like container for instillation of the peritoneal perfusate. A slit in the plastic cover is made to allow access of the surgeon's double-gloved hand to the abdomen and pelvis and manual manipulation of the intra-abdominal contents, thus preventing stasis of the heated perfusate. A smoke evacuator protects operating-room (OR) personnel from aerosolized chemotherapy liberated during the procedure.

A roller pump forces chemotherapy perfusion into the abdomen through the Tenckhoff catheter and extracts it through the drains, with a flow rate ~1 L/min. A heat exchanger keeps the infused fluid at 43–45°C so that the intraperitoneal fluid is maintained at 41–43°C.

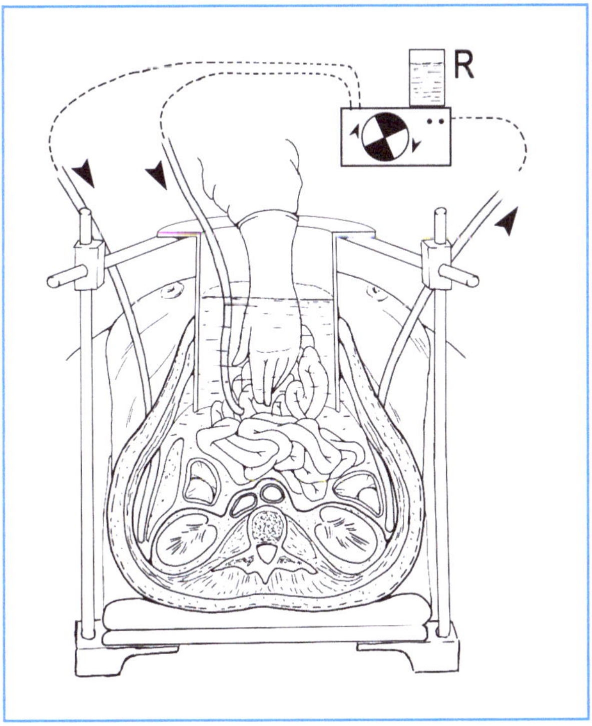

Fig. 10.1 Hyperthermic intraperitoneal chemotherapy (HIPEC): peritoneal cavity expander. (Courtesy of Prof. Angelo Di Giorgio)

The perfusate is first recirculated between the reservoir and the heat exchanger so it can be heated to an adequate temperature. At this point, full circulation of the perfusate in and out of the peritoneal cavity is established until a minimum intraperitoneal temperature of 41.5°C is achieved and maintained. The drug is then added to the circuit, at which stage the perfusion timer is started.

In centers in which bidirectional chemotherapy protocols are used, intravenous infusion of the appropriate drugs is started synchronously with peritoneal chemotherapeutic infusion, although some surgeons prefer to start it 1 h before the actual peritoneal therapy.

Use of the coliseum technique was identified by Elias et al. [7] as the best technique in terms of thermal homogeneity and spatial diffusion. Those benefits are due to the ability to manipulate the intra-abdominal viscera during perfusion, which allows homogeneous exposition of all peritoneal surfaces to the therapy. Furthermore, as excessive heating of normal tissue is associated with a more lasting postoperative ileus and increases the incidence of postoperative perforation or fistula formation, this technique theoretically avoids these complications. The disadvantages of open HIPEC are heat dissipation to the surface of the perfusate, which makes it more difficult to achieve hyperthermia, and possible increased exposure of operative personnel to the chemotherapeutic agent, even if this is as yet only a theoretical risk.

10.4.3 Closed-abdomen Technique

Basically, this technique differs from the open technique only because the skin is sutured following laparotomy so that perfusion is done in a closed, watertight circuit (Fig. 10.2). Patient position varies during perfusion, which is achieved by tilting the surgical table into a Trendelenburg or anti-Trendelenburg position and then laterally in an attempt to promote uniform heat distribution. A larger volume of perfusate is generally needed to establish the circuit compared with during the open technique, and a higher abdominal pressure is achieved during perfusion that, as noted by Jacquet et al. [8], may facilitate drug penetration into tissue.

After hyperthermic perfusion, the abdomen is reopened and anastomoses, stoma, and drain placement are performed. The abdomen is then closed definitively in a standard manner. Otherwise, even when the closed technique is used, anastomoses and stoma are performed before abdominal wall closure. This way, there is no need to reopen the abdomen at the end of HIPEC, and catheters used for perfusion are used as drains during postoperative care.

The major advantage of the closed technique is the rapid achievement and constant maintenance of hyperthermia due to minimal heat loss. Moreover, exposure of OR personnel to aerosolized particles and contact with chemotherapeutic agents is minimized.

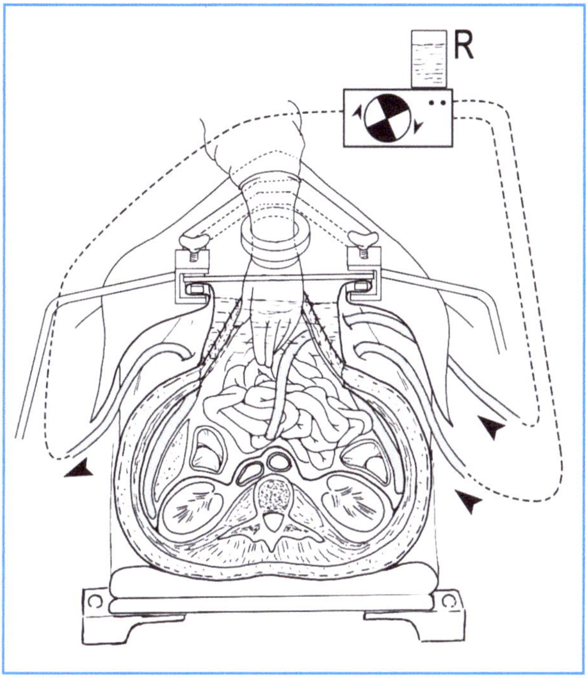

Fig. 10.2 Hyperthermic intraperitoneal chemotherapy (HIPEC): open technique. (Courtesy of Prof. Angelo Di Giorgio)

The lack of uniform distribution of the heated intraperitoneal chemotherapeutic agent is the main disadvantage of closed HIPEC. In fact, Elias et al. [7] reported an uneven distribution of methylene blue after its instillation during the procedure. Theoretically, inadequate circulation of heated intraperitoneal perfusate leads to pooling and accumulation of heat and the chemotherapeutic agent in the lower part of the body. This may result in increased systemic absorption and focal hyperthermic injury, which may prompt postoperative ileus, bowel perforation, and fistula [9]. However, no author has reported any complications that may have been caused by inadequate circulation [10].

10.4.4 Peritoneal Cavity Expander

A variation of the open HIPEC–described by Fujimura et al. and mainly used in Japan for treating or preventing gastric carcinomatosis–is the peritoneal cavity expander (PCE) technique (Fig. 10.3) [11]. The PCE is an acrylic cylinder containing inflow and outflow catheters that is secured over the wound. When filled with heated perfusate, the PCE can accommodate the small bowel, allowing the small intestine to float freely and be manually manipulated in the perfusate. The expander theoretically allows more uniform distribution com-

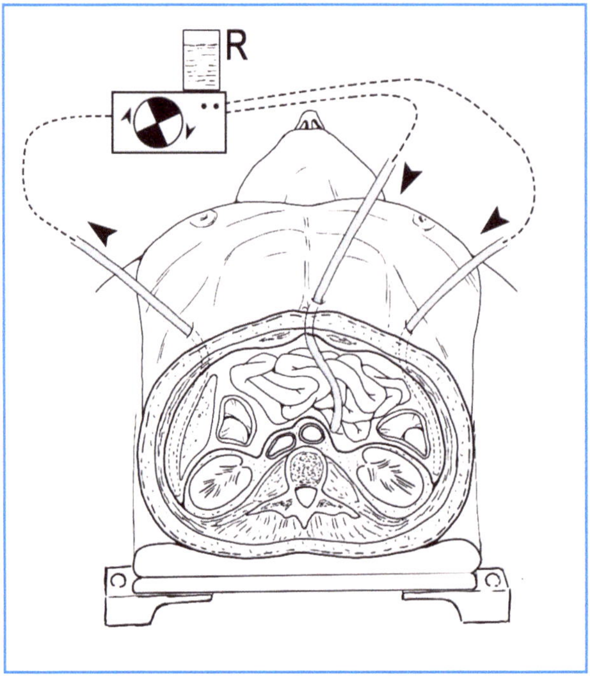

Fig. 10.3 Hyperthermic intraperitoneal chemotherapy (HIPEC): closed technique. (Courtesy of Prof. Angelo Di Giorgio)

pared with the closed technique. Its main disadvantage is the risk of OR personnel exposure to the chemotherapeutic agent, as occurs with the coliseum technique [10].

10.4.6 Semiopen (or Semiclosed) Abdominal Technique

To create a watertight environment, edges of the incision are tightly stapled with a soft abdominal cavity expander supported by a Thompson self-retaining retractor positioned over the abdomen. This permits the level of the liquid to rise above the level of the skin edges. Edges of the anterior-wall peritoneum are constantly exposed to the liquid. Large-amplitude movements become possible: the surgeon can introduce both forearms, even both arms, into the patient's abdomen without causing any liquid loss [12, 13].

10.5 Early Postoperative Intraperitoneal Chemotherapy

A second method of performing perioperative intraperitoneal chemotherapy is early postoperative intraperitoneal chemotherapy (EPIC). This approach is not favored by most surgical centers involved in treating carcinosis (Table 10.1).

Chemotherapeutic agent administration is started immediately after the operation and continued during the first 1–5 postoperative days [14]. The EPIC system is composed of a Tenckhoff catheter or a subcutaneous port placed through the abdominal wall in the approximate area at greatest risk of recurrence following cytoreductive surgery. Closed suction drains are placed in dependant areas in the pelvis and below each hemidiaphragm. EPIC has the advantages of administering multiple chemotherapy cycles and increased exposure of tumor cells to therapy, as the chemotherapeutic drug is not drained for at least 24 h. However, there is greater opportunity for significant systemic absorption and its resultant adverse effects, as the chemotherapeutic agents remains in the peritoneal cavity for such a long period. Using drugs with a high first-pass effect after portal absorption—such as 5-fluorouracil (5-FU), the most common drug used with this technique—partially overcomes this problem [7]. Moreover, other complications related to long-term catheters (infections, bowel obstruction) are reported: EPIC significantly increased the rate of postoperative complications in the large, multicentric retrospective study of 504 patients with colorectal carcinomatosis treated with cytoreductive surgery combined with perioperative intraperitoneal chemotherapy [15].

EPIC efficacy is limited by adhesion formation, which can cause pooling of the chemotherapeutic agent in limited parts of the abdomen, with consequent systemic toxicity; also, this treatment is not performed with hyperthermia. In fact, heat is cytotoxic in vitro at 42.5°C [16], and hyperthermia enhances the antitumor effect of agents such as oxaliplatin, mitomycin, doxorubicin, and cisplatin by augmenting cytotoxicity and increasing drug penetration into tissue [17–19]. Elias et al. compared two similar groups of patients with colorectal peritoneal carcinomatosis, one treated with EPIC using 5-FU and mitomycin C, and one treated with HIPEC using oxaliplatin at 43.8°C (43°C). Mortality, morbidity, peritoneal recurrence, and overall survival rate all favored the HIPEC group. In particular, peritoneal recurrence was reported as being doubled in EPIC group compared with the HIPEC group [20].

Thus, the only acceptable use of EPIC seems to be for treating microscopic residual peritoneal disease following HIPEC. An increased risk of postoperative complications must therefore be taken in account if this combined approach is chosen.

10.6 Drugs, Carrier Solutions, and Temperature

10.6.1 Drugs

When choosing a chemotherapeutic drug, some very important aspects must be considered. Whereas in instillation intraperitoneal chemotherapy all categories of active drugs can be used, in HIPEC procedures, a direct cytotoxic agent (cell cycle nonspecific) is needed; the agent should lack severe direct local toxicity after intraperitoneal administration, have a well-established activity against the malignancy treated, have a heat-synergized cytotoxicity, and should not have to be metabolized systemically into its active form [21]. Intraperitoneally administered drugs inevitably have a variable, although usually limited, systemic absorption, which may, however, lead to toxicity.

Standardized drug dose and carrier-solution volume, assessed according to the patient's body surface area (BSA) (usually 1.5–2 L/m^2), are recommended in order to make exposure and toxicity predictable; drug dosage per liter of perfusate or per body weight usually prevents untoward events secondary to overdosing.

Different single-drug or combination regimens have been employed over the years, as shown in Table 10.1. A dose reduction of 33% should be considered for patients > 60 years, those previously exposed to multiple lines of systemic chemotherapy, those who require granulocyte-macrophage colony-stimulating-factor (GM-CSF) rescue for febrile neutropenia while on systemic chemotherapy, or those who have received radiation therapy to bone-marrow-bearing regions. Typically, centers that associate HIPEC and EPIC use moderate drug doses for HIPEC, whereas those that perform only HIPEC after cytoreductive surgery use much higher doses.

Elias et al. were the first to report using bidirectional HIPEC regimens (concurrent administration of intraperitoneal and IV chemotherapy). In particular, they administer 5-FU and folinic acid IV prior to performing HIPEC with oxaliplatin due to the instability of the mixture of both drugs [22]. The advantage of this strategy was demonstrated by Van der Speeten et al.: after IV administration of 5-FU in a patient undergoing intraperitoneal hyperthermia, the drug unexpectedly accumulated in the peritoneal cavity and in tumor nodules [23].

10.6.2 Carrier Solutions

Different carrier solutions with varying chemical properties have been investigated [24]: 1.5% dextrose isotonic peritoneal dialysis solution is the most commonly used in HIPEC centers rather than the regular crystalloid solutions (normal saline or 5% dextrose in water). Hetastarch (6% hydroxyethyl starch), a high-molecular-weight solution, is regularly employed as carrier for paclitaxel [25].

10.6.3 Temperature

Theoretically, what is the optimal temperature to use during HIPEC? The target range reported in the literature varies from 40° to 45.8°C; however, most

Table 10.1 Different drug regimens applied in different peritoneal surface malignancy centers. (Modified from [26])

Indication	HIPEC: dose/perfusion time	Concomitant IV therapy	EPIC	Center
Appendiceal and colorectal carcinomatosis	Mitomycin C, 15 mg/m^2 doxorubicin, 15 mg/m^2/90 min	5-FU, 400 mg/m^2; LV, 20 mg/m^2	5-FU 4 days	Washington Hospital Center, Washington, DC (USA)
	Oxaliplatin, 130 mg/m^2/60 min	5-FU, 400 mg/m^2; LV, 20 mg/m^2	5-FU 4 days	Washington Hospital Center, Washington, DC (USA)
	Oxaliplatin, 460 mg/m^2/30 min	5-FU, 400 mg/m^2; LV, 20 mg/m^2	No	Gustave Roussy Institute, Villejuif (France)
	Mitomycin C, 35 mg/m^2/60 min	No	No	National Cancer Institute, Amsterdam (The Netherlands)
	Mitomycin C, 3.3mg/m^2/L cisplatin, 25 mg/m^2/L/60 min	No	No	National Cancer Institute, Milan (Italy)
	Mitomycin C,10 mg/mL perfusate/60 minNo	No		Centre hospitalo-universitaire Lyon-sud, Lyon (France)
Gastric cancer	Cisplatin, 50 mg/m^2 doxorubicin, 15 mg/m^2/90 min	5-FU, 400 mg/m^2; LV, 20 mg/m^2	Taxol 4 days	Washington Hospital Center, Washington, DC (USA)
	Mitomycin C,10 mg/mL perfusate/60 min	No	No	Centre hospitalo-universitaire Lyon-sud, Lyon (France)
Peritoneal mesothelioma	Cisplatin, 50 mg/m^2 doxorubicin, 15 mg/m^2/90 min	5-FU, 400 mg/m^2; LV, 20 mg/m^2	Taxol 4 days	Washington Hospital Center, Washington, DC (USA)
	Cisplatin, 43 mg/L doxorubicin ,15.25 mg/mL/90 min	No	No	National Cancer Institute, Milan (Italy)
	Mitomycin C, 0.5 mg/kg cisplatin 0.7 mg/kg/60 min	No	No	Centre hospitalo-universitaire Lyon-sud, Lyon (France)

(*cont.*) →

Table 10.1 *(continued)*

Indication	HIPEC: dose/perfusion time	Concomitant IV therapy	EPIC	Center
	Cisplatin, 250 mg/m²/90 min	No	5-FU Taxol 1 days	National Cancer Institute, Bethesda, MD (USA)
Adverse ovarian cancer	Cisplatin, 50 mg/m² doxorubicin, 15 mg/m²/90 min	5-FU, 400 mg/m²; LV, 20 mg/m²	Taxol 4 days	Washington Hospital Center, Washington, DC (USA)
	Cisplatin, 43 mg/L doxorubicin,15.25 mg/mL/90 min	No	No	National Cancer Institute, Milan (Italy)
	Cisplatin, 20 mg/m²/L/90 min	No	No	Centre hospitalo-universitaire Lyon-sud, Lyon (France)

HIPEC, hyperthermic intraperitoneal chemotherapy; *IV*, intravenous; *5-FU*, 5-fluorouracil; *LV*, leucovorin

authors agree that the desirable range at which to maintain intra-abdominal temperature is 41.5–43°C, which necessitates maintaining an inflow temperature of 46–48°C [26].

To establish the optimal temperature during perfusion, it is useful to consider several aspects, such as the interaction between heat and chemotherapeutic agents, method of temperature control, and risk of side effects. Usually, drug type does not constitute a problem, as all agents typically used for HIPEC are chemically stable at temperatures as high as 50.8°C.

Synergism between various cytotoxic drugs and hyperthermia starts at 39.8°C but is stronger at higher temperatures; according to in vitro studies on culture cells at 45.8°C, agent cytotoxicity is far more intense than at 41°C or 42.8°C; thus it is intuitively reasonable to use the highest level of hyperthermia, restricted only by clinical tolerance. The limiting factor of temperatures as high as 45.8°C is the tolerance level of the small bowel. Only one study addresses thermotolerance, and that study was performed using an animal model (rat). The authors concluded that 44.8°C for 30 min was the maximal, well-tolerated temperature [27].

10.7 Choosing HIPEC Delivery Mode

Each HIPEC perfusion technique has its advantages and disadvantages (Table 10.2). No formal prospective controlled comparison of delivery methods has been performed, and there is no evidence to establish the superiority of one method over the others regarding patient outcomes, morbidity, or safety to surgical staff. Thus, the following factors must be taken into account: (1) the perceived risk of environmental chemotherapy exposure (the real risk is negligible if proper safety measures are followed); (2) concerns regarding possible differences in uniform distribution of the chemotherapeutic agent or heat throughout the peritoneal cavity, which may result in visceral thermal injury; and (3) possible differences in dosage and perfusate volume inherent to the closed method.

Table 10.2 Choosing the hyperthermic intraperitoneal chemotherapy (HIPEC) procedure

Feature	Open	Closed	Semiopen
Uniform heat and chemotherapy distribution	√		√
Minor heat dissipation		√	
No direct contact of surgeon with chemotherapeutic agent		√	
Minimize risk of chemotherapeutic agent exposure to operating-room staff		√	√
Minimize risk of thermal injury	√		√
User friendliness		√	

10.8 Environmental/Surgical-staff Exposure

During HIPEC, a so-called major spill of chemotherapeutic agents (defined by the US Occupational Safety Health Administration as <5 g or 5 mL of undiluted cytotoxic agent) is impossible to imagine, as chemotherapeutic drugs are always diluted, and their doses are in micrograms. Nevertheless, the effects of prolonged, repeated occupational exposure to low doses of chemotherapeutic agents remain unknown. For this reason, all precautions and guidelines for chemotherapy handling should be observed (Box 10.1) [28].

There are two major routes of exposure to chemotherapeutic agents: direct contact, and inhalation of aerosolized or vaporized agent particles. Dermatitis or mucositis are the consequences of direct contact with skin or mucous membranes. Theoretically, systemic effects (bone marrow toxicity, gastrointestinal toxicity, hair loss, and so forth) may be produced by frequent exposure and absorption of low dose of such drugs, but such data are lacking in the literature [29].

Inhalation could occur if cytotoxic drugs vaporize due to the hyperthermia. Using a smoke evacuator under the plastic sheet during HIPEC administration with the coliseum technique, or using acrylic covers in semiopen methods, minimizes this risk. Studies by Stuart et al. and Schmid et al. [30, 31] evaluated personal safety during open HIPEC using the coliseum technique. The studies assessed the level of mitomycin C in urine of members of the operating team and in the air below and above the plastic sheet, and the permeability of sterile gloves commonly used in the operating room. No potential risk of

Box 10.1 Rules for safe administration of hyperthermic intraperitoneal chemotherapy (HIPEC). (Modified from [29])

- Use impervious, disposable drapes; no textile cloth in surgical fields
- Accurate lap-pad count should be obtained before HIPEC initiation
- Operating-room doors closed during HIPEC; signs placed outside the operating room advising that HIPEC is in progress
- Restrict personnel circulation
- Place absorbent towels on the floor around the surgical table in the event of spills
- Use disposable, impervious gown (closed front, long sleeves, closed cuffs)and shoe covers; eye protection (goggles); high-power filtration mask (FFP-3); double, powderless, latex gloving, outer ones elbow length; change of outer gloves should be made every 30 min
- Adequately ventilate the environment
- Use smoke evacuator continuously over surgical field (under plastic drape in coliseum technique)
- Use rigid, leak-proof containers labeled "cytotoxic agents" for every material or bodily fluid discarded during or after HIPEC and during the following 48 h

exposure was found, and all assessments were in compliance with safety standards [30, 31]. A Swedish study detected no platinum in urine or blood of the surgeon or perfusionist during HIPEC with oxaliplatin using the coliseum technique. These studies confirm that, even in the method with a higher chance of chemotherapy exposure for surgical staff, HIPEC is a safe procedure from the occupational risk standpoint when standard protective measures are observed [32].

References

1. Verwaal VJ, van Ruth S, de Bree E et al (2003) Randomized trial of cytoreduction and hyperthermic intraperitoneal chemotherapy versus systemic chemotherapy and palliative surgery in patients with peritoneal carcinomatosis of colorectal cancer. J Clin Oncol 21:3737–3743
2. Gonzalez-Moreno S (2006) Peritoneal surface oncology: A progress report. Eur J Surg Oncol 32:593–596
3. Szafnicki K, Narce C (2006) Towards a crippled-mode operation of an industrial wastewater treatment plant. Water Res 40:579–587
4. Elias DM, Ouellet JF (2000) Intraperitoneal chemohyperthermia: Rationale, technique, indications, and results. Surg Oncol Clin N Am 10:915–933
5. Glehen OMF, Gilly FN (2004) Peritoneal carcinomatosis from digestive tract cancer: New management by cytoreductive surgery and intraperitoneal chemohyperthermia. Lancet Oncol 5:219– 228
6. Sugarbaker PH (2005) Technical handbook for the integration of cytoreductive surgery and perioperative intraperitoneal chemotherapy into the surgical management of gastrointestinal and gynecologic malignancy, 4th ed. Grand Rapids, Michigan, Ludann Company
7. Elias D, Antoun S, Goharin A et al (2000) Research on the best chemohyperthermia technique of treatment of peritoneal carcinomatosis after complete resection. Int J Surg Investig 1:431–439
8. Jacquet P, Averbach A, Stephens AD et al (1998) Heated intraoperative intraperitoneal mitomycin C and early postoperative intraperitoneal 5-fluorouracil: Pharmacokinetic studies. Oncology 55:130–138
9. Stephens AD, Alderman R, Chang D et al (1999) Morbidity and mortality analysis of 200 treatments with cytoreductive surgery and hyperthermic intraoperative intraperitoneal chemotherapy using the coliseum technique. Ann Surg Oncol 16:790–796
10. Glehen O, Cotte E, Kusamura S et al (2008) Hyperthermic intraperitoneal chemotherapy: nomenclature and modalities of perfusion. J Surg Oncol 98.242-246
11. Fujimura T, Yonemura Y, Fushida S et al (1990) Continuous hyperthermic peritoneal perfusion for the treatment of peritoneal dissemination in gastric cancers and subsequent second-look operation. Cancer 65:65–71
12. Rat P, Benoit L, Cheynel N et al (2001) Intraperitoneal chemohyperthermia with overflow open abdomen. Ann Chir 126:669–671
13. Sugarbaker PH (2005) An instrument to provide containment of intraoperative intraperitoneal chemotherapy with optimized distribution. J Surg Oncol 92:142–146
14. Esquivel J, Vidal-Jove J, Steves MA et al (1993) Morbidity and mortality of cytoreductive surgery and intraperitoneal chemotherapy. Surgery 113:631–636
15. Glehen OKF, Sugarbaker PH, Elias D et al (2004) Cytoreductive surgery combined with perioperative intraperitoneal chemotherapy for the management of peritoneal carcinomatosis from colorectal cancer: A multi-institutional study. J Clin Oncol 22:3284–3292
16. Crile G Jr (1963) The effects of heat and radiation on cancers implanted on the feet of mice. Cancer Res 23:372–380

17. Elias D, Ouellet JF (2000) Intraperitoneal chemohyperthermia: Rationale, technique, indications, and results. Surg Oncol Clin N Am 10:915–933
18. Glehen OMF, Gilly FN (2004) Peritoneal carcinomatosis from digestive tract cancer: New management by cytoreductive surgery and intraperitoneal chemohyperthermia. Lancet Oncol 5:219–228
19. Sugarbaker PH (1998) Intraperitoneal chemotherapy and cytoreductive surgery for the prevention and treatment of peritoneal carcinomatosis and sarcomatosis. Semin Surg Oncol 14:254–261
20. Elias D, Benizri E, Di Pietrantonio D et al (2007) Comparison of two kinds of intraperitoneal chemotherapy following complete cytoreductive surgery of colorectal peritoneal carcinomatosis. Ann Surg Oncol 14:509–514
21. de Bree E, Tsiftsis DD (2007) Principles of perioperative intraperitoneal chemotherapy for peritoneal carcinomatosis. Recent Results Cancer Res 169:39-51
22. Elias DM, Bonnay M, Puizillou et al (2002) Heated intra-operative intraperitoneal oxaliplatin after complete resection of peritoneal carcinomatosis: pharmacokinetics and tissue distribution. Ann Oncol 13:267-272
23. Van der Speeten K, Stuart OA, Sugarbaker PH (2009) Pharmacokinetics and pharmacodynamics of perioperative cancer chemotherapy in peritoneal surface malignancy. Cancer J 15:216-224
24. Mohamed F, Sugarbaker PH (2003) Carrier solutions for intraperitoneal chemotherapy. Surg Oncol Clin N Am 12:813-824
25. Mohamed F, Sugarbaker PH (2003) Intraperitoneal taxanes. Surg Oncol Clin N Am 12:825-833
26. Kusamura S, Elias DM, Baratti D et al (2008) Drugs, Carrier Solutions and Temperature in Hyperthermic Intraperitoneal Chemotherapy. J Surg Oncol 98:247–252
27. Shimizu T, Maeta M, Koga S (1991) Influence of local hyperthermia on the healing of small intestinal anastomoses in the rat. Br J Surg 78:57–59
28. Yodaiken RE, Bennett D (1986) OSHA work practice guidelines for personnel dealing with cytotoxic (antineoplastic) drugs. Occupational Safety and Health Administration. Am J Hosp Pharm 43:1193–1204
29. González-Moreno S, González-Bayón L, Ortega-Pérez G (2012), Hyperthermic Intraperitoneal Chemotherapy Methodology and Safety Considerations. Surg Oncol Clin N Am 21:543–557
30. Stuart OA, Stephens AD, Welch L et al (2002) Safety monitoring of the coliseum technique for heated intraoperative intraperitoneal chemotherapy with mitomycin C. Ann Surg Oncol 9:186–191
31. Schmid K, Boettcher MI, Pelz JO et al(2006) Investigations on safety of hyperthermic intraoperative intraperitoneal chemotherapy (HIPEC) with mitomycin C. Eur J Surg Oncol 32:1222–1225
32. Na¨slund Andre´asson S, Anundi H, Tho´ren SB et al (2010) Is platinum present in the blood and urine from treatment givers during hyperthermic intraperitoneal chemotherapy? J Oncol 2010:649–719

The Role of Surgery

11

Marco Lotti, Fausto Catena, Federico Coccolini, Giorgio Ercolani, Antonio Daniele Pinna, and Luca Ansaloni

11.1 Introduction

Peritoneal carcinomatosis (PC) has commonly been considered a terminal disease stage: patients with PC have not been considered candidates for surgical resection and still often receive only palliative surgery, if any, and are committed to systemic chemotherapy (CHT) with minimal improvement in their chances of survival. This attitude arose from the traditional belief that PC is just one of the different forms of cancer metastasis, such as hematogenous or lymphatic metastasis, and is a signal that the disease has become systemic and is no longer curable with surgery. This belief–challenged in recent years by evidence that surgical resection of hepatic or limited pulmonary metastases from colorectal cancer (CRC) is associated with improved survival–is now the subject of an intense debate due to evidence that aggressive surgical treatment of PC–coupled with intraperitoneal chemotherapy (IP-CHT)—is associated with improved survival in patients with peritoneal malignancies such as mesothelioma, pseudomyxoma peritonei (PMP), and PC from colorectal, gastric and epithelial ovarian cancer.

The fact that several patients with gastric cancer and CRC develop PC without any evidence of hepatic, lymphatic, or extra-abdominal metastasis, together with the good results obtained with aggressive surgical treatment of PMP, led to the concept that peritoneal dissemination is a process that involves specific molecular mechanisms that are different from hematogenous or lymphatic dissemination and should still be considered a locoregional rather than a metastatic disease. In recent years, great effort has been made to test molecu-

M. Lotti (✉)
Department of General and Emergency Surgery, "Papa Giovanni XXIII" Hospital, Bergamo, Italy
e-mail: mlotti@hpg23.it

A. Di Giorgio, E. Pinto (Eds), *Treatment of Peritoneal Surface Malignancies*, Updates in Surgery
DOI: 10.1007/978-88-470-5711-1_11,

lar markers to identify patients at risk for PC and peritoneal recurrence, further clarifying the role of specific gene mutations in determining detachment of free cells from the serosal surface of gastric [1] and colorectal [2] tumors, their seeding in the peritoneal cavity, and their adhesion to the peritoneum and penetration into peritoneal surface lymphatics [3, 4]. There is now little, if any, doubt that PC should be considered in a quite different light: the risk of peritoneal dissemination should be evaluated in the preoperative staging of cancer, and PC, if present, should be described in a precise manner and considered for multimodal treatment that involves systemic chemotherapy and a surgical strategy to obtain local control of peritoneal dissemination [5].

11.2 Model for Surgery: Pseudomyxoma Peritonei

PMP is a rare and low-grade malignancy developing usually from a ruptured mucinous neoplasm of the appendix: the release of slowly growing mucin-producing cells in the peritoneal cavity leads to the characteristic mucinous ascites, with progressive symptoms of bowel obstruction and starvation [6]. PMP with hematogenous or lymphatic metastasis is a rare occurrence: for this reason, the traditional treatment of PMP consisted of repeated debulking surgery procedures, which is a strategy still used in some centers, with a reported 5-year overall survival (OS) rate of 50 %. This strategy is almost always followed by recurrence, with increasing difficulty in performing debulking surgery due to adhesions and small-bowel injury, and patients ultimately die because of surgical complications, bowel obstruction, or severe starvation [7]. Systemic CT for PMP is ineffective because systemically delivered drugs have only limited peritoneal barrier penetration and do not reach effective intraperitoneal concentrations. For this reason, in the 1980s, a new multimodal strategy was introduced combining an aggressive surgical procedure aimed at reaching a zero macroscopic residual tumor [cytoreductive surgery (CRS)] and the delivery of cytotoxic drugs directly into the peritoneum (IP-CHT), with a dramatic increase in 10-year OS from 20–30 % to 70 % [8]. The positive results achieved with this multimodal strategy made PMP a "model disease" for treating PC from other malignancies.

Studies on the pharmacokinetics and pharmacodynamics of IP chemotherapeutics further clarified the importance of surgery in reducing residual tumor to a minimum due to the limited depth of penetration of the chemotherapeutics into neoplastic nodules [9, 10]. All subsequent studies showed that the efficacy of this multimodal strategy is maximal when complete removal of PC is achieved by CRS and that the capability of surgery to obtain a zero residual tumor is directly influenced by the IP tumor load.

11.3 Defining Intraperitoneal Tumor Load: PCI Score

The Peritoneal Cancer Index (PCI) score is used to clearly define PC extent [11]. This score, proposed by Jacquet and Sugarbaker [11], quantitatively assesses cancer distribution and implant size throughout the abdomen and pelvis. The abdomen and pelvis are divided by lines into nine regions (regions 0–8). The small bowel is then divided into four regions: 9 and 10 define upper and lower portions of the jejunum, respectively; 11 and 12 define upper and lower portions of the ileum. In each region, lesion size (LS) of the largest implant is scored as follows: LS-0, no implants seen; LS-1, implants up to 0.5 cm are visible; LS-2, nodules > 0.5 cm and up to 5 cm; LS-3, implants >5 cm or to confluent nodules. Measurement is made after a complete adhesiolysis and complete inspection of all parietal and visceral peritoneal surfaces. LS values for each region can be summed as a numerical score (PCI score varying from 1 to 39) describing tumor load in the peritoneal cavity as a whole. This score allows estimation of the probability of complete cytoreduction (Fig. 11.1).

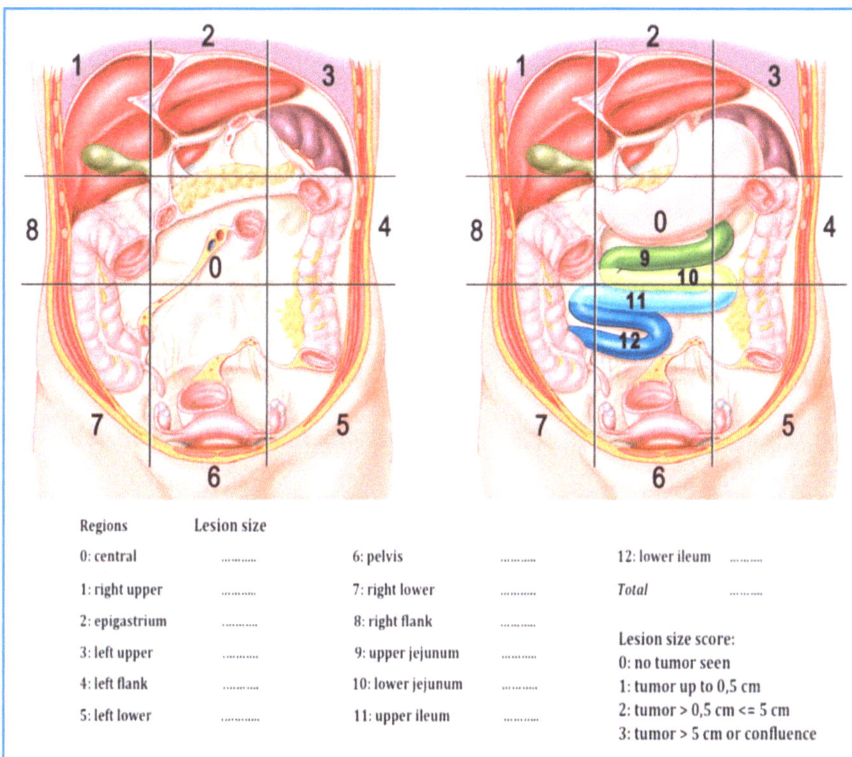

Fig. 11.1 Peritoneal Cancer Index (PCI) scoring system

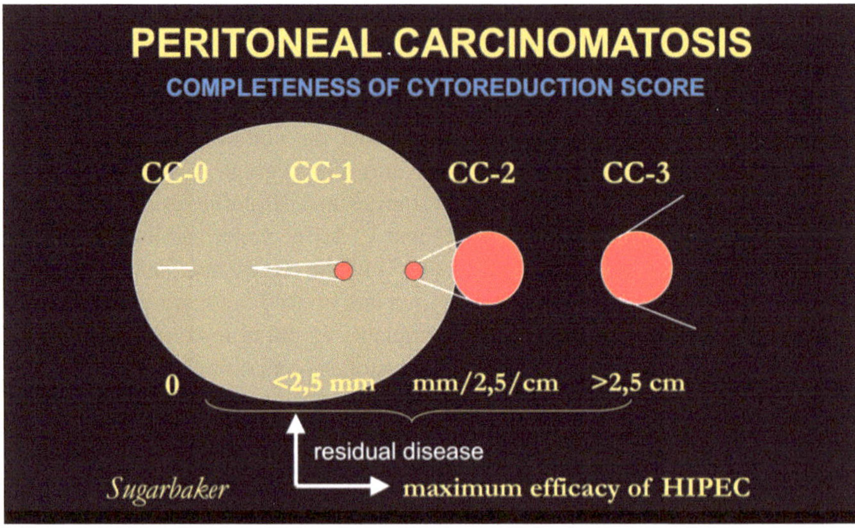

Fig. 11.2 Completeness of Cytoreduction (CC) scoring system. *HIPEC,* hyperthermic intraperitoneal chemotherapy. (Modified from [12])

11.4 Defining Completeness of Cytoreduction: CC score

Completeness of cytoreduction is the most important prognostic factor after CRS. Residual disease after CRS is properly described using the Completeness of Cytoreduction (CC) score [12] (Fig. 11.2):

- CC-0, no visible residual tumor
- CC-1, residual tumor nodules < 2.5 mm
- CC-2, residual tumor nodules between 2.5 mm and 2.5 cm
- CC-3, residual tumor > 2.5 cm

Adequate cytoreduction is defined as CC-0 or 1 because only microscopic or minimal residual nodules are targeted by IP-administered drugs; IP-CHT is not indicated if a CC-2 or 3 score is obtained after CRS. The probability of adequate cytoreduction is correlated with the extent of PC, as described by the PCI.

11.5 How can Surgery Achieve Complete Cytoreduction? CRS, Peritonectomy, and Sugarbaker Procedures

The techniques required to accomplish complete surgical resection of PC were detailed by Sugarbaker [13, 14] and consist of six different peritonectomy procedures (aimed at resecting peritoneal surfaces that contain tumor implants) and visceral dissections, with maximal surgical effort to remove as much macroscopic tumor as possible, followed by direct instillation of hyperthermic

Table 11.1 Sugarbaker peritonectomy procedures

1	Greater omentectomy, right parietal peritonectomy, right colon resection
2	Left upper quadrant peritonectomy, splenectomy, and left parietal peritonectomy
3	Right upper quadrant peritonectomy and Glissonian capsule resection
4	Lesser omentectomy, cholecystectomy, stripping of omental bursa, and antrectomy
5	Pelvic peritonectomy with sigmoid colon resection with or without hysterectomy and bilateral salpingo-oophorectomy
6	Other intestinal resection and/or abdominal mass resection
7	Bowel anastomosis

intraperitoneal chemotherapy (HIPEC) to address microscopic residual disease (Table 11.1).

The need to perform one or more CRS procedures to achieve complete cytoreduction and the subsequent risk of postoperative complications is strictly related to disease extent described by PCI score. Postoperative complication and mortality rates after CRS range from 20 % to 50 % and from 2 % to 12 %, respectively, so that proper patient selection and careful evaluation of disease extent of are required prior to CRS [14]. In general, a PCI score > 20 is accepted as indicative of poor chances of obtaining adequate cytoreduction [15]. For PC from gastric cancer, some authors suggest a PCI ≤ 12 as a threshold for expecting a CC-0 surgery with minimal complication rates [11, 16]. The role of adequate surgical technique and surgeon skill in reducing complications and obtaining adequate cytoreduction is emphasized by several authors, as is the importance of the learning curve for this complex surgical procedure. With adequate experience, surgeons can achieve adequate cytoreduction with acceptable risk, even in selected patients with PCI > 20 [17].

11.6 Cytoreduction Completeness and Patient Survival

When interpreting results of the CRS plus IP-CHT strategy, the relative contribution of each CRS and IP-CHT in determining survival benefit remains unclear. Nevertheless, there is uniform agreement that cytoreduction completeness is the only variable clearly associated with increased survival rates, with optimal results being achieved when a CC-0 is accomplished [18]. Even in PC from CRC and gastric cancer, the impact of CC-0 surgery on survival benefit clearly emerged from randomized controlled trials (RCTs). In PC from CRC, an impressive 22–43 % 5-year survival rate was observed in CC-0 patients after CRS plus HIPEC [19], with those results being maintained even after a long-term follow-up [20].

Even without IP-CHT or HIPEC, an aggressive surgical strategy for obtaining a zero-residual tumor is a mainstay of therapy in patients with advanced ovarian cancer, with systemic CHT being considerably less effective in women with macroscopic residual tumor after surgery [21, 22]. In order to reduce the IP cancer load before surgery and increase chances for adequate cytoreduction, systemic neoadjuvant CHT has been proposed in ovarian and gastric cancer patients. In some centers, IP-CHT is also administered together with systemic CHT in a neoadjuvant setting for gastric PC [23]. In treating PC from gastrointestinal and ovarian cancer, CRS, IP-CHT, HIPEC, and systemic CHT become part of a multimodal treatment strategy: all cases should be discussed in a multidisciplinary team including surgeon, clinical oncologist, radiotherapist, pathologist, radiologist, and anesthesiologist in order to target therapy and select patients suitable for a CC-0 surgery with a low risk for complications and the greatest chance to benefit from this complex strategy.

11.7 Selecting Patients for CRS

There is much controversy among clinical oncologists and surgeons around this subject, many of the former being convinced that the positive results obtained with CRS and IP-CHT are mainly due to patient selection. There is no doubt, however, that in selected patients (i.e., patients with PC load amendable by surgery), CRS + IP-CHT, eventually followed by systemic CHT, provides better results than systemic CHT alone [18].

PC patients are often denied surgery and sent for multiple cycles of systemic CHT, which shows only limited effects. They are referred to the surgeon only in case of bowel obstruction or perforation and are proposed for CRS plus IP-CHT only after the failure of several cycles of systemic CHT, by which time the cancer load is massive and patients are usually physically wasted: in this setting, there is little chance of obtaining a CC-0 operation; patients often require multiple peritonectomy procedures and multiorgan resections and are at maximum risk for perioperative complications [24]. Early referral to surgery should thus be encouraged, so that the tumor load is limited, a CC-0 resection is still possible with a reduced need for multiorgan resections, and the risk for complications is minimal. In this scenario, patients recover better after surgery and are eventually fit for adjuvant systemic CHT, if indicated. On the other hand, patients with massive PC (PCI > 20) who are not suitable for optimal cytoreduction should not be treated with CRS plus IP-CHT, because they often require extensive surgical resections and experience a high risk of complications and mortality, with little chance of improving their survival and quality of life [14].

11.8 Reducing Complications after CRS

Patient selection and surgical quality are the most important factors in preventing postoperative complications [24]. Several factors are associated with risk of complications, including the number of anastomoses performed, the need for diaphragmatic resection, scald injuries to the bowel due to HIPEC, the toxicity of IP-CHT itself, and the number of blood transfusions required. In preventing complications, a skilled anesthesiologist is required for careful intraoperative patient management: during CRS plus HIPEC, patients face several dangers, such as hyperthermia, abdominal hypertension, electrolyte abnormalities, coagulopathies, increased cardiac index, reduced oxygen consumption, and decreased systemic vascular resistance [25]. In the postoperative period, anastomotic leakage, bowel obstruction due to adhesions, bowel perforation due to scald injury, or direct toxicity of chemotherapeutic drugs are the most anticipated complications. In most centers, a diverting stoma is performed when there is need for multiple anastomoses or rectal anastomosis. When complications develop, it is often difficult to differentiate between morbidity resulting from surgery and that attributable to IP-CHT or HIPEC: in order to optimize the reporting of postoperative complications, the NCI-CTCAE classification should be adopted [24, 26].

11.9 Learning Curve

Recent reports suggest that the initial high morbidity and mortality rates seen with CRS and HIPEC decreases with increasing surgeon experience [27-29]. This is evident in specialized centers and includes improvements in patient selection, surgical expertise and postoperative management. This increased information base is culminating in a global learning curve and reduced complications rates (Table 11.2).

11.10 Conclusions and Directions

A well-trained surgical team can achieve a CC-0 resection in patients with extensive PC, and better results are thus anticipated in preventing the development or recurrence of PC in patients at risk.

Table 11.2 Mortality according to increasing experience using cytoreduction and HIPEC for peritoneal carcitomatosis

	% Perioperative Mortality		
Study [Reference]	**Initial**	**Intermediate**	**Recent**
Moran [27]	18	3	3
Smeenk et al. [28]	8	6	4
Yan et al. [29]	7	-	1

In patients with gastric cancer, careful preoperative staging, including endoscopic ultrasonography and computed tomography (CT) scan and adoption of explorative laparoscopy and diagnostic peritoneal washing, helps in identifying patients at risk for PC: these patients are eventually treated with HIPEC at the time of surgical resection [30].

In patients with CRC, second-look surgery has been proposed in those at higher risk for peritoneal recurrence (i.e., bowel obstruction or perforation or synchronous ovarian metastases): in these patients, the chance of finding PC 1 year after the first surgical procedure ranges from 33 % to 75 %, even if CT scan is negative. When present, PC could be treated with CRS plus HIPEC, which achieves optimal results in terms of survival [31].

A single-center case–control study analyzed the role of HIPEC for preventing peritoneal metastases after primary surgery in patients with CRC at high risk for peritoneal spread. That study demonstrated that when such patients were treated with a more aggressive surgical approach plus HIPEC, a statistically significant difference in disease-free and overall survival can be achieved [33].

In patients with ovarian cancer, HIPEC is often performed only after recurrence. Some evidence exists that better results could be achieved when performing HIPEC as a first-line treatment for advanced ovarian cancer, and an RCT is ongoing [33].

Much research is being conducted pertaining to molecular mechanisms for PC development: identifying specific gene mutations could lead to the availability of specific molecular biomarkers for selecting patients at risk for PC. While awaiting those results, surgeons are invited to participate in a multidisciplinary team, together with all other specialties involved in treating patients with cancers at risk for PC, and to encourage early patient referral to centers highly experienced in CRS plus IP-CHT.

References

1. de Cuba EM, Kwakman R, van Egmond M et al (2012) Understanding molecular mechanisms in peritoneal dissemination of colorectal cancer : future possibilities for personalised treatment by use of biomarkers. Virchows Arch 461:231-243
2. Tang B, Peng Z-h, Yu P-W, Yu G et al (2013) Aberrant Expression of Cx43 Is Associated with the Peritoneal Metastasis of Gastric Cancer and Cx43-Mediated Gap Junction Enhances Gastric Cancer Cell Diapedesis from Peritoneal Mesothelium. PLoS ONE 8:e74527
3. Yonemura Y, Kawamura T, Bandou E (2007) The natural history of free cancer cells in the peritoneal cavity Recent Results Cancer Res 169:11-23
4. Shimotsuma M, Shirasu M, Hagiwara A, Takahashi T (1996) Role of omentum-associated lymphoid tissue in the progression of peritoneal carcinomatosis. Cancer Treat Res 82:147-154
5. Witkamp AJ, de Bree E, Van Goethem R, Zoetmulder FA (2001) Rationale and techniques of intra-operative hyperthermic intraperitoneal chemotherapy. Cancer Treat Rev 27:365-374
6. McBride K, McFadden D, Osler T (2012) Improved survival of patients with pseudomyxoma peritonei receiving intraperitoneal chemotherapy with cytoreductive surgery: a systematic review and meta-analysis. J Surg Res 183:246-252

7. Andreasson H, Graf W, Nygren P et al (2012) Outcome differences between debulking surgery and cytoreductive surgery in patients with pseudomyxoma peritonei. Eur J Surg Oncol 38:962-968
8. Sørensen O, Flatmark K, Reed W, Wiig JN (2012) Evaluation of complete cytoreductive surgery and two intraperitoneal chemotherapy techniques in Pseudomyxoma peritonei. Eur J Surg Oncol 38:969-976
9. Van der Speeten K, Stuart OA, Sugarbaker PH (2012) Pharmacology of perioperative intraperitoneal and intravenous chemotherapy in patients with peritoneal surface malignancy. Surg Oncol Clin N Am 21:577-597
10. Hasovits C, Clarke S (2012) Pharmacokinetics and pharmacodynamics of intraperitoneal cancer chemotherapeutics. Clin Pharmacokinet 51:203-224
11. Cotte E, Passot G, Gilly FN, Glehen O (2010) Selection of patients and staging of peritoneal surface malignancies World J Gastrointest Oncol 2:31-35
12. Esquivel J, Sticca R, Sugarbaker P, Levine E, Yan TD, Alexander R, Baratti D, Bartlett D, Barone R, Barrios P, Bieligk S, Bretcha-Boix P, Chang CK, Chu F, Chu Q, Daniel S, de Bree E, Deraco M, Dominguez-Parra L, Elias D, Flynn R, Foster J, Garofalo A, Gilly FN, Glehen O, Gomez-Portilla A, Gonzalez-Bayon L, Gonzalez-Moreno S, Goodman M, Gushchin V, Hanna N, Hartmann J, Harrison L, Hoefer R, Kane J, Kecmanovic D, Kelley S, Kuhn J, Lamont J, Lange J, Li B, Loggie B, Mahteme H, Mann G, Martin R, Misih RA, Moran B, Morris D, Onate-Ocana L, Petrelli N, Philippe G, Pingpank J, Pitroff A, Piso P, Quinones M, Riley L, Rutstein L, Saha S, Alrawi S, Sardi A, Schneebaum S, Shen P, Shibata D, Spellman J, Stojadinovic A, Stewart J, Torres-Melero J, Tuttle T, Verwaal V, Villar J, Wilkinson N, Younan R, Zeh H, Zoetmulder F, Sebbag G; Society of Surgical Oncology Annual Meeting (2007) Cytoreductive surgery and hyperthermic intraperitoneal chemotherapy in the management of peritoneal surface malignancies of colonic origin: a consensus statement. Society of Surgical Oncology. Ann Surg Oncol 14:128-133
13. Sugarbaker PH (1995) Peritonectomy procedures. Ann Surg 221:29-42
14. Bao P, Bartlett D (2009) Surgical techniques in visceral resection and peritonectomy procedures Cancer J 15:204-211
15. Sugarbaker PH (2012) Cytoreductive surgery plus hyperthermic perioperative chemotherapy for selected patients with peritoneal metastases from colorectal cancer: a new standard of care or an experimental approach? Gastroenterol Res Pract 2012:309417
16. Glehen O, Gilly FN, Arvieux C, Cotte E, Boutitie F, Mansvelt B, Bereder JM, Lorimier G, Quenet F, Elias D; Association Française de Chirurgie (2010) Peritoneal carcinomatosis from gastric cancer: a multi-institutional study of 159 patients treated by cytoreductive surgery combined with perioperative intraperitoneal chemotherapy. Ann Surg Oncol 17:2370-2377
17. Kusamura S, Baratti D, Hutanu I et al (2012) The importance of the learning curve and surveillance of surgical performance in peritoneal surface malignancy programs. Surg Oncol Clin N Am 21:559-576
18. Coccolini F, Gheza F, Lotti M et al (2013) Peritoneal carcinomatosis. World J Gastroenterol 19:6979-6994
19. Weber T, Roitman M, Link KH (2012) Current Status of Cytoreductive Surgery With Hyperthermic Intraperitoneal Chemotherapy in Patients With Peritoneal Carcinomatosis. Clinical Colorectal Cancer 11:167-176
20. Verwaal VJ, Bruin S, Boot H et al (2008) 8-year follow-up of randomized trial: cytoreduction and hyperthermic intraperitoneal chemotherapy versus systemic chemotherapy in patients with peritoneal carcinomatosis of colorectal cancer. Ann Surg Oncol 15:2426-2432
21. Shih KK, Chi DS (2010) Maximal cytoreductive effort in epithelial ovarian cancer surgery. J Gynecol Oncol 21:75-80
22. Schorge JO, McCann C, Del Carmen MG (2010) Surgical debulking of ovarian cancer: what difference does it make? Rev Obstet Gynecol 3:111-117
23. Yonemura Y, Elnemr A, Endou Y et al (2010) Multidisciplinary therapy for treatment of patients with peritoneal carcinomatosis from gastric cancer. World J Gastrointest Oncol 2:8597
24. Jaehne J (2009) Cytoreductive procedures-strategies to reduce postoperative morbidity and

management of surgical complications with special emphasis on anastomotic leaks. J Surg Oncol 100:302-305
25. Webb CA, Weyker PD, Moitra VK, Raker RK (2013) An overview of cytoreductive surgery and hyperthermic intraperitoneal chemoperfusion for the anesthesiologist. Anesth Analg 116:924-931
26. Cancer Therapy Evaluation Program, Common Terminology Criteria for Adverse Events, Version 3.0, DCTD, NCI, NIH, DHHS; published date: August 9, 2006. http://ctep.cancer.gov.
27. Moran BJ (2006) Decision-making and technical factors account for the learning curve in complex surgey. J Public Health 28:375-378
28. Smeenk RM, Verwaal VJ, Zoetmulder FA (2007) Learnig curve of combined modality treatment in peritoneal surface disease. Br J Surg 94:1408-1414
29. Yan TD, Links M, Fransi S et al (2007) Learning curve for cytoreductive surgery and perioperative intraperitoneal chemotherapy for peritoneal surface malignancy–a journey to becoming a Nationally Funded Peritonectomy Center. Ann Surg Oncol 14:2270-2280
30. Coccolini F, Cotte E, Glehen O et al (2014) Intraperitoneal chemotherapy in advanced gastric cancer. Meta-analysis of randomized trials. Eur J Surg Oncol 40:12-26
31. Honoré C, Goéré D, Souadka A et al (2013) Definition of patients presenting a high risk of developing peritoneal carcinomatosis after curative surgery for colorectal cancer: a systematic review. Ann Surg Oncol 20:183-192
32. Sammartino P, Sibio S, Biacchi D et al (2014) Long-term results after proactive management for locoregional control in patients with colonic cancer at high risk of peritoneal metastases. Int J Colorectal Dis [Epub ahead of print] PMID 24980687
33. Ansaloni L, De Iaco P, Frigerio L (2012) Re: "cytoreductive surgery and hyperthermic intraperitoneal chemotherapy as upfront therapy for advanced epithelial ovarian cancer: multi-institutional phase II trial." - Proposal of a clinical trial of cytoreductive surgery and hyperthermic intraperitoneal chemotherapy in advanced ovarian cancer, the CHORINE study. Gynecol Oncol 125:279-281

The Role of Systemic Chemotherapy 12

Patrizia Trenta, Sara Giovannoni, Emanuela Risi,
and Enrico Cortesi

12.1 Introduction

Development of peritoneal carcinomatosis (PC) in metastatic solid tumors is associated with poor prognosis and is usually more frequent in gynecological and gastrointestinal (GI) malignancies. No standard systemic or local treatment can eradicate PC definitively, and chemotherapy (CHT) and surgery alone seem unable to improve patient survival, so that PC is usually considered a terminal condition [1]. PC is commonly observed in ovarian cancer (OC), in which the spread of disease is primarily locoregional and then to visceral sites. In this pathology, complete PC removal is associated with improved survival. In GI tumors, such as gastric and colorectal cancer (CRC), PC is seen less frequently, and its cytoreduction is not considered mandatory due to the high percentage of short-term recurrence and no effect on survival rates [2]. Systemic CHT has a limited impact on the peritoneum, probably because the peritoneal cavity is a "pharmacological sanctuary" in which intravenously administered drug diffusion is difficult. This is due to a blood–peritoneal barrier, composed of stromal tissues between mesothelial and endothelial cells, of ~90-μm thickness, which is difficult to overcome by many systemic agents [3]. Given this low effectiveness of systemic therapies or surgery alone and the necessity to improve the local action of drugs, in recent decades, new multimodal approaches have been developed based on the association of cytoreductive surgery (CRS) with intravenous (IV) (neoadjuvant or adjuvant) and/or intraperitoneal (IP) administration of CHT (IP-CHT). Different combinations and integrations of these treatments have been proposed and evaluated in randomized or nonrandomized tri-

P. Trenta (✉)
Department of Radiology, Oncology, and Human Pathology, Sapienza University
of Rome, Rome, Italy
e-mail: trentapatrizia@libero.it

A. Di Giorgio, E. Pinto (Eds), *Treatment of Peritoneal Surface Malignancies*,
Updates in Surgery
DOI: 10.1007/978-88-470-5711-1_12,

als in many cancer types.

IP-CHT enables delivery of high concentrations of drugs onto peritoneal masses, thus providing an expected higher percentage of volume reduction compared with IV treatments. Indeed, chemotherapeutic agents have a high molecular weight and are generally hydrophilic, so they easily remain in the peritoneal space for a considerable length of time. This advantage of IP-CHT is expressed by the area under the curve (AUC) ratios of IP versus plasma exposure: in particular, cisplatin, paclitaxel, docetaxel, gemcitabine, 5-fluorouracil, and doxorubicin can be the best candidates for IP-CHT because of their high AUC ratio [4]. The ability to penetrate deep into the peritoneal surface and the diffusion distance of each drug (up to 1–2 mm) are other important parameters to consider. Of course, the superiority of IP over IV delivery of chemotherapeutic agents is limited to patients with very little peritoneal-tumor residual volumes [5]. Moreover, IP-CHT has an optimal chance of succeeding if it immediately follows surgery, if exposure of the entire peritoneal surface at risk is guaranteed, and if IP hyperthermia is created. In fact, some drugs increase in activity when combined with mild hyperthermia, and temperatures of ~41–43°C are able alone to favor cell death until thermal tolerance develops due to activation of the heat-shock protein pathway [6, 7]. These concepts are at the basis of the combination between CRS and the hyperthermic intraperitoneal chemotherapy (HIPEC) technique, which shows good results in many cancer types. IP chemotherapy combined with heat penetrates up to 3–6 mm into PC nodules, so even HIPEC acts better on small peritoneal cancer volumes after optimal CRS.

In this chapter, we report data regarding the integration of systemic CHT with CRS and HIPEC, particularly in patients with PC from gynecological, GI, and peritoneal tumors.

12.2 Neoadjuvant and Adjuvant Systemic Chemotherapy, Cytoreductive Surgery, and HIPEC

The combination of CRS and HIPEC has shown improved survival rates and quality of life (QoL) over CHT alone for selected patients with PC [8]. The role of neoadjuvant and adjuvant CHT in managing patients with PC, both before and after CRS plus HIPEC, is not yet well recognized as a standard treatment due to the lack of significant clinical trials focused on evaluating whether adding systemic CHT to these locoregional treatments is effective. The potential advantages of IV-CHT prior to surgery plus HIPEC include a reduction of tumor volume with a greater chance of obtaining complete surgical removal and organ preservation with no macroscopic residual tumor. To quote Sugarbaker: "Advances in powerful chemotherapies and the use of neoadjuvant therapies are also contributing to the procedure's evolving effectiveness" [9]. It is therefore conceivable that CHT can contribute to making CRS more effective by shrinking tumors before surgery, thereby increasing the outcome of HIPEC treatment.

At the same time, neoadjuvant systemic CHT is useful in preventing extraperitoneal metastases and can favor prognosis and effectiveness of locoregional therapies. Chemotherapeutic agents used for PC before HIPEC vary depending primary on tumor type and extension. There is no standard duration for CHT before surgery: the number of therapy cycles depends on tumor type, initial tumor burden, and the patient's clinical condition [2, 10–12]. A multidisciplinary agreement is essential to identify the appropriate moment at which patients' benefit maximally from surgical and locoregional approaches. Few prospective and some retrospective data about neoadjuvant CHT before CRS plus HIPEC are at our disposal for many cancer types.

However, little information is available about the effectiveness of adjuvant CHT after CRS plus HIPEC. This is because the most PC trials have focused on demonstrating the superiority of HIPEC combined with CRS in comparison with surgery or CHT alone [8, 11]. We know that CHT is not sufficient for treating PC, independent of the primary tumor, but we still do not know whether managing peritoneal disease could be improved with adjuvant systemic treatments after CRS plus HIPEC. We must consider that, as we are dealing with the advanced stage of the illnesses, systemic treatment should be undertaken as well: HIPEC is an effective therapy for treating peritoneal but not systemic disease, whereas IV-CHT is able to prevent recurrence in other organs, which is critical for patient survival. In some trials on CRS plus HIPEC, some patients underwent adjuvant CHT, even if generally this was not well predefined in the study design and the effect of this systemic treatment was not well focused. Some other trials investigated the efficacy of adjuvant CHT after CRS; thus, no specific data regarding HIPEC are available. For these reasons, there are still no selection criteria to determine which patients with PC could benefit from adjuvant treatment after surgery plus HIPEC, regardless of the type of primary tumor. The oncologist's choice should be personalized case by case. Prospective and randomized trials are therefore needed to better establish the algorithm of integrated treatments (systemic and locoregional) for patients with PC in different cancer types. Probably, as indicated by Franko et al. in 2010, surgery plus HIPEC and systemic CHT should not be considered competitive but, rather, complementary techniques [13].

12.2.1 Ovarian Cancer

Epithelial OC is one of the main causes of death from gynecological tumors in the Western world. It represents 80– %90 % of all ovarian malignancies. The disease most often presents in advanced stage [Fédération Internationale de Gynécologie et Obstétrique (FIGO) stage III or IV], but dissemination is often confined to the peritoneal cavity [14]. Current standard treatment for patients with FIGO III or IV and predominant peritoneal disease consists of optimal CRS to residual nodules < 1 cm and systemic CHT with IV administration of paclitaxel and carboplatin. Six to eight cycles of this regimen are recommended for patients with stage III epithelial OC on the basis of two prospective randomized trials: the Gynecologic Oncology Group (GOG) 158 and AGO-OVAR 3 trials [15, 16]. Even with optimal CRS and the best systemic CHT, 60–70 % of patients experienced disease progression. Recurrent OC very often involves only the peritoneum and adjacent intra-abdominal organs. Systemic therapy could be ineffective for PC due to the blood–peritoneal barrier: even with high-dose CHT, the response rate does not exceed 22 %.

Peritoneal recurrence from OC is the preferred—probably more so than in other malignancies—context for locoregional treatments such as IP-CHT. IV/IP-CHT regimens were proven to increase survival rates for women with advanced OC in three phase III trials: GOG 104, GOG 114, and GOG 172 [17–19]. In the latter study, survival was increased from 49 months in the control arm (cisplatin/paclitaxel given IV) to 65 months in the experimental arm (cisplatin/paclitaxel given IP combined with paclitaxel given IV). A limitation of the study was the control arm, which today is not considered a standard: carboplatin/paclitaxel given IV would be the appropriate comparator. The survival advantage in GOG 172 came at the expense of increased toxicity, catheter-related complications, and reduced quality of life: patients in the IP group suffered more with fatigue, pain, hematologic, GI, and metabolic and neurologic toxic effects than the others [19]. This is why IV/IP-combined CHT regimen does not have a widespread consensus among oncologists. It could be useful to better select patients who benefit the most from IV/IP-CHT. This was the objective of an ancillary data analysis of GOG trials published by Landrum et al. The study indicates that young age at time of diagnosis, mucinous- or clear-cell histology, and minimal residual disease after CRS are independent predictors of good prognosis in stage III OC patients treated with IP-CHT [20].

PC from OC is also the most promising field of application of CRS plus HIPEC, having the advantage in terms of progression-free (PFS) and overall (OS) survival both in patients with PC at diagnosis and in those with a relapse after primary treatments [2, 10, 21–23]. The first report on HIPEC for OC was published in 1995 [24]. Since that time, there has been a large volume of studies evaluating this modality in conjunction with CRS. The published reports are mainly case series and early phase II studies. Patients are in variable stages of their disease, with HIPEC used as frontline, interval debulking, or adjuvant treatment in recurrent disease. The use of HIPEC as frontline therapy following CRS is presented in several studies, but the total number of patients is only around 50. Rufian at al. reported data of 19 patients treated at the time of first CRS with paclitaxel for 60 min at 41–43°C. Patients treated for primary OC with optimal cytoreduction obtained survival rates up to 63 % at 5 years (if negative lymph nodes) [25]. Similar results were demonstrated by Deraco et al. several years later in 26 patients [26]. In both series, patients underwent systemic CHT after HIPEC. Because of the small number of patients and the use of subsequent IV-CHT, these trials are not able to determine the advantage of using frontline

HIPEC after CRS compared with CRS followed by systemic CHT only.

In clinical practice, neoadjuvant systemic CHT in OC is considered, in case of nonoperable tumors, to favor debulking and complete cytoreduction: data about survival advantage are conflicting, and it seems that when radical surgery is performed, there are no differences between pre- and postoperative systemic therapy [27, 28]. There are, however, no definitive and prospective specific data focusing on the efficacy of neoadjuvant CHT before CRS plus HIPEC.

The first report of the HYPER-O registry showed no significant differences in survival between patients treated with CRS plus HIPEC versus CRS plus HIPEC following neoadjuvant systemic therapy [29]. Ryu et al. reported a retrospective observation of 57 patients who received HIPEC at the time of interval debulking or second-look surgery after IV-CHT and 60 patients receiving CHT and CRS only (conventional treatment). Considering stage III OC patients only, the survival rate was 53.8 % in the HIPEC group versus 33.3 % for conventional treatment ($p = 0.0015$). However, results of this trial did not focus on neoadjuvant CHT but on HIPEC efficacy, which was found to be an independent prognostic factor at multivariate analysis [hazard ratio (HR) 0.496, $p = 0.0176$)] [30]. At the time this chapter was written, there was an ongoing phase III trial randomizing patients with stage IIIC unresectable OC to receive CRS plus HIPEC (cisplatin plus paclitaxel) versus CRS alone after three cycles of first-line CHT (carboplatin/paclitaxel) [31].

Data regarding adjuvant systemic CHT after primary CRS plus HIPEC are even more fragmentary and certainly not exhaustive. In 2011, Fagotti et al. published the results of a study on OC that assessed 41 patients with platinum-sensitive recurrence. They were treated with CRS and platinum-based HIPEC, followed by six cycles of systemic CHT. The study concluded that CRS plus HIPEC safely increases survival rate in this setting compared with CHT or surgery alone, but the role of adjuvant treatment was not analyzed [32]. Carrabin et al. conducted a nonrandomized trial on 22 patients with advanced OC who underwent CRS plus HIPEC with no adjuvant CHT. The authors concluded that HIPEC with no other systemic therapy could be feasible and safe with encouraging survival results, even though randomized trials are needed to establish better this concept [33]. Of course, no definitive conclusion could be drawn from a nonrandomized trial with so few patients.

HIPEC is an interesting and promising treatment in recurrent OC at the time of secondary cytoreduction. A substantial number of studies reported good survival outcomes, especially for patients optimally treated with cytoreduction : Helm et al. registered a DFS of 10 months with an OS of 31 months and a perioperative mortality rate of 6 %; Cotte et al. described data on 81 patients achieving a DFS of 19 months, a median OS of 28 months, and an OS of up to 55 months in those with < 0.25 cm residual disease [34, 35]. Di Giorgio published data on 47 patients with advanced or recurrent (25) OC treated with CRS (peritonectomy) plus HIPEC plus systemic CHT in a phase II nonrandomized study: they achieved a median OS and DFS of 24 and 20 months, respectively, and a 5-

year survival rate of 17%. Patients treated with optimal cytoreduction had an OS of 26 months [23]. Bakrin et al. retrospectively selected 566 patients with PC from OC who were treated with CRS plus HIPEC. This combined treatment yielded a median OS of 45.7 months for recurrent OC [10]. Ansaloni et al. collected data from a prospective phase II trial assessing 39 patients with primary or recurrent peritoneal OC carcinomatosis receiving cytoreductive surgery plus HIPEC. Median DFS was 14 months; microscopically complete cytoreduction was achieved for 35 patients (90 %) [36].

Despite the lack of extensive evidence, CRS plus HIPEC is associated with increased survival chances with a manageable toxicity profile in patients with advanced or recurrent and prevalent peritoneal disease, in particular for patients with no macroscopic residual disease. Data are still heterogeneous, optimal CRS is not well defined, and randomized trials integrating systemic CHT in homogeneous populations are needed to better define timing and efficacy of this multimodal treatment.

12.2.2 Gastric Cancer

Peritoneal dissemination is the principal cause of death and most frequent (30 %) kind of recurrence in patients with gastric cancer (GC), and the probability of its appearance is higher when primary tumor invades serosa (30–60 %), even if it appears also in tumors not invading the gastric surface (5–11 %) [1, 37]. Medical and surgical treatments alone have only palliative effects. New multimodal and multidisciplinary strategies have been tested in an attempt to improve survival rates in these patients, even though there remains a lack of trials specifically assessing patients with PC.

IV-CHT alone has little effect on survival rates in patients with PC, even if it can reduce the peritoneal cancer burden in responders: its combination with CRS plus HIPEC seems to be more useful, especially when complete cytoreduction is obtained [38], but the role of neoadjuvant CHT before these procedures is yet to be well defined in large series, and actual clinical evidence is heterogeneous [2]. A phase II trial by Hultman et al. evaluated the feasibility and effectiveness of neoadjuvant CHT plus HIPEC in a study evaluating 18 patients; the authors concluded that preoperative therapy is not associated with prolonged OS in patients with extensive PC from GC over radical surgery alone. The authors did no recommend neoadjuvant treatment considering also the increased risk of postoperative complications [39]. Costa et al. published data on ten patients treated with three cycles of neoadjuvant docetaxel, 5-Fluorouracil (5-FU), plus cisplatin (DCF) therapy followed by gastric resection with D2 lymphadenectomy plus HIPEC with mitomycin and by adjuvant systemic CHT (three cycles) with the same regimen. No data on survival are available due to the short follow-up, but the conclusion of the authors emphasized the feasibility of the association between perioperative CHT, gastric resection, and D2 lymphadenectomy plus HIPEC [40]. The role of neoadjuvant CHT with 5-FU, oxaliplatin, and docetaxel (FLOT) followed by surgery plus HIPEC; adjuvant systemic treatment was tested in 26 patients with PC from GC. Median OS was 19 months, with 38 % of patients alive at 2 years. Regression analysis showed that a Peritoneal Cancer Index (PCI) > 12 was a negative prognostic factor. The authors concluded that neoadjuvant CHT with FLOT followed by surgery plus HIPEC increases OS of patients with PC from GC, but this treatment seems not to be recommended in cases of extensive peritoneal involvement and a PCI > 12 [41].

Yonemura et al. proposed a new type of neoadjuvant multimodal treatment for PC in GC called neoadjuvant intraperitoneal and systemic (NIPS) therapy. This bidirectional CHT acts on PC from both sides of the peritoneum—from the peritoneal cavity and from blood vessels— before CRS. A total of 96 GC patients with PC and no other sites of disease were treated with both systemic and IP-CHT administered through a peritoneal port system (BARD). Patients received TS-1 (composed of tegafur, gimestat, and otostat potassium) orally twice daily for 21 of 28 days; on days 1, 8, and 15, they received 30 mg/mq of docetaxel and 30 mg/mq of cisplatin were introduced through the peritoneal port. A laparotomy was then performed in 82 patients without disease progression at the end of the combined treatment. Total gastrectomy was performed in 67 patients, and 33 underwent visceral peritonectomy: 70.7 % (58) achieved complete cytoreduction. Patients who underwent CRS lived longer than those who did not (14.4 versus 9 months, $p = 0.032$), as did patients who obtained complete cytoreduction (CC 0) versus patients who did not (CC 1–3) (21.1 vs. 8.4 months, $p < 0.001$). In that study, 2.1 % and 1 % of patients with grades 3 and 4 toxicities, respectively, were registered; overall operative mortality rate related to multiple organ failure, hepatic coma, or sepsis was 3.7 % (3/82) [42]. NIPS and minimal residual PC after surgery were evaluated as good independent prognostic factors for GC patients treated with CRS plus HIPEC [43]. Given the efficacy of this multimodal strategy, better patient selection (i.e., patients who could truly benefit) and improved surgeon expertise to avoid toxicities is necessary.

The role of adjuvant systemic CHT after CRS plus HIPEC has not been evaluated in clinical trials; however, early postoperative intraperitoneal chemotherapy (EPIC) may be another option for GC patients undergoing CRS for PC. This protocol should be started early after surgery, when tumor burden is minimal. The greatest clinical experience was reported for 248 patients randomized to receive surgery alone, or surgery and then a combination of IP-delivered mitomycin C and 5-FU. The latter group had a better OS, which was statistically significant for patients with gross serosal invasion and lymph node metastasis. The authors concluded that EPIC should be recommended for treating patients with stage 3 or 4 advanced GC and T3 or N+ [44]. A systematic review of randomized controlled trials showed that a significant improvement in survival rates after CRS was associated with HIPEC alone (HR = 0.60; 95 % CI = 0.43–0.83; $p = 0.002$) or HIPEC combined with EPIC (HR = 0.45; 95 % CI = 0.29–0.68; $p = 0.0002$), even though IP-CHT was also found to be associated with higher risk of intra-abdominal abscess [relative risk (RR) = 2.37; 95 % CI = 1.32–4.26; p = 0.003) and neutropenia (RR = 4.33; 95 % CI = 1.49–12.61; p = 0.007) [45].

In GC, HIPEC has even been tested for preventing PC: 82 patients with gross serosal invasion but without peritoneal metastases were randomized to receive surgery plus mitomycin-C-based HIPEC or surgery alone. The 5-year OS rate for the first group was 64.2 % versus 52.5 % for the control arm, but this difference was not statistically significant. There was a trend toward lower mortality rates for PC in patients treated with HIPEC (p = 0.0854), whereas peritoneal recurrence was more frequent in the surgery-alone group [46]. Yonemura et al. randomized 139 patients with GC to receive surgery alone (47) or surgery plus HIPEC with mitomycin and cisplatin (48) or surgery plus IP-delivered perfusion (44) with the same drugs. Five-year OS rates were 42 %, 61 %, and 43 %, respectively; patients with nodal or serosal invasion showed a statistically significant improvement in OS when treated with HIPEC, whereas IP-delivered perfusion provided no survival benefit. HIPEC was an independent positive prognostic factor, so its use seems to be advisable for patients with high-risk resectable GC [47].

Further prospective data are required to establish more definitively the efficacy of IV and IP treatments in patients with PC and GC, to test new combinations of cytotoxic drugs and/or biological agents, and to better define patient selection and optimal timing for multimodal treatments.

12.2.3 Colorectal Cancer

PC is a frequent site of progression in patients with CRC. Abdominal failure is very frequent, in particular when bowel-wall penetration increases; peritoneal seeding occurs in up to 30 % of patients with CRC and is the second highest cause of death after liver metastases [48]. Because of its poor prognosis, PC in CRC is considered a terminal condition in which surgery and CHT alone are palliative only because they cannot completely eradicate peritoneal disease.

Over the past two decades, new and alternative therapeutic approaches have developed based on the combination of different strategies, such as surgery, CHT, and IP-delivered treatments, thus improving chances of survival for selected patients with PC and CRC; even curative aims can sometimes be achieved. Some clinical trials compared the efficacy of CHT versus CRS plus HIPEC in patients with PC and CRC. Verwaal et al. randomized 105 patients to receive systemic CHT with 5-FU with or without surgery (standard arm) or aggressive CRC plus HIPEC followed by systemic therapy (experimental arm). Median survival rate of patients in the first group was 12.6 months versus 22.4 months for those who received the more aggressive treatment (p = 0.032). The mortality rate in the HIPEC group was 8 % (four patients); extent of peritoneal involvement and number of peritoneal regions involved during CRS were prognostic factors. The efficacy of cytoreduction was also important, because patients with no residual macroscopic disease had better prognosis than those with greater residual peritoneal involvement ($p < 0.0001$). Despite these significant results, it must be recognized that this trial had some limitations, such as the fact that the chemotherapeutic regime used is not an actual gold standard for treating advanced CRC (not including irinotecan and oxaliplatin or biologic agents), the HIPEC protocol was based only on mitomycin C perfusion, and the role of surgery in the control arm was unclear [49].

Other prospective randomized trials comparing the same regimen were closed due to lack of accrual and survival advantage in the HIPEC arm, so it remains difficult to draw conclusions or to report a good level of evidence regarding the usefulness of this treatment for patients with CRC [50, 51].

Some retrospective or case–control series reported good results. In 2010, Elias et al. described the outcome of 523 patients with CRC and PC treated with CRS and IP-CHT with or without hyperthermia. OS time was 30.1 months, 5-year survival rate was 27 %, and 5-year DFS rate was 10 %; patients in whom complete cytoreduction was obtained (84 %) had a median survival rate of 33 months. Postoperative mortality rate was 3 %, and grade 3–4 early morbidities occurred in 31 % of patients. Positive independent prognostic factors in multivariate analysis were complete CRS, limited PC, use of adjuvant CHT, and absence of nodal involvement; disease grade or liver metastases were not prognostic [52]. A retrospective comparison between palliative CHT (based on 5-FU, oxaliplatin, and irinotecan) and CRS plus HIPEC was published by Elias et al. in 2009. Median survival was 23.9 months in the standard group versus 62.7 months in the HIPEC group ($p < 0.05$); 5-year OS rate was 51 % for the HIPEC group and 13 % for the standard group [53]. Chua et al. retrospectively evaluated the outcome of 294 patients with PC treated with supportive care or palliative CHT versus perioperative CHT (with both modern chemotherapeutic agents and biological drugs), associated or not with HIPEC (with mitomycin C) and EPIC, comparing a palliative versus a curative approach. The results showed that curative strategy is able to grant a total median survival of 38 months (95 % CI 30.2–45.2) versus 9 months of the palliative strategy (95 % CI 5.9–12.8) ($p < 0.001$) and confirmed that limited peritoneal involvement is a good prognostic factor for patients receiving multimodal and more aggressive treatment ($p = 0.002$) [54]. All these data suggest that an optimal CRS associated with HIPEC may play an important role in managing patients with PC from CRC, especially in well-selected patients (according to lymph node involvement, comorbidities, performance status, age, complete cytoreduction, and PCI value) [55].

The role of neoadjuvant CHT before CRS plus HIPEC is still not well defined due to the lack of targeted trials. A study published by Rivard et al. who assessed 68 patients with PC from CRC showed no advantage in terms of OS between patients treated with preoperative CHT followed by surgery plus HIPEC and patients who received no neoadjuvant treatment [56]. Several trials included target therapies before CRS plus HIPEC but were inconclusive in evaluating its usefulness as neoadjuvant therapy. Eveno et al. randomized 182 patients to receive CHT with or without bevacizumab followed by surgery plus HIPEC. Patients treated with bevacizumab showed a significant increase in postoperative complications (doubled risk of morbidity), including death ($p = 0.04$), whereas the clinical benefit of bevacizumab before HIPEC remains to be determined [12].

An ongoing (at the time of this writing) phase II German study by Glockzin et al. was designed to determine whether systemic neoadjuvant CHT with cetuximab [monoclonal anti-epithelial-growth-factor-receptor (anti-EGFR) antibody)] followed by cytoreductive surgery plus HIPEC with oxaliplatin would be effective in patients with PC from colorectal KRAS wild-type tumor [57]. No specific data are available regarding adjuvant IV-CHT after CRS plus HIPEC in patients with PC from CRC. The lack of valid confirmation regarding the efficacy of CRS plus HIPEC, of a clear algorithm for patient selection (before and after surgery), and of integration of systemic treatments still makes CRS and IP-administered treatments a nonstandard approach for PC in CRC. Prospective clinical trials are awaited.

12.2.4 Peritoneal Mesothelioma and Pseudomyxoma Peritonei

12.2.4.1 Peritoneal Mesothelioma

Malignant mesothelioma is an aggressive primary neoplasm arising from pleural, peritoneal, pericardiac, or tunica vaginalis lining. Diffuse malignant peritoneal mesothelioma (DMPM) is a very rare disease, often associated with asbestos exposure and macroscopically characterized by multiple tumor nodules, which may coalesce to form plaques or masses extending to the entire peritoneal surface.

The first case of DMPM was described by Miller et al. in 1908; nevertheless, few therapeutic advances have occurred in the last century mainly because of the rarity of the disease and the subsequent difficulty recruiting patients for randomized trials with endpoints of safety and efficacy [58]. Historically, DMPM was treated with systemic CHT, palliative surgery, and abdominal radiotherapy. Patient prognosis was poor: median survival was only 12 months [59, 60]. In the early 2000s, the combination of CRS plus HIPEC was proposed for DMPM. The rationale for this treatment was the prevalent abdominal localization of DMPM and the inefficacy of CRS alone, especially in the presence of diffusion on the intestinal surface.

Several observational studies report on CRS plus HIPEC, but no randomized controlled or comparative trials exist. In 2007, Yan et al. published a systematic review of seven observational studies. The objective of their review was to evaluate the efficacy of CRS with perioperative IP-CHT for treating DMPM. The IP regimen comprised HIPEC and/or EPIC; 240 patients were evaluated. Median survival ranged from 34 to 92 months and the 3-year survival rate from 65 % to 43 %. Two studies also reported the 7-year survival rate:

39 % and 33 %. Perioperative morbidity varied from 25 % to 40 %, and mortality rate was < 8 % [61].

In 2009, a multi-institutional retrospective review was published assessing 405 patients affected by DMPM and treated with CRS plus HIPEC. The most common HIPEC regimen was cisplatin/doxorubicin. Overall median survival was 53 months, the 3-year survival rate was 60 %, and the 5-year survival rate was 47 %. In the study four independent prognostic factors associated with a good prognosis were identified: epithelial subtype, absence of lymph node metastasis, optimal cytoreduction, plus HIPEC administration [62].

The efficacy of neoadjuvant CHT before surgery plus HIPEC was evaluated in a retrospective study published by Deraco et al. The effects of perioperative systemic therapy on short-term surgical and long-term oncological results in patients with malignant peritoneal mesothelioma were evaluated. Of 116 patients, 60 received neoadjuvant treatment (platinum plus pemetrexed), 30 received adjuvant CHT, and 26 received no chemotherapeutic treatment. No differences in OS, morbidity, and completeness of cytoreduction were detected [63]. The rarity of DMPM is the main impediment to the feasibility of conducting a randomized clinical trial. Nevertheless, the combination of CRS plus HIPEC provides a benefit in terms of survival, passing—on average—from 12 to 60 months, with acceptable toxicity. This makes CRS plus HIPEC the treatment of choice in selected patients with peritoneal mesothelioma.

12.2.4.2 Pseudomyxoma Peritonei

Pseudomyxoma peritonei (PMP) is a rare disease affecting the abdominal cavity, with an incidence of two to three cases per million per year, which generally originates from an appendiceal neoplasm. The condition, characterized by mucinous ascites and multifocal peritoneal epithelial implants, is called PMP syndrome [64]. PMP tends to remain confined within the peritoneal cavity, so therapy mainly consists of regional treatments: traditional debulking procedures are associated with a 5-year survival rate between 53 % and 75 % and a 10 year DFS rate of 3–4 % [65].

The introduction of CRS combined with HIPEC changed the history of PMP. There are no randomized controlled trials or comparative studies to demonstrate the efficacy of this treatment; however, CRS plus HIPEC is considered the best option for treating this disease. In 2007, Yan TD et al. published a systematic review regarding the efficacy of CRS and perioperative IP-CHT. Ten observational studies were reviewed for a total of 863 patients with PMP. IP regimens included HIPEC and/or EPIC, and median survival ranged from 51 to 156 months. The 5-year survival rate was 52–96 %, and overall morbidity and mortality were 33–56 % and 0–18 %, respectively [66]. An important consideration coming from this analysis is that optimal CRS (residual peritoneal nodules < 2.5 mm after CRS) is primarily responsible for improved survival rates. The study by Deraco et al., included in the systematic review, reported a surprising 10-year survival rate of 78.9 % for patients affected by PMP who were treated with optimal CRS; however, for patients receiving incomplete cytoreduction, the 10-year survival rate was zero [67]. In 2012, Chua et al. published the results of a retrospective multicenter registry that involved 2,998 patients, all of whom underwent CRS, which was combined with HIPEC in 89 % of the overall population. Median survival rate was 16.3 years and median PFS was 8.2 years. Overall 5- and 10-year survival rates were 74 % and 59 %, respectively. HIPEC was associated with an improved PFS, and mortality and morbidity rates were 2 % and 24 %, respectively [68].

In conclusion, considering these good results, improved survival rates, and low morbility and mortality rates, CRS plus HIPEC can be considered the standard of care for PMP. An accurate preoperative understanding of each patient and the disease, and the experience of the unit personnel, may predict and influence outcomes.

12.3 Conclusions

Systemic treatment alone may be no longer appropriate for patients with PC and no other sites of disease because of its low impact on the peritoneum and survival rates. IP therapies, in particular, HIPEC, associated with good CRS, shows promising results and the ability to control successfully PC, even though the impact on patient prognosis is not always clear, probably due to extraperitoneal recurrence. Given the limits of both IV-administered drugs and locoregional approaches when used alone, their integration could be the right solution for combining local control granted by surgery and IP treatments, with the systemic protection of chemotherapeutic agents.

Determining the best way to maximize the efficacy of both systemic and local treatments by combining them in a multidisciplinary therapy algorithm in which the right method is used at the right time for the right patient. Given the complexity of conducting dedicated studies on PC, especially for rare cancers, an effort is necessary to create prospective trials that definitively answer open questions and improve collaboration among different institutions regarding patient enrollment. Creating specialized centers for patients with PC from different cancer types could improve the performance of surgeons and oncologists alike in treating this condition and could help reduce the heterogeneity of clinical results that makes it difficult to understand the precise efficacy of locoregional and systemic treatments.

Overcoming actual limits and improving patient outcomes requires a great effort toward a multidisciplinary approach. Better knowledge of peritoneal dissemination biology is desirable.

References

1. Chu DZ, Lang NP, Thompson C et al (1989) Peritoneal carcinomatosis in nongynecologic malignancy. A prospective study of prognostic factors. Cancer 63:364-367
2. Coccolini F, Gheza F, Lotti M et al (2013) Peritoneal carcinomatosis. World J Gastroenterol 19:6979–6994
3. Jacquet PH, Sugarbaker PH (1996) Peritoneal-plasma barrier. In: Sugarbaker PH, editor. Peritoneal Carcinomatosis: Principles of Management. Boston: Kluwer Academic Publisher, pp 53-63
4. Sugarbaker PH, Mora JT, Carmignani P et al (2005) Update on chemotherapeutic agents utilized for perioperative intraperitoneal chemotherapy. Oncologist 10:112-122
5. Los G, Mutsaers PH, van der Vijgh WJ et al (1989) Direct diffusion of cis-diamminedichloroplatinum(II) in intraperitoneal rat tumors after intraperitoneal chemotherapy: a comparison with systemic chemotherapy. Cancer Res 49:3380-3384
6. Sticca RP, Dach BW (2003) Rationale for hyperthermia with intraoperative intraperitoneal chemotherapy agents. Surg Oncol Clin N Am 12:689-701
7. Mohamed F, Marchettini P, Stuart OA et al (2003) Thermal enhancement of new chemotherapeutic agents at moderate hyperthermia. Ann Surg Oncol 10:463-468
8. Roviello F, Caruso S, Marrelli D et al (2011) Treatment of peritoneal carcinomatosis with cytoreductive surgery and hyperthermic intraperitoneal chemotherapy. G Chir 32:211-233
9. http://medstarhealthphysicians.org/body.cfm?id=559148
10. Bakrin N, Bereder JM, Decullier E et al (2013) Peritoneal carcinomatosis treated with cytoreductive surgery and Hyperthermic Intraperitoneal Chemotherapy (HIPEC) for advanced ovarian carcinoma: a French multicentre retrospective cohort study of 566 patients. Eur J Surg Oncol 9:1435-1443
11 Gervais MK, Dubè P, McConnell Y et al (2013) Cytoreductive surgery plus hyperthermic intraperitoneal chemotherapy with oxaliplatin for peritoneal carcinomatosis arising from colorectal cancer.J Surg Oncol 108:438-443
12. Eveno C, Passot G, Goéré D et al (2013) Bevacizumab Doubles the Early Postoperative Complication Rate after Cytoreductive Surgery with Hyperthermic Intraperitoneal Chemotherapy (HIPEC) for Peritoneal Carcinomatosis of Colorectal Origin. Ann Surg Oncol [Epub ahead of print]
13. Franko J, Ibrahim Z, Gusani NJ et al (2010) Cytoreductive surgery and hyperthermic intraperitoneal chemoperfusion versus systemic chemotherapy alone for colorectal peritoneal carcinomatosis. Cancer 116:3756-3762
14. Randall TC, Rubin SC (2001) Cytoreductive surgery for ovarian cancer. Surg Clin North Am 81:871–883
15. Ozols RF, Bundy BN, Greer BE et al (2003) Phase III trial of carboplatin and paclitaxel compared with cisplatin and paclitaxel in patients with optimally resected stage III ovarian cancer: a Gynecologic Oncology Group study. J Clin Oncol 21:3194–200
16. Du Bois A, Lück H-J, Meier W et al (2003) A randomized clinical trial of cisplatin/paclitaxel versus carboplatin/ paclitaxel as first-line treatment of ovarian cancer. J Natl Cancer Inst 95:1320–1330
17. Alberts DS, Liu DY, Hannigan EV et al (1996) Intraperitoneal cisplatin plus intravenous cyclophosphamide versus intravenous cisplatin plus intravenous cyclophosphamide for stage III ovarian cancer. New Engl J Med 335:1950-1955
18. Markman M, Bundi BM, Alberts DS et al (2001) Phase III trial of standard-dose intravenous cisplatin plus paclitaxel versus moderately high-dose carboplatin followed by intravenous paclitaxel and intraperitoneal cisplatin in small-volume stage III ovarian carcinoma: an intergroup study of the Gynecologic Oncology Group, Southwestern Oncology Group, and Eastern Cooperative Oncology Group. J Clin Oncol 19:1001-1007
19. Armstrong DK, Bundy B, Wenzel L et al (2006) Intraperitoneal cisplatin and paclitaxel in ovarian cancer. N Engl J Med 354:34–43

20. Landrum LM, Java J, Mathews CA et al (2013) Prognostic factors for stage III epithelial ovarian cancer treated with intraperitoneal chemotherapy: A Gynecologic Oncology Group study. Gynecol Oncol 130:12-18
21. Gonzalez Bayon L, Steiner MA, Vasquez Jimenez W et al (2013) Cytoreductive surgery and hyperthermic intraperitoneal chemotherapy for the treatment of advances epitheliasl ovarian carcinoma: upfront therapy, at first recurrence or later? Eur J Surg Oncol 39:1109-1115
22. Chan DL, Morris DL, Rao A, Chua TC (2012) Intraperitoneal chemotherapy in ovarian cancer: a review of tolerance and efficacy. Cancer Manag Res 4:413-422
23. Di Giorgio A, Naticchioni E, Biacchi D et al (2008) Cytoreductive surgery (peritonectomy procedures) combined with hyperthermic intraperitoneal chemotherapy (HIPEC) in the treatment of diffuse peritoneal carcinomatosis from ovarian cancer. Cancer 113:315–325
24. Loggie BW, SterchiJM, Rogersetal AT (1995) Intraperitoneal hyperthermic chemotherapy for advanced gastrointestinal and ovarian cancers. Regional Cancer Treatment 7:78–81
25. Rufian S, Munoz-Casares FC, Briceno J et al (2006) Radical surgery—peritonectomy and intra-operative intra- peritoneal chemotherapy for the treatment of peritoneal carcinomatosis in recurrent or primary ovarian cancer. Journal of Surgical Oncology 94:316–324
26. Deraco M, Kusomura S, Virzi S et al (2011) Cytoreductive surgery and hyperthermic intraperitoneal chemotherapy as up front therapy for advanced. EOC: multi-institutional phase II study. Gynecologic Oncology 122:215–220
27. Ma DY, Tan BX, Li XF et al (2013) A meta-analysis: neoadjuvant chemotherapy versus primary surgery in ovarianc cancer FIGO stage III and IV . World J Surg Oncol 11:267-271
28. Sehouli J, Sawatis K, Braicu EI et al (2010) Primary versus interval debulking surgery in advanced ovarian cancer: results from a systemic single-center analysis. Int J Gynecol Cancer 20:1331-1340
29. Helm CW, Richard SD, Pan J et al (2010) HIPEC in ovarian cancer: first report of HYPER-O registry. International Journal of Gynecological Cancer 20:61–69
30. Ryu KS, Kim JH, Ko HS et al (2004) Effects of intraperitoneal hyperthermic chemotherapy in ovarian cancer. Gynecol Oncol 94:325–332
31. http://clinicaltrials.gov/ct2/results?term=NCT01628380&Search=SearchNCT01628380
32. Fagotti A, Costantini B, Vizzielli G et al (2011) HIPEC in recurrent ovarian cancer patients: morbidity-related treatment and long-term analysis of clinical outcome. Gynecol Oncol 122:221–225
33. Carrabin N, Mithieux, Meeus P et al (2010) Hyperthermic intraperitoneal chemotherapy with oxaliplatin and without adjuvant chemotherapy in stage IIIC ovarian cancer. Bull. Du Cancer 97:E23-32
34. Helm CW, Randall-Whitis L, Martin RS et al (2007) Hyperthermic intraperitoneal chemotherapy in conjunction with surgery for the treatment of recurrent ovarian carcinoma. Gynecol Oncol 105:90–96
35. Cotte E, Glehen O, Mohamed F et al (2007) Cytoreductive surgery and intraperitoneal chemohyperthermia for chemo-resistant and recurrent advanced epithelial ovarian cancer: prospective study of 81 patients. World J Surg. 31:1813–1820
36. Ansaloni L, Agnoletti V, Amadori A et al (2012) Evaluation of extensive cytoreductive surgery and hyperthermic intraperitoneal chemotherapy (HIPEC) in patients with advanced epithelial ovarian cancer. J Gynecol Cancer 22:778-785
37. Roviello F, Marrelli D, de Manzoni G et al (2003) Prospective study of peritoneal recurrence after curative surgery for gastric cancer. Br J Surg 90:1113–1119
38. Sugarbaker PH, Yonemura Y (2000) Clinical pathway for the management of resectable gastric cancer with peritoneal seeding: Best palliation with a ray of hope of cure. Oncology 58:96–107
39. Hultman B, Lind P, Glimelius B et al (2013) Phase II study of patients with peritoneal carcinomatosis from gastric cancer treated with preoperative systemic chemotherapy followed by peritonectomy and intraperitoneal chemotherapy. Acta Oncol 52:824-830
40. Costa WL, Coimbra FJ, Ribeiro FS et al (2012) Safety and preliminary results of periopera-

tive chemotherapy and hyperthermic intraperitoneal chemotherapy (HIPEC) for high-risk gastric cancer patients. World J Surg Oncol 10:195
41. Müller H, Hotopp TH, Tofeili A, Wutke K Systemic chemotherapy using FLOT - regimen combined with cytoreductive surgery plus hipec for treatment of peritoneal metastasized gastric cancer.
http://www.onkochirurgie.de/content/public/local/systemic_chemotherapy_using_flot.html
42. Yonemura Y, Elnemr A, Endou Y et al (2012) Effects of neoadjuvant intraperitoneal/systemic chemotherapy (bidirectional chemotherapy) for the treatment of patients with peritoneal metastasis from gastric cancer. Int J Surg Oncol 2012:148420
43. Yonemura Y, Elnemr A, Endou Y et al (2010) Multidisciplinary therapy for treatment of patients with peritoneal carcinomatosis from gastric cancer. World J Gastrointest Oncol 2:85-97
44. Yu W, Whang I, Chung HY et al (2001) Indications for earl postoperative intraperitoneal chemotherapy of advanced gastric cancer: results of a prospective randomized trial. World J Surg 25:985-990
45. Yan TD, Black D, Sugarbaker PH et al (2007) A systematic review and metaanalysis of the randomized controlled trials on adjuvant intraperitoneal chemotherapy for resectable gastric cancer. Ann Surg Oncol 14:2702-2713
46. Hamazoe R, Maeta M, Kaibara N (1994) Intraperitoneal thermochemotherapy for prevention of peritoneal recurrence of gastric cancer. Final results of a randomized controlled study. Cancer 73:2048-2052
47. Yonemura Y, de Aretxabala X, Fujimura T et al (2001) Intraoperative chemohyperthermic peritoneal perfusion as an adjuvant to gastric cancer: final results of a randomized controlled study. Hepatogastroenterology 48:1776-1782
48. Minsky BD, Mies C, Rich TA et al (1988) Potentially curative surgery of colon cancer: Patterns of failure and survival. J Clin Oncol 6:106-118
49. Verwaal VJ, van Ruth S, de Bree E et al (2003) Randomized trial of cytoreduction and hyperthermic intraperitoneal chemotherapy versus systemic chemotherapy and palliative surgery in patients with peritoneal carcinomatosis of colorectal cancer. J Clin Oncol 21:3737–3743
50. Elias D, Delperro JR, Sideris L et al (2004) Treatment of peritoneal carcinomatosis from colorectal cancer: impact of complete cytoreductive surgery and difficulties in conducting randomized trials. Ann Surg Oncol 11:518–521
51. Avital I, Brucher BL, Nissan A, Stojadinovic A (2012) Randomized clinical trials for colorectal cancer Peritoneal carcinomatosis and peritoneal surface malignancy. Surg Oncol Clin N Am 21:665–688
52. Elias D, Gilly F, Boutitie F et al (2010) Peritoneal colorectal carcinomatosis treated with surgery and perioperative intraperitoneal chemotherapy: retrospective analysis of 523 patients from a multicentric French study. J Clin Oncol 28:63–68
53. Elias D, Lefevre JH, Chevalier J et al (2009) Complete cytoreductive surgery plus intraperitoneal chemohyperthermia with oxaliplatin for peritoneal carcinomatosis of colorectal origin. J Clin Oncol 27:681-685
54. Chua TC, Morris DL, Saxena A et al (2011) Influence of modern systemic therapies as adjunct to cytoreduction and perioperative intraperitoneal chemotherapy for patients with colorectal peritoneal carcinomatosis: a multicenter study. Ann Surg Oncol 18:1560–1567
55. Riss S, Mohamed S, Dayal S et al (2013) Peritoneal metastases from colorectal cancer : patient selection for cytoreductive surgery and hyperthermic intraperitoneal chemotherapy. Eur J Surg Oncol 39:931-937
56. Rivard JD, McConnell YJ, Temple WJ, Mack LA (2014) Cytoreduction and heated intraperitoneal chemotherapy for colorectal cancer: Are we excluding patients who may benefit? J Surg Oncol 109:104-109
57. Glockzin G, Rochon J, Arnold D et al (2013) A prospective multicenter phase II study evaluating multimodality treatment of patients with peritoneal carcinomatosis arising from appendiceal and colorectal cancer: the COMBATAC trial. BMC Cancer 13:67
58. Miller J, Wynn H (1908) A malignant tumor arising from the endothelium of the peritoneum and producing a mucoid ascitic fluid. J Pathol Bacteriol 12:267

59. Chailleux E, Dabouis G, Pioche D et al (1988) Prognostic factors in diffuse malignant pleural mesothelioma. A study of 167 patients. Chest 93:159–162
60. Eltabbakh GH, Piver MS, Hempling RE et al (1999) Clinical picture, response to therapy,and survival of women with diffuse malignant peritoneal mesothelioma. J Surg Oncol 70:6–12
61. Yan TD, Welch L, Black D et al (2007) A systematic review on the efficacy of cytoreductive surgery combined with perioperative intraperitoneal chemotherapy for diffuse malignancy peritoneal mesothelioma. Ann Oncol 18:827–834
62. Yan TD, Deraco M, Baratti D (2009) Cytoreductive surgery and hyperthermic intra- peritoneal chemotherapy for malignant peritoneal mesothelioma: multi- institutional experience. J Clin Oncol 27:6237e42
63. Deraco M, Baratti D, Hatanu I et al (2013) The role of perioperative systemic chemotherapy in diffuse malignant peritoneal mesothelioma patients treated with cytoreductive surgery and hyperthermic intraperitoneal chemotherapy. Ann Surg Oncol 20:1093-1100
64. Smeenk RM, van Velthuysen ML, Verwaal VJ et al (2008) Appendiceal neo- plasms and pseudomyxoma peritonei: a population based study. Eur J Surg Oncol 34:196–201
65. Gough DB, Donohue JH, Schutt AJ et al (1994) Pseudomyxoma peritonei: long-term patient survival with an aggressive regional approach. Ann Surg 219:112e9.
66. Yan TD, Black D, Savady R et al (2007) A sistematic review on the efficacy of cytoreductive surgery and perioperative intraperitoneal chemotherapy for pseudomyxoma peritonei. Ann Surg Oncol 14:484-492
67. Deraco M1, Kusamura S, Laterza B et al (2006) Cytoreductive surgery and hyperthermic intra-peritoneal chemotherapy (HIPEC) in the treatment of pseudomyxoma peritonei: ten years experience in a single center. In Vivo 20:773-776
68. Chua TC, Moran BJ, Sugarbaker PH (2012) Early- and long-term outcome data of patients with pseudomyxoma peritonei from appendiceal origin treated by a strategy of cytoreductive surgery and hyper- thermic intraperitoneal chemotherapy. J Clin Oncol 30:2449-2456

Patient Selection for Treatment

13

Paolo Sammartino, Fabio Accarpio, Bianca Maria Sollazzo, Alessio Impagnatiello, Tommaso Cornali, and Daniele Biacchi

13.1 Introduction

Appropriate patient selection is of primary importance to successful cytoreductive surgery (CRS) plus hyperthermic intraperitoneal chemotherapy (HIPEC). Given the high morbidity rate associated with these combined procedures, we need to select patients who will derive maximum benefits from treatment and who carry lower risks of postoperative complications and mortality. The high morbidity and mortality rates, especially in treatment groups approaching this type of surgery for the first time, have raised concern and often criticism [1, 2]. At the same time, besides problems linked to postoperative complications, criteria for selecting patients to undergo integrated treatment must take into account preoperative factors predicting a favorable oncologic outcome. Hence, we need to know which tumors causing peritoneal spread this combined treatments should target and to define the extent of peritoneal spread to use as a cut-off beyond which these procedures are contraindicated. To rationalize this topic, even though schematizing has its limitations, we divided selection criteria according to whether they most directly address patients' characteristics, the site and histology underlying peritoneal spread, and the extent of peritoneal and extraperitoneal malignant spread.

13.2 Patient Selection

Given that CRS plus HIPEC is an aggressive method for managing peritoneal

P. Sammartino (✉)
Department of Surgery "Pietro Valdoni", Sapienza University of Rome, Rome, Italy
e-mail: paolo.sammartino@uniroma1.it

A. Di Giorgio, E. Pinto (Eds), *Treatment of Peritoneal Surface Malignancies*, Updates in Surgery
DOI: 10.1007/978-88-470-5711-1_13, © Springer-Verlag Italia 2015

surface malignancy (PSM), with an operation lasting ≥ 6–10 h, patients' general condition plays a crucial role, reflecting possible intraoperative and postoperative complications. The presence of associated disease (cardiovascular, renal, pulmonary comorbidity) will influence decision making and, if malfunction cannot be corrected, CRS plus HIPEC may be contraindicated. The performance status can be quantified using various scoring systems. The most commonly used are the Eastern Cooperative Oncology Group Performance Status (ECOG PS) and the Karnofsky Index. In a series of patients who underwent CRS plus HIPEC for colonic adenocarcinoma or pseudomyxoma peritonei (PMP), Reuter et al. show that patients with ECOG PS ≥ 2 had a higher complication rate than those with ECOG PS of 0 or 1 (89 % vs. 26 % [3]. In a report by Shen et al., preoperative ECOG PS correlated significantly with survival [4], but in other series [3]—even though patients with lower ECOG PS tended to have better survival—the difference failed to reach statistical significance. Subsequent reports confirmed ECOG PS as among the independent variables predicting major morbidity and overall survival (OS) [5, 6].

Most prospective clinical trials in cancer either underrepresented or excluded elderly patients, a population at increased risk for postoperative morbidity [7, 8]. These data notwithstanding, age cannot be considered an absolute contraindication for CRS plus HIPEC. Nevertheless this combined treatment modality should be offered only to a subset of elderly patients and only after stringent patient selection based on type of primary tumor, possibility of achieving complete CRS, and patient nutritional and performance status [9].

Obesity is a risk factor for a variety of cancers and diabetes, and obese patients usually have nonalcoholic steatohepatitis and cardiovascular disease. A recent report found no difference in overall major and minor morbidity rates between obese and nonobese patients undergoing CRS plus HIPEC for PSM. Obese patients were more likely than the nonobese cohort, however, to have a late (31–90 days) readmission. Survival was similar for obese and nonobese patients who underwent CRS plus HIPEC for PSM from colon cancer (CRC) or high-grade appendiceal cancer. Subanalysis based on the degree of obesity disclosed a significantly worse prognosis for severely obese patients with low-grade appendiceal cancer [10].

In PSM management, the extent of prior resection before definitive CRS plus HIPEC has a negative impact on survival. Surgery opens tissue planes in which the raw surface is a favored site for cancer-cell adherence (cancer-cell entrapment phenomenon): the greater the surgery before definitive combined treatment, the poorer the results of carcinomatosis treatment. The Prior Surgical Score (PSS) proposed by Sugarbaker (Chap. 5) quantifies the extent of surgery before definitive combined treatment, and a previous report showed that PSS has a high prognostic impact [11]. Whereas reported results from many tertiary centers with expertise in PSM treatment show a substantial improvement in prognosis and quality of life, many patients undergoing CRS plus HIPEC will experience tumor recurrence [12]. Most failures after CRS plus HIPEC exclusively involve intra-abdominal sites. This finding supports the knowledge that a subset of patients exists who will manifest intra-abdominal disease without manifesting hematogenous metastases. Many investigators assume that in selected patients a second CRS procedure combined with a second HIPEC may be of value. Iterative procedures combining CRS and HIPEC are feasible and allow long-term survival but may increase morbidity and mortality rates. Patients must be carefully selected according to favorable tumor biology, duration of recurrence-free survival, performance status, and the possibility of achieving complete cytoreduction [13–15].

13.3 Origin of Peritoneal Spread

Tumor site and histology are important selection criteria. Indications for CRS plus HIPEC are now validated for several diseases [pseudomyxoma peritonei (PMP)], malignant peritoneal mesothelioma (MPM), carcinomatosis from appendiceal and colorectal cancer (CRC). CRS plus HIPEC is now under evaluation in the treatment of peritoneal spread from gastric (GC), ovarian (OC), and neuroendocrine tumors, whereas few reported series refer to CRS plus HIPEC for carcinomatosis from breast cancer, desmoplastic small-round-cell tumors, and Frantz tumor of the pancreas [16–19].

PMP has been considered the classic indication for using CRC plus HIPEC in PSM. PMP is a rare disease, and most PMP arise from appendiceal tumors. The main prognostic factor is histopathologic subtype classification according to Ronnett et al.'s or Bradley et al.'s criteria [20, 21]. In a study of 2,298 patients collected from 16 specialized units and with a treatment-related mortality of 2 % and a major operative complications rate of 24 %, CRS plus HIPEC achieved a 10-year OS rate of 63 % and a 15-year OS rate of 59 % [22]. A multivariate analysis with a Cox regression model showed that older age, major postoperative complications, macroscopic residual disease [Completeness of Cytoreduction (CC) scores 2–3], prior chemotherapy treatment, and peritoneal mucinous carcinomatosis (PMCA) subtype were independent variables predicting poorer OS [22].

The prognosis for patients with diffuse MPM (DMPM) has been improved by CRS plus HIPEC, and as with other PSM, survival benefit is maximal when surgery achieves complete surgical cytoreduction. From a prospective database of 108 patients with DMPM undergoing complete cytoreduction (CC0/CC1) plus HIPEC with cisplatin and doxorubicin, several patient-, tumor-, and treatment-related variables were assessed by multivariate analysis with respect to OS and progression-free survival (PFS) [23]. Median OS was 63.2 months and PFS 25.1 months; epithelial histological subtype, negative lymph nodes, and Ki67-positive cells < 10 % correlated with increased OS and PFS. That study suggested that 7-year actual survival defines cure for at least 43.6 % of patients with DMPM after CC and HIPEC [23].

Peritoneal carcinomatosis (PC) from CRC has long been regarded as a terminal condition with a dismal prognosis and a median life expectancy ranging between 5.2 and 7 months after systemic chemotherapy [24]. Following the disappointing results of systemic chemotherapy in patients with PC from CRC, some investigators suggested that these patients could undergo aggressive therapeutic regimens (CRS plus HIPEC) [25–27]. A prospective randomized trial conducted by Verwaal et al. in 2003 documented a significantly increased median survival for patients with CRC and PC treated by CRS plus HIPEC and postoperative systemic chemotherapy compared with those treated by systemic chemotherapy alone with or without palliative surgery [28]. Long-term results for the same study population clearly showed that patients with no residual disease after CRS plus HIPEC reached a median survival of 48 months and a 5-year survival of 45 % [29]. These results received confirmation from several multicenter studies [30–33].

Peritoneal dissemination from GC is common and arose in 5–20 % of patients who underwent exploratory laparotomy for potentially curative resection [34]. Despite efforts to apply CRS plus HIPEC in patients with PC from GC, the median survival rate remains disappointing (< 12 months); only in patients who undergo surgery leaving no residual disease does the 5-year survival rate increase to 30 % [35–37]. In an attempt to improve outcomes, Yonemura et al. introduced a bidirectional strategy (intraperitoneal normothermic plus systemic chemotherapy) before CRS plus HIPEC in patients with PC from GC but obtained less beneficial results than expected [38].

Complete cytoreduction (CC) is a fundamental issue in surgery for peritoneal spread from OC [39], and given the high recurrence rate after surgery (65 %), HIPEC assumes a theoretical role for treating invisible residual disease. Although ample evidence establishes that CRS plus HIPEC is a feasible option in advanced OC, timing (upfront, consolidation, or at recurrence) and survival benefit are not yet clarified [40]. CRS plus HIPEC has mainly been used in PC from recurrent OC, and according to Bakrin et al. reporting on a French multicenter retrospective cohort study, chemosensitive and chemoresistant patients gained an equal survival rate [41].

13.4 Extent of Disease

By far the most influential prognostic factor in patients with PSM is the completeness of cytoreduction (CC). Hence, the main obstacle facing the surgeon is the malignant mass at surgery. Because the diagnostic methods used for quantifying the extent of malignant disease in the peritoneum and eventually in other extra-abdominal sites are specifically addressed elsewhere in this book (Chaps. 5 and 6), they are not discussed here. Although the presence of extra-abdominal metastases limits survival in patients with PC and influences outcome [42], the presence of widespread extra-abdominal malignant disease, including the frequent pleural involvement (pleural effusion) found in patients with advanced OC, does not preclude treatment. In these cases [Fédération Internationale de Gynécologie et Obstétrique//Union Internationale Contre le Cancer (FIGO-UICC) stage IV], especially after neoadjuvant chemotherapy, the percentage of optimal cytoreduction achieved and the long-term prognosis, despite being considerably lower than for IIIc tumors, seems to guarantee previously unhoped-for results [43].

In patients with PSM, the extent of abdominal disease is generally scored with the Sugarbaker Peritoneal Cancer Index (PCI), as extensively described in previous chapters. An especially high PCI severely reduces the likelihood that the surgeon will achieve CC. Depending on the origin of the primary tumor, we can consider a cutoff beyond which it would be inadvisable to continue PC treatment. A French retrospective study of 523 patients with PC from CRC and treated with CRS plus HIPEC showed that when the PCI exceeded 20, long-term survival was no longer than that obtained with systemic chemotherapy alone [31]. This cutoff certainly holds true for CRC but is less valid for biologically less aggressive tumor types or those more responsive to systemic chemotherapy, such as PMP and advanced OC. In patients with low-grade PMP, a PCI > 20 will not influence the prognosis as long as CC can be achieved [22, 44].

Besides assessing overall peritoneal spread using the PCI, the presence of disease in certain critical anatomical areas regardless, of size, can provide a selection criterion that can preclude complete CRS. These particular anatomic circumstances can themselves be the borderline between obtaining or not obtaining CC. They also involve other problems, such as the surgical team's technical expertise, making this factor a further selection criteria. In a patient with PC chosen as a candidate to CRS plus HIPEC, an uninvolved small bowel offers the best chance of CC. Conversely, if the small bowel is involved by gross disease at the mesentery root or partial obstruction at several segmental sites, surgery is no option [45].

Patients with a biliary or ureteral obstruction or both are usually considered unresectable [46]. However, when biliary or ureteral obstruction depends simply on compression by large tumor masses, particularly in patients with PMP, these masses can be resected without segmental ureteral or bile duct resection. When Votanopoulos et al. analyzed results in a series of patients with PC who were candidates to CRS plus HIPEC, all of whom had coexisting urinary tract involvement, they did not consider urologic procedures as a contraindication in patients with resectable PSM [47]. Disease affecting the lesser omentum and gastrohepatic ligament should be managed with lesser omentectomy, cholecystectomy, clearance of the hepatoduodenal ligament, and omental bursa-floor stripping. During greater omentectomy, the right and left gastroepiploic vessels are often resected, and if—as often is the case—disease necessitates splenectomy, the blood supply to the stomach can be guaranteed only by preserving the lesser omental arcade or at least the left gastric vessels. The surgeon's ability to complete these site-specific cytoreduction maneuvers is itself a selection criterion (Figs. 13.1 and 13.2).

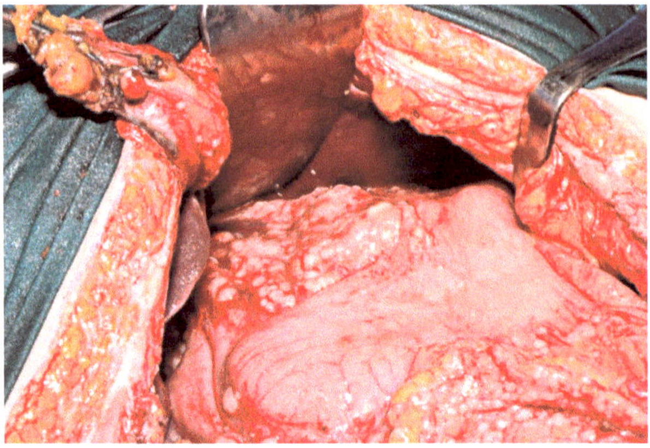

Fig. 13.1 Peritoneal carcinomatosis from ovarian cancer: involvement of lesser omentum and hepatoduodenal ligament

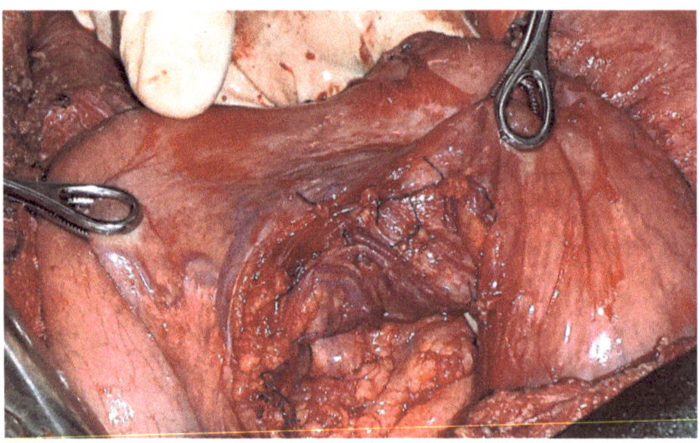

Fig. 13.2 Lesser omentectomy and stripping of the omental bursa floor

Another challenging problem, especially in patients with CRC, concerns coexisting PC with liver metastases. A meta-analysis conducted by Dutch investigators showed a trend toward lower OS after curative resection plus HIPEC in patients with CRC metastases in the liver, as well as in the peritoneum, than in patients with peritoneal metastases alone after the same treatment [48]. Although this approach can be used to treat PC and liver metastases during the same procedure in selected patients, only patients who have limited peritoneal spread (PCI < 12) and a limited extent of liver disease (liver metastases < 3) really benefit from this approach, with a median survival of 40 months [49].

13.5 Decision Making

In his "Presidential Address to the Society of Surgical Oncology," Blake Cady stated that tumor biology is the king, patient selection is the queen, and technical procedure the prince, of the kingdom. Only rarely does the prince usurp the kingdom [50]. These considerations perfectly illustrate the problem being addressing. Patient selection criteria must maintain the balance between opposing forces. On the one side is a frequently unfavorable and undoubtedly aggressive tumor biology; on the other side is a surgeon convinced that technical efforts will snatch the patient away from an ineluctable destiny. Ideal selection criteria should indicate patients for whom surgery is most likely to have a successful outcome and therefore in whom technical, organizational, and economic efforts, necessitated by these procedures, should be invested.

Research over the past few years, limited to PC from CRC, has developed a staging classification intended chiefly for preoperative use [Peritoneal Surface Disease Severity Score (PSDSS)], which analyzes separately the entity of patient symptoms, the extent of peritoneal disease (PCI), and the histopathologic tumor features (including lymphatic spread), yielding a specific score and then subdivided into four stages (Fig. 13.3) [32]. The American Society of Peritoneal Surface Malignancies conducted a retrospective review of 609 patients who underwent CRS plus HIPEC after PSDSS staging. Their findings show that the PSDSS, assessed before surgery, can define a popula-

Peritoneal Surface Disease Severity Score (PSDSS) of colorectal cancer with peritoneal spread

Clinical symptoms	Extent of carcinomatosis CT-PCI	Histology
No symptoms 0	PCI>10 (Low) 1	G1 G2 N-L-V 1
Mild symptoms 1	PCI>10-20 (Medium) 3	G2 N+ and/or L+ and/or V+ 3
Severe symptoms 6	PCI>20 (High) 7	G3 Signet ring 9

Score	Stage
2-3	Stage I
4-7	Stage II
8-10	Stage III
>10	Stage IV

Clinical symptoms

Mild symptoms = weight loss <10% of body weight mild abdominal pain, some ascites

Severe sympt. = weight loss >10% of body weight unremitting pain, bowel obstruction, symptomatic ascites

Peritoneal Cancer Index (PCI)

By imaging (CT, PET, MRI) or exploration (laparoscopy or evalutation at time of first operation in synchronous peritoneal carcinomatosis)

Fig. 13.3 Peritoneal Surface Disease Severity Score (PSDSS). (Reproduced from [52], with permission)

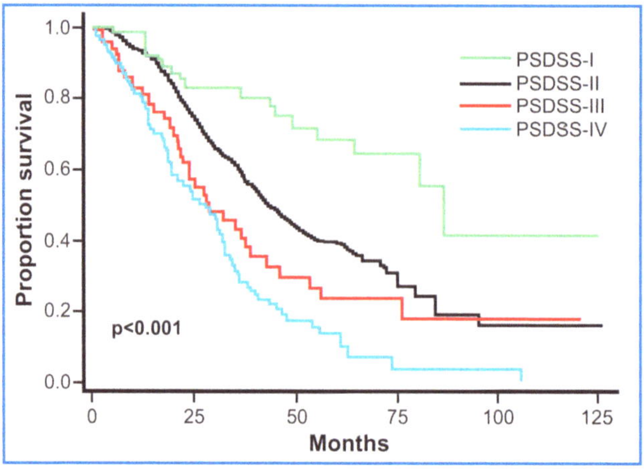

Fig. 13.4 Long-term survival according to the Peritoneal Surface Disease Severity Score (PSDSS). (Reproduced from [52], with permission)

tion with a statistically high or notably low likelihood of long-term survival (Fig. 13.4) [51].

Regardless, whatever the pros and cons of one scoring system or another, the intellectual rationale for selecting patients as candidates for CRS plus HIPEC procedures never concerns the surgeon alone. The decision inevitably requires a multidisciplinary contribution involving many specialists and includes the patients themselves so as to offer an individualized treatment option. Especially important is the need to alert the medical community (medical oncologists, the message is for you) that PSM is not by definition incurable. Quite the contrary: CRS plus HIPEC offers many of these patients a real chance of cure. Only keeping these management options firmly in mind will increase the number of patients referred to expert centers for treatment, help identify patients with PSM at earlier stages and thus simplify patient selection.

References

1. Mohamed F, Moran BJ (2009)Morbidity and mortality with cytoreductive surgery and intraperitoneal chemotherapy: the importance of a learning curve. Cancer J 15:196-199
2. Herzog TJ (2012) The role of heated intraperitoneal chemotherapy (HIPEC) in ovarian cancer: hope or hoax? Ann Surg Oncol 19:3998-4000
3. Reuter NP, Macgregor JM, Woodall CE et al (2008) Preoperative performance status predicts outcome following heated intraperitoneal chemotherapy. Am J Surg 196:909-913
4. Shen P, Hawksworth J, Lovato J et al (2004) Cytoreductive surgery and intraperitoneal hyperthermic chemotherapy with mitomycin C for peritoneal carcinomatosis from nonappendiceal colorectal carcinoma. Ann Surg Oncol 11:178-186
5. Levine EA, Stewart JH, Shen P et al (2014) Intraperitoneal chemotherapy for peritoneal surface malignancy: experience with 1,000 patients. J Am Coll Surg 218:573-585
6. Baratti D, Kusamura S, Mingrone E et al (2012) Identification of a subgroup of patients at

highest risk for complications after surgical cytoreduction and hyperthermic intraperitoneal chemotherapy. Ann Surg 256:334-341
7. Hutchins LF, Unger JM, Crowley JJ et al (1999) Underrepresentation of patients 65 years of age or older in cancer-treatment trials. N Engl J Med 341:2061-2067
8. Polanczyk CA, Marcantonio E, Goldman L et al (2001) Impact of age on perioperative complications and length of stay in patients undergoing noncardiac surgery. Ann Intern Med 134:637-643
9. Votanopoulos KI, Newman NA, Russell G et al (2013) Outcomes of Cytoreductive Surgery (CRS) with hyperthermic intraperitoneal chemotherapy (HIPEC) in patients older than 70 years; survival benefit at considerable morbidity and mortality.Ann Surg Oncol 20:3497-503
10. Votanopoulos KI, Swords DS, Swett KR et al (2013) Obesity and peritoneal surface disease: outcomes after cytoreductive surgery with hyperthermic intraperitoneal chemotherapy for appendiceal and colon primary tumors. Ann Surg Oncol 20:3899-904
11. Sugarbaker PH, Chang D (1999) Results of treatment of 385 patients with peritoneal surface spread of appendiceal malignancy. Ann Surg Oncol 6:727-731
12. Bijelic L, Yan TD, Sugarbaker PH (2008) Treatment failure following complete cytoreductive surgery and perioperative intraperitoneal chemotherapy for peritoneal dissemination from colorectal or appendiceal mucinous neoplasms. J Surg Oncol 98:295-299
13. Golse N, Bakrin N, Passot G et al (2012) Iterative procedures combining cytoreductive surgery with hyperthermic intraperitoneal chemotherapy for peritoneal recurrence: postoperative and long-term results. J Surg Oncol 106:197-203
14. Votanopoulos KI, Ihemelandu C, Shen P et al (2012) Outcomes of repeat cytoreductive surgery with hyperthermic intraperitoneal chemotherapy for the treatment of peritoneal surface malignancy. J Am Coll Surg 215:412-417
15. Sardi A, Jimenez WA, Nieroda C et al (2013) Repeated cytoreductive surgery and hyperthermic intraperitoneal chemotherapy in peritoneal carcinomatosis from appendiceal cancer: analysis of survival outcomes. Eur J Surg Oncol 39:1207-1213
16. Elias D, Goéré D, Dumont F et al (2014) Role of hyperthermic intraoperative peritoneal chemotherapy in the management of peritoneal metastases. Eur J Cancer 50:332-340
17. Cardi M, Sammartino P, Framarino ML et al Treatment of peritoneal carcinomatosis from breast cancer by maximal cytoreduction and HIPEC: a preliminary report on 5 cases. Breast 22:845-849
18. Hayes-Jordan A, Green HL, Lin H et al (2014) Complete cytoreduction and HIPEC improves survival in desmoplastic small round cell tumor. Ann Surg Oncol 21:220-224
19. Honore C, Goere D, Dartigues P et al (2012) Peritoneal carcinomatosis from solid pseudopapillary neoplasm (Frantz's tumour) of the pancreas treated with HIPEC. Anticancer Res 32:1069-1073
20. Ronnett BM, Zahn CM, Kurman RJ et al (1995) Disseminated peritoneal adenomucinosis and peritoneal mucinous carcinomatosis. A clinicopathologic analysis of 109 cases with emphasis on distinguishing pathologic features, site of origin, prognosis, and relationship to "pseudomyxoma peritonei". Am J Surg Pathol 19:1390-1408
21. Bradley RF, Stewart JH, Russell GB et al (2006) Pseudomyxoma peritonei of appendiceal origin: a clinicopathologic analysis of 101 patients uniformly treated at a single institution, with literature review. Am J Surg Pathol 30:551-559
22. Chua TC, Moran BJ, Sugarbaker PH et al (2012) Early- and long-term outcome data of patients with pseudomyxoma peritonei from appendiceal origin treated by a strategy of cytoreductive surgery and hyperthermic intraperitoneal chemotherapy. J Clin Oncol 30:2449-2456
23. Baratti D, Kusamura S, Cabras AD et al (2013) Diffuse malignant peritoneal mesothelioma: long-term survival with complete cytoreductive surgery followed by hyperthermic intraperitoneal chemotherapy (HIPEC). Eur J Cancer 49:3140-3148
24. Sadeghi B, Arvieux C, Glehen O et al (2000) Peritoneal carcinomatosis from non-gynecologic malignancies: results of the EVOCAPE 1 multicentric prospective study. Cancer 88:358-363

25. Sugarbaker PH, Schellinx ME et al (1996) Peritoneal carcinomatosis from adenocarcinoma of the colon. World J Surg 20:585-591
26. Glehen O, Cotte E, Schreiber V et al (2004) Intraperitoneal chemohyperthermia and attempted cytoreductive surgery in patients with peritoneal carcinomatosis of colorectal origin. Br J Surg 91:747-754
27. Elias D, Raynard B, Farkhondeh F et al (2006) Peritoneal carcinomatosis of colorectal origin. Gastroenterol Clin Biol 30:1200-1204
28. Verwaal VJ, van Ruth S, de Bree E et al (2003) Randomized trial of cytoreduction and hyperthermic intraperitoneal chemotherapy versus systemic chemotherapy and palliative surgery in patients with peritoneal carcinomatosis of colorectal cancer. J Clin Oncol 21:3737-343
29. Verwaal VJ, Bruin S, Boot H et al (2008) 8-year follow-up of randomized trial: cytoreduction and hyperthermic intraperitoneal chemotherapy versus systemic chemotherapy in patients with peritoneal carcinomatosis of colorectal cancer. Ann Surg Oncol 15:2426-2432
30. Glehen O, Kwiatkowski F, Sugarbaker PH et al (2004) Cytoreductive surgery combined with perioperative intraperitoneal chemotherapy for the management of peritoneal carcinomatosis from colorectal cancer: a multi-institutional study. J Clin Oncol 22:3284-3292
31. Elias D, Gilly F, Boutitie F et al Peritoneal colorectal carcinomatosis treated with surgery and perioperative intraperitoneal chemotherapy: retrospective analysis of 523 patients from a multicentric French study. J Clin Oncol 28:63-68
32. Chua TC, Morris DL, Esquivel J (2010) Impact of the peritoneal surface disease severity score on survival in patients with colorectal cancer peritoneal carcinomatosis undergoing complete cytoreduction and hyperthermic intraperitoneal chemotherapy. Ann Surg Oncol 17:1330-1336
33. Cavaliere F, De Simone M, Virzì S et al (2011) Prognostic factors and oncologic outcome in 146 patients with colorectal peritoneal carcinomatosis treated with cytoreductive surgery combined with hyperthermic intraperitoneal chemotherapy: Italian multicenter study S.I.T.I.L.O. Eur J Surg Oncol 37:148-1454
34. Kuramoto M, Shimada S, Ikeshima S et al (2009) Extensive intraoperative peritoneal lavage as a standard prophylactic strategy for peritoneal recurrence in patients with gastric carcinoma. Ann Surg 250:242-246
35. Cheong JH, Shen JY, Song CS et al (2007) Early postoperative intraperitoneal chemotherapy following cytoreductive surgery in patients with very advanced gastric cancer. Ann Surg Oncol 14:61-68
36. Glehen O, Gilly FN, Arvieux C et al (2010) Peritoneal carcinomatosis from gastric cancer: a multi-institutional study of 159 patients treated by cytoreductive surgery combined with perioperative intraperitoneal chemotherapy. Ann Surg Oncol 17:2370-2377
37. Yang XJ, Huang CQ, Suo T et al (2011) Cytoreductive surgery and hyperthermic intraperitoneal chemotherapy improves survival of patients with peritoneal carcinomatosis from gastric cancer: final results of a phase III randomized clinical trial. Ann Surg Oncol 18:1575-15781
38. Canbay E, Mizumoto A, Ichinose M et al (2014) Outcome data of patients with peritoneal carcinomatosis from gastric origin treated by a strategy of bidirectional chemotherapy prior to cytoreductive surgery and hyperthermic intraperitoneal chemotherapy in a single specialized center in Japan. Ann Surg Oncol 21:1147-1152
39. Chang SJ, Bristow RE, Ryu HS (2012) Impact of complete cytoreduction leaving no gross residual disease associated with radical cytoreductive surgical procedures on survival in advanced ovarian cancer. Ann Surg Oncol 19:4059-4067
40. Helm CW (2012) Current status and future directions of cytoreductive surgery and hyperthermic intraperitoneal chemotherapy in the treatment of ovarian cancer. Surg Oncol Clin N Am 21:645-663
41. Bakrin N, Bereder JM, Decullier E et al (2013) Peritoneal carcinomatosis treated with cytoreductive surgery and Hyperthermic Intraperitoneal Chemotherapy (HIPEC) for advanced ovarian carcinoma: a French multicentre retrospective cohort study of 566 patients. Eur J Surg Oncol 39:1435-1443

42. Esquivel J, Sticca R, Sugarbaker P et al (2007)Cytoreductive surgery and hyperthermic intraperitoneal chemotherapy in the management of peritoneal surface malignancies of colonic origin: a consensus statement. Society of Surgical Oncology. Ann Surg Oncol 14:128-133
43. Perri T, Ben-Baruch G, Kalfon S et al (2013) Abdominopelvic cytoreduction rates and recurrence sites in stage IV ovarian cancer: is there a case for thoracic cytoreduction? Gynecol Oncol 131:27-31
44. Moran B, Baratti D, Yan TD et al (2008) Consensus statement on the loco-regional treatment of appendiceal mucinous neoplasms with peritoneal dissemination (pseudomyxoma peritonei). J Surg Oncol 98:277-282
45. Elias D, Benizri E, Vernerey D et al (2005) Preoperative criteria of incomplete resectability of peritoneal carcinomatosis from non-appendiceal colorectal carcinoma. Gastroenterol Clin Biol 29:1010-1013
46. Verwaal VJ, Kusamura S, Baratti D et al (2008) The eligibility for local-regional treatment of peritoneal surface malignancy. J Surg Oncol 98:220-223
47. Votanopoulos KI, Randle RW et al (2014) Significance of urinary tract involvement in patients treated with cytoreductive surgery (CRS) and hyperthermic intraperitoneal chemotherapy (HIPEC). Ann Surg Oncol 21:868-874
48. De Cuba EM, Kwakman R, Knol DL et al (2013) Cytoreductive surgery and HIPEC for peritoneal metastases combined with curative treatment of colorectal liver metastases: Systematic review of all literature and meta-analysis of observational studies. Cancer Treat Rev 39:321-327
49. Maggiori L, Goéré D, Viana B et al (2013) Should patients with peritoneal carcinomatosis of colorectal origin with synchronous liver metastases be treated with a curative intent? A case-control study. Ann Surg 258:116-121
50. Cady B (1990) The Society of Surgical Oncology at a crossroads: thoughts for the future. Presidential address. Arch Surg 125:153-157
51. Esquivel J, Lowy AM, Markman M et al (2014) The American Society of Peritoneal Surface Malignancies (ASPSM) Multiinstitution Evaluation of the Peritoneal Surface Disease Severity Score (PSDSS) in 1,013 Patients with Colorectal Cancer with Peritoneal Carcinomatosis. Ann Surg Oncol [Epub ahead of print]

Morbidity and Mortality

14

Antonio Macrì, Francesco Fleres, Eugenio Cucinotta,
and Edoardo Saladino

14.1 Introduction

Mortality and morbidity rates remain the most comprehensive measures used to assess short-term outcomes of a specific procedure. Surgical complications are frequently the main reason to modify patient treatment and ultimately attain wide acceptance for a particular procedure by the medical community. Nevertheless, these two outcome measures remain hard to asses and identify by the surgical literature due to lack of standardization and underreporting. For this reason, in the surgical field, there is an absence of a clear system to classify complications. These considerations are valid for cytoreductive surgery (CRS) plus hyperthermic intraperitoneal chemotherapy (HIPEC), which is not an exception to the rule. In fact, appreciable effort has been developed by surgeons performing CRS plus HIPEC to relate morbidity and mortality to the procedure. However, the issue is relatively complex because the appearance of postoperative complications related to intraoperative manipulation can be confounded with toxic side effects of the intraperitoneally administered chemotherapy (IP-CHT).

14.2 Classification Systems

Among the numerous classification systems used to report surgical complications, some investigators preferred to use the Clavien system (Table 14.1) [1], others the Feldman or modified Clavien system (Table 14.2) [2], and still oth-

A. Macrì (✉)
Department of Human Pathology, University of Messina,
Messina, Italy
e-mail: amacri@unime.it

A. Di Giorgio, E. Pinto (Eds), *Treatment of Peritoneal Surface Malignancies*,
Updates in Surgery
DOI: 10.1007/978-88-470-5711-1_14, © Springer-Verlag Italia 2015

Table 14.1 Classification of complications according to Clavien et al. [1]

Grade I: Events carrying minor risks; complication, if left untreated, resolves spontaneously or at most requires a simple bedside procedure. Analgesics, antipyretics, antiemetics, antibiotics orally, and antidiarrheals are permitted
Grade II: Potentially life threatening; requires some form of intervention. Grade IIa requires drugs other than above, parental nutrition, or transfusions. Grade IIb requires invasive procedures (radiological or endoscopic) or reoperation
Grade III: Events with residual or lasting disability, including organ resection
Grade IV: Complications result in death

Table 14.2 Classification of complications according to Feldman et al. [2]

Grade I: Minor complications; resolves spontaneously if left untreated or requires a simple bedside procedure. Analgesics, antipyretics, antiemetics, antibiotics orally, and antidiarrheals are permitted. Examples include superficial surgical-site infection, urinary retention, lower urinary tract infection, ileus requiring nasogastric tube
Grade II: Potentially life threatening; requires intervention that carries some risks. Grade IIa requires other drugs, parental nutrition, or transfusions. Examples include pneumonia, arrhythmia, or acute pancreatitis. Grade IIb requires invasive procedures (radiological or endoscopic) or reoperation. Examples include computed-tomography-guided abscess drainage
Grade III: Events with residual or lasting disability or organ loss; includes cerebrovascular events with residual disability and iatrogenic splenectomy. All complications categorized as cardiac, respiratory, gastrointestinal, urinary, local, or other
Grade IV: Complications result in death

ers the Elias classification (Table 14.3) [3], the Bozzetti classification (Table 14.4) [4], or the National Cancer Institute Common Terminology Criteria for Adverse Events (NCI-CTCAE) [5] to report on both morbidity and toxicity. This heterogeneity in the adopted systems impedes comparison between treatment-related complication rates among the various reports. All these classifications systems, although different from each other, are not intended to account for toxicities related to the use of chemotherapy during CRS plus HIPEC. For this reason, Kusamura et al. [6] proposed using the World Health Organization (WHO) toxicity scale (Table 14.5). This is a relatively simple four-grade scale that comprises 12 categories for toxicity, with predetermined cutoff values within each category by which to grade the adverse event. Others authors, such as Elias et al. [3], Smeenk et al. [7], and Glehen et al. [8] prefer to use CTCAE version 3.0 to relate toxicity to the procedure [5]. This classification, used to record medication toxicity in randomized control trials, is a five-scale system regrouping 310 types of complications within 28 categories based on anatomy and/or pathophysiology of the complication. The main advantage of this classification is that it can be used to determine both toxicity and surgical morbidity. Until now, accurate evaluation of the various classification systems raises the

Table 14.3 Classification of complications according to Elias et al. [3]

Grade 0: No complication
Grade I: Complications requiring either no or minor intervention, such as antibiotics orally, bowel rest, or basic monitoring
Grade II: Complications requiring moderate interventions, such medication intravenously (e.g., antibiotics or antiarrhythmics), total parental nutrition, prolonged tube feeding, or chest-tube insertion
Grade III: Complications requiring hospital readmission, surgical intervention, or radiological intervention
Grade IV: Complications producing chronic disability, organ resection, or enteric diversion
Grade V: Complications result in death

Table 14.4 Classification of complications according to Bozzetti et al. [4]

Grade I: No complication
Grade II: Minor complications; wound infection, urinary tract infection, pancreatitis, ileus, deep vein thrombosis
Grade III: Major complications; requiring reoperation on intensive care admission or interventional radiology treatment
Grade IV: In-hospital or intensive care unit mortality

Table 14.5 Categories in the World Health Organization (WHO) toxicity scale [6]

Hematological disorders	Infections
Gastrointestinal disorders	Hair disorders
Renal–bladder disorders	Cardiac disorders
Pulmonary–allergic disorders	Neurotoxicity disorders
Cutaneous disorders	Constipation disorders
Fever, drug disorders	Pain

following considerations: all classifications are different in terms of total number of classes (four or five grades); there is no correspondence between grades; in all the systems analyzed, grade can be grouped in two main groups, minor and major complications. Hence, in light of these considerations, in 2006, during the Fifth International Workshop on Peritoneal Surface Malignancy, CTCAE version 3.0 was adopted by an international panel of experts as the definitive classification system for complications resulting from CRS plus HIPEC. The rationale is that a numeric grading system seems to be the most appropriate way to report complications related to this aggressive procedure and thus potentially standardize results. In 2009, an updated version, 4.0, of CTCAE was published [9].

14.3 Risk Factors

Many risk factors associated with the appearance of adverse events during CRS plus HIPEC are described by many authors. However it is not possible to compare the various series due to the numerous variables used by the different authors. Consequently, we report the most representative series: Kusamura et al. [6], using univariate analysis, found the following variables have a statistically significant correlation with major morbidity: male gender ($p = 0.016$), Eastern Cooperative Oncology Group (ECOG) performance status ($p = 0.05$), no previous systemic chemotherapy ($p = 0.004$), carcinomatosis extent ($p = 0.027$), number of bowel anastomoses > 2 ($p = 0.028$), procedure duration ($p = 0.014$), extent of cytoreduction ($p = 0.019$), and cisplatin (CDDP) dose for intraperitoneal hyperthermic perfusion > 240 mg ($p = 0.02$). However, in multivariate analysis, no previous systemic chemotherapy [odds ratio (OR) 2.719; 95% confidence interval (CI) 0.984–7.512; $p = 0.054$], extent of cytoreduction (OR 2.877; 95% CI 1.292–6.404; $p = 0.01$), and CDDP dose > 240 mg (OR 3.128; 95% CI 1.239–7.900; $p = 0.016$) were independent risk factors for major morbidity. Glehen et al. [9] carried out only a univariate analysis in which they found that major morbidity was statistically linked with carcinomatosis stage ($p = 0.016$), duration of surgery ($p = 0.005$), and number of resections and peritonectomy procedures ($p = 0.042$). Hansson et al., [10], in their multivariate analysis, observed the adverse events were associated with stoma formation, duration of surgery, perioperative blood loss, and Peritoneal Cancer Index (PCI). Casado-Adam et al. [11], in their univariate analysis, found a statistically significant correlation between morbidity, histological grade ($p = 0.0166$), PCI ($p = 0.0049$), small-bowel resections ($p = 0.0493$), colorectal anastomosis ($p = 0.0430$), and the number of anastomoses performed per patient ($p = 0.0288$). However, multivariate analysis showed that PCI was the only independent risk factor for gastrointestinal complications ($p = 0.0586$). Finally, Mizumoto et al. [12], in their univariate analysis, showed that PCI > 20, operation time > 5 h, and blood loss > 2.5 L were significant risk factors for postoperative complications. On the other hand, the complication rate in patients who received HIPEC was significantly lower than in patients treated without HIPEC. Gender, age >/< 65 years old, origin of peritoneal carcinomatosis (PC), and completeness of cytoreduction were not related to morbidity. Multivariate analysis showed that PCI higher than 20 was the only significant factor that increased the occurrence of postoperative complications. PCI > 20 was associated with 2.8 times increased risk of postoperative complications. In multivariate analysis, patients who received HIPEC showed significantly lower mortality and morbidity rates than patients who did not.

14.4 Analysis of the Literature

Peritoneal carcinomatosis has been regarded as an inoperable condition and treated by systemic chemotherapy or palliative therapies. Based on the theory that PC is a locoregional disease, CRS plus HIPEC has been applied in selected patients with this pathology. It is clear, however, that the effects of this regional chemotherapy are not limited to the peritoneal space. The profound effect that these treatments have on wound healing is shown by the increased incidence of gastrointestinal events. However Chua et al. [13], in a systematic review, showed that morbidity and mortality rates of CRS plus HIPEC were similar to other major gastrointestinal interventions. Literature reports major morbidity rates ranging from 12 % to 57 % in high-volume treatment centers [13, 14], even if, in recent publications, overall grades III–IV morbidity rates are reported to be between 7 % and 41% [6, 8, 10–12, 15]. These results are due to the high surgeon learning curve demonstrated in the expanded application of CRS plus HIPEC. In fact, the literature reports that 130–140 cases are necessary to minimize mortality and morbidity rates after the procedure [16, 17].

Among gastrointestinal events, small-bowel perforations and anastomotic leaks are the most common and clinically significant complications reported [6, 8, 10–12, 15, 18]; mortality is reported to range from 0.9 % to 11 % [13, 14, 19]. Comparing various data of the main literature reports that calculated the incidence of gastrointestinal events grades III–IV, Kusamura et al. [6] conducted a study on 205 patients treated by CRS plus HIPEC with the closed abdomen technique, in which overall postoperative morbidity rate, including all grades III–IV, was 12 %. They reported 17 anastomotic leaks, six digestive perforations, one biliary fistula, two pancreatic fistulas, and four cases of ileus/gastric stasis. The most severe complications in their series were intestinal leakages due to anastomotic insufficiency and/or intestinal perforation. This morbidity constituted ~ 70% of all cases with major morbidity. Glehen et al. [8] reported on 207 patients treated by CRS plus HIPEC with the closed abdomen technique, finding an overall postoperative morbidity rate, including all grades III–IV, of 24.5 %. They reported 14 digestive fistulas, 11 cases of prolonged ileus, and five intraperitoneal abscesses. Hansson et al. [10] conducted a study of 123 patients in which they observed an overall postoperative morbidity rate, including all grades III–IV, of 41 %. Among gastrointestinal events, seven were anastomotic leaks, 11 digestive-tract perforations, one pancreatitis, one bile leak, and three cases of prolonged ileus. Youssef et al. [15] reported on 456 patients with pseudomyxoma peritonei (PMP) syndrome of appendiceal origin, finding grades III–IV morbidity of 7 %: seven anastomotic leaks, five pancreatic complications, and eight intestinal fistulas. Casado-Adam [11], reporting on 147 patients with appendiceal and colorectal carcinomatosis, found an incidence of grades III–IV events of 8 %: five nausea/vomiting, three anastomotic failures, three fistulas, one pancreatic fistula, one case of pancreatitis, one bile leak, and one small-bowel obstruction. In the report of Mizumoto et al. [12], conducted on 284 patients with appendiceal, colon cancer, and gastric cancer carcinomatosis, grades III–IV morbidity rate was 17 %, with 12 intra-abdominal abscesses, 13 gastric/ileus perforations, five cases of postoperative ileus, six anastomotic leakages, one urinary disturbance, three intestinal fistulas, six cases of postoperative bleeding, one case of respiratory distress, and one diaphragmatic hernia.

14.5 Italian Multicenter Experience

A retrospective multicenter study from eight Italian centers* was performed [20]. From November 2000 to January 2014, 683 patients underwent CRS plus HIPEC. To satisfy statistical criteria, only 507 patients were enrolled. Morbidity was evaluated in accordance with the NCI-CTCAE 4.0. [9]

Morbidity and mortality predictors [age, gender, body mass index (BMI), primary tumour site, American Association of Anesthesiologists (ASA) score, ECOG score, ascites, neoadjuvant chemotherapy (NACT), HIPEC, PCI, operative time, Completeness of Cytoreduction (CC) score] were evaluated with univariate and multivariate analysis; p values < 0.05 were considered statistically significant.

Mean patient age was 56.6 years [standard deviation (SD ± 11.5)], and 83 % were women. There were 461 patients with peritoneal carcinomatosis: 293 of ovarian, 106 of colon, and 62 of gastric origin; 46 patients had other peritoneal malignancies. ECOG score was 0 for 193 patients (38.1 %), 1 for 150 (29.6 %), 2 for 136 (26.8 %), and 3 for 28 (5.5 %); 174 patients (50.7 %) had ascites. The average PCI was 12 (SD ± 9.4). The closed-abdomen technique was used in 396 cases (78.1 %) and the Coliseum technique in 111 (21.9 %); 387 (76.3 %) patients did not have visible residual disease (CC-0), 73 (14.4 %) had residual disease ≤ 2.5 mm (CC-1), 29 (5.7 %) had residual disease between 2.5 mm and 2.5 cm (CC-2), and 18 (3.6 %) had residual disease > 2.5 cm (CC-3). Average operative time was 504 min (SD ± 156.2). Grades II–IV morbidity occurred in 280 patients (55.2 %), and mortality occurred in 18 cases (3.6 %). In univariate analysis, older age ($p = 0.027$), ECOG score 3 vs. 0 ($p = 0.016$), greater PCI ($p = 0.014$) and CC score 2 vs. 0 ($p = 0.044$) were correlated with a higher mortality rate, whereas older age ($p < 0.01$), presence of ascites ($p < 0.01$), ovarian origin ($p < 0.01$), closed-abdomen technique ($p = 0.015$), greater PCI ($p = 0.014$), longer operative time ($p < 0.01$), and CC-score 1 vs. 0 ($p = 0.022$)

*Macrì A[1], Arcoraci V[1], Belgrano V[2,3] Caldana M[3], Cioppa T[4], Costantini B[5], Cucinotta E[1], De Cian F[2], De Iaco P[6], De Manzoni G[3], Di Giorgio A[7], Muffatti F[8], Orsenigo E[8], Pinna AD[6], Roviello F[4], Sammartino P[7], Scambia G[5], Saladino E[1]. [1] University of Messina; [2] University of Genoa; [3] University of Verona; [4] University of Siena; [5] Catholic University of Sacred Heart, Rome; [6] S. Orsola-Malpighi Hospital, Bologna; [7] Sapienza University, Rome; [8] San Raffaele Scientific Institute, Milan.

and 2 vs. 0 ($p = 0.043$) were predictors of higher morbidity rates. In multivariate analysis, older age ($p = 0.047$) and greater PCI ($p = 0.026$) were correlated with a higher mortality rate; older age ($p < 0.01$), ovarian origin ($p < 0.01$), presence of ascites ($p = 0.011$), closed-abdomen technique ($p < 0.01$), and longer operative time ($p < 0.01$) were predictors of higher morbidity rates.

In light of these results, to improve outcomes, patient selection, especially with reference to age; ECOG score; and PCI, is necessary to improve treatment outcomes.

References

1. Clavien PA, Sanabria JR, Strasberg SM (1992) Proposed classification of complications of surgery with examples of utility in cholecystectomy. Surgery 111:518-526
2. Feldman L, Barkun J, Barkun A et al (1997) Measuring postoperative complications in general surgery patients using an outcomes-based strategy: Comparison with complications presented at morbidity and mortality rounds. Surgery 122:711-719
3. Elias D, Matsuhisa T, Sideris L et al (2004) Heated intra-operative intraperitoneal oxaliplatin plus irinotecan after complete resection of peritoneal carcinomatosis: Pharmacokinetics, tissue distribution and tolerance. Ann Oncol 15:1558-1565
4. Bozzetti F, Braga M, Gianotti L et al (2001) Postoperative enteral versus parenteral nutrition in malnourished patients with gastrointestinal cancer: A randomised multicentre trial. Lancet 358:1487-92
5. https://webscape.ctep.nci.nih.gov/webobjs/ctc/webhelp/welcome_to_ctcae.htm
6. Kusamura S, Younan R, Baratti D et al (2006) Cytoreductive surgery followed by intraperitoneal hyperthermic perfusion: Analysis of morbidity and mortality in 209 peritoneal surface malignancies treated with closed abdomen technique. Cancer 106:1144-1153
7. Smeenk RM, Verwaal VJ, Zoetmulder FA (2006) Toxicity and mortality of cytoreduction and intraoperative hyperthermic intraperitoneal chemotherapy in pseudomyxoma peritonei-A report of 103 procedures. Eur J Surg Oncol 32:186-190
8. Glehen O, Osinsky D, Cotte E et al (2003) Intraperitoneal chemohyperthermia using a closed abdominal procedure and cytoreductive surgery for the treatment of peritoneal carcinomatosis: Morbidity and mortality analysis of 216 consecutive procedures. Ann Surg Oncol 10:863-869
9. https:ctep.cancer.gov/protocolDevelopment/electronic_applications/ctc.htm
10. Hansson J, Graf W, Pahlman L, et al (2009) Postoperative adverse events and long-term survival after cytoreductive surgery and intraperitoneal chemotherapy. European Journal of Surgical Oncology 35:202–208
11. Casado-Adam A, Alderman R, Stuart OA, et al (2011) Gastrointestinal complications in 147 consecutive patients with peritoneal surface malignancy treated by cytoreductive surgery and perioperative intraperitoneal chemotherapy. Int J Surg Oncol 2011:468698
12. Mizumoto A, Canbay E, Hirano M et al (2012) Morbidity and mortality outcomes of cytoreductive surgery and hyperthermic intraperitoneal chemotherapy at a single institution in Japan. Gastroenterol Res Pract 2012:836425
13. Chua TC, Yan TD, Saxena A, Morris DL (2009) Should the treatment of peritoneal carcinomatosis by cytoreductive surgery and hyperthermic intraperitoneal chemotherapy still be regarded as a highly morbid procedure? A systematic review of morbidity and mortality. Annals of Surgery 249:900–907
14. Stewart JH IV, Shen P, Levine EA (2008) Intraperitoneal hyperthermic chemotherapy: an evolving paradigm for the treatment of peritoneal surface malignancies. Expert Rev Anticancer Ther 8:1809–1818

15. Youssef H, Newman C, Chandrakumaran K et al (2011) Operative findings, early complications, and long-term survival in 456 patients with pseudomyxoma peritonei syndrome of appendiceal origin. Diseases of the Colon and Rectum 54:293–299
16. Smeenk RM, Verwaal VJ, Zoetmulder FA (2007) Learning curve of combined modality treatment in peritoneal surface disease. British Journal of Surgery 94:1408–1414
17. Kusamura S, Baratti D, Deraco M (2012) Multidimensional analysis of the learning curve for cytoreductive surgery and hyperthermic intraperitoneal chemotherapy in peritoneal sur- face malignancies. Annals of Surgery 255:348–356
18. Younan R, Kusamura S, Baratti D et al (2005) Bowel complications in 203 cases of peritoneal surface malignancies treated with peritonectomy and closed-technique intraperitoneal hyperthermic perfusion. Annals of Surgical Oncology 12:910–918
19. Verwaal VJ, van Ruth S, de Bree E et al (2003) Randomized trial of cytoreduction and hyperthermic intraperitoneal chemotherapy versus systemic chemotherapy and palliative surgery in patients with peritoneal carcinomatosis of colorectal cancer. J Clin Oncol 21:3737–3743
20. Macrì A, Arcoraci V, Belgrano V et al (2014) Short-term outcome of cytoreductive surgery and hyperthermic intraperitoneal chemotherapy: preliminary analysis of a multicenter study. Anticancer Research. Vol. 34 [In press]

15 Organizational Problems, Costs, and Data Collection

Carlo Vallicelli, Simone Sibio, Maurizio Cardi, Davide Cavaliere, and Giorgio Maria Verdecchia

15.1 Introduction

The combined procedure of cytoreductive surgery and chemohyperthermic intraperitoneal perfusion with antiblastic solutions (CRS plus HIPEC) is a promising approach to the treatment of peritoneal carcinomatosis (PC). Experienced surgical skills and multidisciplinary team working are required to perform this complex and integrated procedure in dedicated surgical oncology units of highly specialized centers. Ongoing and future studies will be able to suggest this as the next standard of care for many patients with PC. This promising landscape emphasizes the importance of standardizing procedures, providing adequate technology and treatment centers, and increasing surgeons' learning curve and awareness of the results of this procedure. Common protocols are needed to ensure the maximum organizational efficiency and safety in the operating room (OR). Centers at which this type of treatment is performed began to elaborate personal protocols and opened the way to such work.

Furthermore, CRS plus HIPEC is a very expensive procedure, and the hospital discharge form does not adequately evaluate its economic component. Therefore, hospitals treating patients with PC must bear this economic deficit. Study protocols involving multiple experienced centers are needed to improve evidence in the literature regarding CRS plus HIPEC results.

C. Vallicelli (✉)
Department of Surgery and Advanced Oncological Therapies,
"G.B. Morgagni- L. Pierantoni" Hospital,
Forlì, Italy
e-mail: carlovallicelli@hotmail.it

A. Di Giorgio, E. Pinto (Eds), *Treatment of Peritoneal Surface Malignancies*,
Updates in Surgery
DOI: 10.1007/978-88-470-5711-1_15,

15.2 Accredited Centers

The combined procedure of CRS plus HIPEC requires a high level of scientific knowledge and proven surgical skills. Furthermore, the complexity of the procedure demands integrated postoperative care. Therefore, patients with PC must be treated in qualified centers. Surgeons who treat these patients must attain a specific learning curve, as must all personnel involved in the patient's care. Enhancing the cultural background and practical experience of a center and achieving overall excellence, including in terms of organization, is mandatory for successfully performing such complex procedures. Glehen et al. report data collected from a multi-institutional study (25 institutions) related to a curative treatment of 1,290 patients with PC from nonovarian origin using CRS plus HIPEC. The authors noted that surgical center greatly affects not only survival but also morbidity and mortality rates. The study found that center environment is an independent predictor for postoperative complications ($p < 0.0001$) and influences prognosis: institutions or centers in which practitioner experience exceeds 7 years produce better survival rates ($p < 0.001$) [1]. Surgical studies of major scientific relevance come from high-volume-activity centers [2–5]. Efficiency and efficacy of centers treating peritoneal surface malignancies (PSM) are also based on availability of advanced technologies and multidisciplinary teamwork. Hospitals that attain a high level of trained experience must be considered as referral centers (hub units) by other local or national hospitals in order to ensure standardized and verified treatment protocols and avoid local differences in treatment delivery. Data collection from hub centers in national shared databases is highly recommended to enrich single-center experiences and to match results. Appropriate health-care planning by regional or local authorities is needed to promote strategic integration in clinical and oncological networks and to improve activity volume and quality in accredited PSM treatment centers.

15.3 Treating Peritoneal Carcinomatosis

Treating primary or secondary PC from ovarian (OC), colorectal (CRC), gastric (GC) cancers, and cancer of other origins is a relatively young experience compared with other well-standardized surgical procedures. Significant skills and standardized working protocols can be gained after the first 100 procedures: Approximately 140–150 cases are deemed to be necessary for the treating physician to acquire competence in CRS plus HIPEC with adequate radicality and acceptable safety; 80–100 cases are also deemed necessary to assure short-term prognostic gains in rare PSM [6]. Health-care personnel, both physicians and nurses, involved in this procedure must be adequately trained and qualified through internships in specific centers with proven experience. A multidisciplinary surgical oncological approach to PC is essential, because treatment requires a strictly integrated collaboration between surgeon and oncologist, who together must coordinate all treatment phases and the other involved specialists.

Multidisciplinary meetings in which each individual case is studied and discussed and in which the patient must also be involved are mandatory to reach the correct therapeutic decision. Patient participation to the final strategy workup is essential because only very close cooperation ensures patient compliance to what are sometimes very long-lasting and intensive treatment protocols. A close relationship and awareness must exist among units (anesthesiology, medical oncology, intensive care, surgery, pathology, pharmacy) in the same hospital. The choice of chemotherapeutic drug is based on primary cancer type. Specific programs calculate the dose and perfusate volume based on the patient's body surface area (BSA). Preparation and delivery of these items by the hospital pharmacy is subject to confirmation by the surgical team according to cytoreduction score obtained from results of surgery [7, 8]. Data must be carefully collected from patients and procedures and should always include personal identification data; surgical procedure [date, duration, Peritoneal Cancer Index (PCI), Completeness of Cytoreduction (CC) score, number and type of surgical procedures, number of anastomoses performed, whether or not an ostomy was created, previous surgery for laparoscopy staging]; the primary neoplasm; post-surgery recovery (length of hospital stay, grade of any complications, relative treatment); follow-up (adjuvant therapy, global survival rate, disease-free survival rate, relapse, treatment). If possible, chemosensitivity tests are useful [9].

Standardized, optimized preoperative patient assessment protocols are mandatory and must be evaluated with other specialists and units in every hospital. In recent years, PSM centers have established dedicated, well-standardized preoperative diagnostic and assessment methods for treating these patients. Diagnosis and treatment start in the centralized surgical day service. Preoperative evaluation includes blood count and blood chemistry, including renal function and tumor markers. Full-body computed tomography (CT) with integrated positron emission tomography (PET) scan and—on a case-by-case basis—abdominopelvic magnetic resonance imaging (MRI) and gastrointestinal (GI) endoscopy are performed. Laparoscopic staging and PCI assessment are highly recommended before surgery. Heart and respiratory functions are carefully evaluated, and an echocardiogram is always performed. If necessary, psychological support is also provided. When needed, and enterostomy specialist provides adequate support to guarantee ostomy toleration and autonomous management by the patient. The day before surgery, bowel preparation is achieved.

Specific antibiotic and antimycotic prophylaxis must be delivered to the patient before surgery, and specific protocols have been developed in agreement with infectious disease specialists. The following drugs are administered on the day prior to surgery: fluconazole 400 mg orally, Ceftazidime 2 g IV at 8 a.m. and 8 p.m., metronidazole 500 mg at 8 a.m. and 8 p.m., colimycin 2 million IU three times a day, tobramycin 75 mg three times a day. On the days of surgery and after surgery, the following is administered: fluconazole 400 mg, ceftazidime 2 g at 8 a.m. and 8 p.m., metronidazole 500 mg four times a day. Prophylaxis for thromboembolic injury includes low-molecular-weight heparin (enoxaparin sodium 4,000 IU) administered on the eve of surgery and continued for 30 days after discharge. While still in the OR, the patient is fitted with intermittent-pressure compression boots, which will be removed when the patient is mobile. At least 4 U of blood and 3 U of plasma must be available for the procedure.

On the day of surgery, preoperative preparation includes central venous catheter (CVC) placement and bilateral mono-J ureteral stent placement when the pelvis is massively involved and upstream ureter lumen dilated, especially in patients with OC. Ureteral stents are removed after surgery. During surgery, in addition to antibiotics provided by the protocol, methylprednisolone 4 g is administered [10]. CRS includes multiple visceral resections and peritonectomies conducted according to Sugarbaker criteria [11, 12]. Immediate postoperative care includes an initial stay in the intensive care unit (ICU) for at least 24–72 h. The patient receives hypercaloric total parenteral nutrition by CVC and/or enteral nutrition when needed. All patients are assessed by the clinical nutrition service to create a tailored diet. Respiratory physiotherapy is begun early. The patient enters a medical and oncological treatment follow-up of at least 5 years.

15.4 HIPEC: Perioperative Procedure and Safety

We developed a checklist to improve patient safety and reduce perioperative morbidity and mortality rates [13] by adapting government guidelines to the specificity of CRS plus HIPEC because of surgical complexity and duration. Complexity pertains to the surgical procedures connected with peritonectomy and the integrated locoregional treatment, which requires using different surgical devices. Duration may entail a personnel change because of shifts. This requires creating and using a checklist of specific questions during the sign-in and time-out phases and documenting that the information is passed on to the next shift in the OR. Therefore, gauzes and surgical instruments are counted at the end of the cytoreductive procedure, before perfusion and when anastomoses are performed after HIPEC, before laparotomy suture. Sign out is essential. It is the third and the last phase in the checklist, the phase in which information is passed to personnel who will treat the patient in the postsurgical phase. Any problems in the performance of major surgical devices in CRS plus HIPEC are reported. Therefore, testing the perfusion device the night before is essential.

Several perfusion techniques have been described in relation to HIPEC, but the most frequently used are the open and closed coliseum techniques [14]. During HIPEC, it is mandatory to monitor temperature continuously to adjust the incoming temperature and perfusate volume. Perfusion duration and chemotherapy drug type depend on the patient's diagnosis; contemporary administration of kidney-function-preserving drugs, such as amifostine, may be useful [15]. Maintaining the patient's thermal homeostasis during the entire surgery, particularly during the HIPEC phase, is of critical importance. Following

HIPEC induction, heat loss must be reduced using low-flow fresh gas and actively warming up the patient by infusing heated liquids and using a thermal drape. Thirty minutes prior to hyperthermic perfusion, active warming up is suspended. During hyperthermic perfusion, if needed, the patient's temperature may be lowered with a refrigerated helmet, cold infusions, and refrigerated packs placed on the carotid arteries. If body temperature reaches 38°C, the surgical team is alerted; at 40°C, suspending the procedure is mandatory. The closed technique is preferred for a more uniform thermal conservation, the need for fewer personnel, minimizing environmental exposure to chemotherapeutic drugs and fumes, for increasing tissue drug penetration, and distribution provided by perfusate pressure.

Despite many centers preferring the coliseum technique for optimal thermal consistency and spatial distribution [16, 17], there is no general agreement or guidelines regarding this issue. One of the disadvantages of the open technique is that the open abdomen inevitably causes heat dissipation, making it more difficult to reach hyperthermia with high temperatures. Also, surgical personnel are more exposed to the chemotherapy drug, although no trial has reported an increased risk of drug exposure [18–20]. Regardless, there is the clear need to implement all possible precautions to avoid any environmental or personnel contamination. Precautionary measures must be taken in preparing the operating theater. We use nonwoven fabric towels and disposable Mayor pillowcases. A Steri-Drape is positioned to prevent the patient's skin coming into contact with the chemotherapy drug. Before starting the HIPEC procedure, a fluid-collection bag is placed under the drainage tubes. The scrub nurse and operating-room nurse perform a partial count of gauzes and surgical instruments, cover the serving trays with disposable towels, and ensure that all personnel in the OR are wearing protective gowns.

HIPEC in the open modality is performed by one of the operating surgeons. Other personnel are positioned away from the surgical table. If perfusion lasts longer than 30 min, the surgeon performing this procedure is replaced by another. The surgeon performs intra-abdominal manipulation of the antiblastic mixture wearing protection devices that include nonwoven fabric disposable head covering and footwear, goggles with side protection, filtering face mask, disposable sterile gown with reinforced sleeves and front, disposable closure, disposable sterile long-sleeve gloves, all of which must be free of dust, deproteinized, and be specific for antiblastic handling. The surgeon performing the procedure wears two pairs of gloves, which are replaced every 30 min. Environmental protection devices include the Coliseum cover in PVC to create an artificial enclosed chamber. In our center, we routinely use an electric scalpel connected with a suction system during the entire cytoreductive phase and a fumes aspiration system during the entire abdominal chemotherapy perfusion. We use a disposable, single-patient filter. Therefore, the fumes aspirator placed close to the Coliseum cover draws the vapors from the antiblastic mixture that comes up from the laparotomy. The fumes aspirator is enough in terms of environment

Table 15.1 Common recommendations for operating room safety during hyperthermic peritoneal chemotherapy (HIPEC)

Procedural safety recommendations	
Surgical field	Use of disposable drapes (not textile cloth)
Operating room	Closed door, access restriction, prevent of possible spills
Caregivers	Disposable impervious gown and shoe covers; double gloves, the outer to be changed every 30 min; eye goggles; high-power filtration mask
Environment	Ventilation, smoke evacuator over surgical field
Residue	Rigid dedicated containers during and 48-h after HIPEC

protection because the vapors of the antiblastic drug rise to < 5 cm from the edge of the cut. At the end of the procedure, the remaining chemotherapy drug is disposed of in a closed-circuit system or by aspirators equipped with a disposable container. The residue, including antiblastic material and the final flush, are disposed of in ad hoc containers. OR personnel who are not involved in chemotherapy perfusion never come in contact with devices and/or substances containing antiblastic medication.

Following HIPEC, patient blood and body fluids are considered contaminated for 48 h. Body fluids and postsurgery drain fluids are treated with the same precautions used during the procedure. Drainage and urine collection bags are disposed of in ad hoc containers. In case of accidental personnel contamination, protocols provide for specific procedure and emergency response is determined if chemotherapy drug diffusion occurs. The OR is equipped with an emergency kit containing all that is needed to safely remove the chemotherapy drug and reclaim the environment. Environmental and biological sampling to determine the presence of antiblastic chemotherapy drugs from items such as gloves, air, urine, or blood of OR personnel may be considered in order to determine the safety of working conditions.

Many recent studies contributed to confirm that chemotherapy exposure during CRS plus HIPEC is absent or of acceptable limkits according established safety standards in the United States and Europe [20–22]. Recommendations regarding OR safety during HIPEC reported by Gonzales Moreno et al. [23] may useful and are summarized in Table 15.1.

15.5 Costs

The *International Classification of Diseases*, 9th revision, Clinical Modification (ICD-9-CM) does not include the many surgical procedures distinctive of peritonectomy, except visceral resections. Neither does it include coding for abdominal-cavity hyperthermic perfusion with antiblastic drugs. Therefore, the

Hospital Discharge Form, a data-collection tool for patients discharged from public and private health-care structures in Italy, does not adequately evaluate the economic commitment of CRS plus HIPEC. Furthermore, the form reports no more than six procedures, and in many cases, it is difficult to prioritize procedures, which most of the time exceed six. In specialized literature, interest in HIPEC costs is significantly lower than interest in its medical outcome, although issues concerning this matter have been raised in recent years. Baratti et al. [24] assessed the cost of > 380 CRS plus HIPEC procedures performed at the Milan National Cancer Institution from 1995 to 2008, comparing it to reimbursement obtained in the last 2 years. The authors calculated that the average cost for each individual hospitalization was €36,015.89 (range €28,435.24–82,189.08), with a total cost in 2007–2008, of €2,665,185.29. Total reimbursement in those 2 years was €804,483.30, resulting in a loss of €1,861,301.99. It is therefore clear that in Italy, a project for treating PC does not receive adequate financial and institutional support.

In fact, the Italian Classification of Diagnosis-Related Groups (DRGs) does not include CRS or HIPEC. Therefore, hospitals that treat patients with PC must bear this economic deficit. We analyzed the costs in our hospital and determined the cost of the material needed for CRS was €2,792.51 per procedure (without considering staplers), for a diagnostic laparoscopy was €553.14, and for the kit for a single HIPEC procedure was €1,098. Considering mean operative times, the cost of OR personnel (surgeons, anesthesiologist, nurses) was €3,434.12. Moreover, the cost of the OR itself, excluding personnel, and the sterilization procedure was €2,048.86. Evaluating mean ICU and hospital stay, the cost was €13,247.45 per patient. Finally, the cost of preoperative examination of each patient was €1,229.45. The hospital must assume this economic deficit. In France, where the health system is similar to Italy, a similar test was conducted [25]. The authors calculated that the average cost for a single hospitalization was €39,358 (costs for HIPEC administration were excluded). Reimbursement from the health system was €20,485 on average, with a loss of €18,873 per patient. Over a period of 2 years, the deficit was €1,400,000, which is significantly lower than the deficit calculated for Italy. Costs are closely connected to surgery but also to the duration of the hospital stay and therefore to any postoperative complication [25].

The CRS plus HIPEC technique is sometimes criticized, despite expanding scientific evidence of its value, because of its high costs. An Australian analysis [26] compared the cost of CRS plus HIPEC with the cost of lifetime palliative care for PC patients. The analysis of the cost per life-year saved allowed the authors to consider HIPEC as a cost-effective treatment for patients with PC from appendiceal tumor, CC, pseudomyxoma peritonei (PMP), and malignant peritoneal mesothelioma (MPM), and possibly also from other etiologies. Cost analyses also emphasize the need to centralize treatments in tertiary referral centers. In analyzing the per CRS plus HIPEC procedure costs for PC from advanced OC origin in centers with more or less experience, Bristow et al. indicated that there is an incremental cost-effectiveness ratio of US $17,149 per quality-adjusted life year gained with referral to an experienced center [27].

15.6 Data Collection and Study Protocols

HIPEC is now the standard of care in treating PMP, MPM, and CRC with limited peritoneal involvement [28]. With regard to colorectal carcinomatosis, there are different attitudes in international guidelines: the US National Cancer Institute (NCI) does not even mention HIPEC among treatment options, whereas French guidelines recommend it. An ongoing randomized trial, protocol IOV-CAR-CRC-1-2012, in Italy evaluates the role of CRS plus HIPEC compared with systemic chemotherapy in resectable CRC PC. HIPEC is in the evaluation phase for PC from OC and GRC, but it is probably useful in particular settings [28]. Two ongoing trials in Italy are evaluating the effectiveness of CRS plus HIPEC in PC from OC: The CHORINE study (Cytoreduction and HIPEC in the treatment of OvaRIaN cancer) is a prospective randomized trial that evaluates stage III unresectable epithelial ovarian/tubal cancer with partial or complete response after first-line neoadjuvant chemotherapy with three cycles of carboplatin (CBDCA) and paclitaxel. The trial compares CRS versus CRS plus HIPEC, both treatment modalities being followed by three cycles of CBDCA and paclitaxel. The Italian Hyperthermic Intra-peritoneal Chemotherapy in Ovarian Cancer Recurrence (HORSE) trial is a prospective randomized study that compares CRS with or without HIPEC in the first recurrence of OC, if platinum sensitive. Further trials are necessary to improve evidence.

Most trials supporting the importance of CRS plus HIPEC are multi-institutionally based [29–35]. This indicates the importance of study protocols for data collection. A protocol must be adequately organized, structured, and shared by the various participating centers. The objective is to evaluate what impact this treatment has on patient survival in terms of disease-free (DFS) and overall (OS) survival. A fundamental and specific element of the HIPEC research protocol is timing the investigation of the procedure. For example, in order to assess the effectiveness of CRS plus HIPEC in patients with OC, this therapy may be studied in the various stages of the cancer's natural history. Patient inclusion and exclusion criteria for the study must be shared among the various centers. Sampling size required to achieve the specified objectives must be established. Therefore, the minimum number of cases each center has to present for data collection should be established. Data to be reported and made available in the patient's medical history file must be established and shared. Presurgery data (past treatment, histological diagnosis, any relapse), intrasurgery data (PCI, CC score, procedures performed, chemotherapy drug used for HIPEC), and post-surgery data (morbidity and mortality, follow-up) must be assessed.

The informed consent issue is of critical importance. Patients must be provided with a thorough oral explanation and with written documentation. The patient must be fully aware of the study objectives and the reason he/she was selected to be enrolled. Enrollment shall take place only after the informed consent is signed, and all patient agreement must be on a voluntary basis. It must be specified that if the patient does not want to be enrolled in the study, he/she will still receive the best possible medical treatment based on available scientific evidence. Data confidentiality must be guaranteed, and it must be made clear to the patient that the study protocol was assessed and approved by an ethics committee.

References

1. Glehen O, Gilly FN, Boutitie F et al (2010) Toward curative treatment of peritoneal carcinomatosis from non-ovarian origin by cytoreductive surgery combined with perioperative intraperitoneal chemotherapy: a multi-institutional study of 1290 patients. Cancer 116:5608-5618
2. Deraco M, Kusamura S, Laterza B et al (2006) Cytoreductive surgery and hyperthermic intra-peritoneal chemotherapy (HIPEC) for the treatment of pseudomixoma peritonei: ten years experience in a single center. In Vivo 20:773-776
3. Baratti D, Kusamura S, Nonaka D et al (2009) Pseudomixoma peritonei: biological features are the dominant prognostic determinants after complete cytoreduction and hyperthermic intraperitoneal chemotherapy. Ann Surg 249:243-249
4. Verwaal VJ, van Ruth S, de Bree E et al (2003) Randomized trial of cytoreduction and hyperthermic intraperitoneal chemotherapy versus systemic chemotherapy and palliative surgery in patients with peritoneal carcinomatosis of colorectal cancer. J Clin Oncol 21:3737-3743
5. Elias D, Lefevre JH, Chevalier J et al (2009) Complete cytoreductive surgery plus intraperitoneal chemohyperthermia with oxaliplatino for peritoneal carcinomatosis of colorectal origin. J Clin Oncol 27:681-685
6. Kusamura S, Baratti D, Hutanu I et al. (2012) The importance of the learning curve and surveillance of surgical performance in peritoneal surface malignancy programs. Surg Oncol Clin N Am 21:559-576
7. Jacquet P, Sugarbaker PH (1996) Current methodologies for clinical assessment of patients with peritoneal carcinomatosis. J Exp Clin Cancer Res 15:49-58
8. Sugarbaker PH (1996) Complete parietal and visceral peritonectomy of the pelvis for advanced primary and recurrent ovarian cancer. In: Sugarbaker P, editor. Peritoneal carcinomatosis: drugs and diseases. Boston, Kluwer Academic Publishers, pp. 75–86
9. Arienti C, Tesei A, Verdecchia GM et al (2013) Role of conventional chemosensitivity test and tissue biomarker expression in predicting response to treatment of peritoneal carcinomatosis from colon cancer. Clin Colorectal Cancer 12:122-127
10. Sumida M, Inaba H, Isawa E et al (1999) Prevention by Methylprednisolone of increased circulating tumor necrosis factor-α and lung injury associated with systemic infiammatory response syndrome due to intraperitoneal hyperthermia. Anesth Analg 88:771-776
11. Sugarbaker PH (1995) Peritonectomy procedures. Ann Surg 21:29–42
12. Sugarbaker PH (1999) Management of peritoneal-surface malignancy: the surgeons role. Langenbecks Arch Surg 384:576–587
13. www.salute.gov.it
14. Glehen O, Cotte E, Kusamura S et al (2008) Hyperthermic intraperitoneal chemotherapy: nomenclature and modalities of perfusion. J Surg Oncol 98:242-246
15. Vaira M, Barone R, Aghemo B et al (2001) Renal protection with amifostine during intraoperative peritoneal chemiohyperthermia with cisplatin (CDDP) for peritoneal carcinomatosis. Phase I trial. Minerva Med 92:207-211
16. Elias D, Goere D, Blot F et al (2007) Optimization of hyperthermic intraperitoneal chemotherapy with oxaliplatin plus irinotecan at 43 degrees C after complete cytoreductive surgery: mortality and morbidity in 106 consecutive patients. Ann Surg Oncol 14:1818-1824

17. Stephens AD, Alderman R, Chang D et al (1999) Morbidity and mortality analysis of 200 treatments with cytoreductive surgery and hyperthermic intraperitoneal chemotherapy using the coliseum technique. Ann Surg Oncol 6:790-796
18. Stuart OA, Stephens AD, Welch L et al (2002) Safety monitoring of the Coliseum technique for heated intraoperative chemotherapy with mitomycin C. Ann Surg Oncol 9:186-191
19. Guerbet M, Goulle JP, Lubrano J (2007) Evaluation of the risk of contamination of surgical personnel by vaporization of Oxaliplatin during the intraoperative hyperthermic intraperitoneal chemotherapy. Eur J Surg Oncol 33:623-626
20. Schmid K, Boettcher MI, Pelz JO et al (2006) Investigations on safety of hyperthermic intraoperative intraperitoneal chemotherapy (HIPEC) with mitomycin C. Eur J Surg Oncol 32:1222-1225
21. Stuart OA, Stephens AD, Welch L et al (2002) Safety monitoring of the coliseum technique for heated intraoperative intraperitoneal chemotherapy with mytomicin C. Ann Surg Oncol 9:186-191
22. Naslund Andreasson S, Anundi H, Thoren SB et al (2010) Is platinum present in the blood and urine from treatment givers during hypothermic intraperitoneal chemotherapy? J Oncol 2010:649-719
23. Gonzales Moreno S, Gonzales Bayon L, Ortega Perez G (2012) Hyperthermic Intraperitoneal Chemotherapy. Methodology and safety considerations. Surg Oncol Clin N Am 21:543-557
24. Baratti D, Scivales A, Balestra MR et al (2010) Cost analysis of the combined procedure of cytoreductive surgery and hyperthermic intraperitoneal chemotherapy (HIPEC). Eur J Surg Oncol 36:463-469
25. Bonastre J, Jan P, de Pouvourville G et al (2005) Cost of an intraperitoneal hyperthermia related to cytoreductive surgery. Ann Chir 130:553-561
26. Chua TC, Martin S, Saxena A et al (2010) Evaluation of the cost-effectiveness of cytoreductive surgery and hyperthermic intraperitoneal chemotherapy (peritonectomy) at the St George Hospital peritoneal surface malignancy program. Ann Surg 251:323-329
27. Bristow RE, Santillan A, Diaz-Montes TP et al (2007) Centralization of care for patients with advanced-stage ovarian cancer: a cost-effectiveness analysis. Cancer 109:1513-1522
28. Elias D, Goerè D, Dumont F et al (2014) Role of hyperthermic intraoperative peritoneal chemotherapy in the management of peritoneal metastasis. Eur J Cancer 50:332-340
29. Kuijpers AMJ, Mirck B, Aalbers AGJ et al (2013) Cytoreduction and HIPEC in the Netherlands: nationwide long-term outcome following the Dutch protocol. Ann Surg Oncol 20:4224-4230
30. Glehen O, Gilly FN, Boutitie F et al (2010) Toward curative treatment of peritoneal carcinomatosis from non-ovarian origin by cytoreductive surgery combined with perioperative intraperitoneal chemotherapy: a multi-institutional study of 1290 patients. Cancer 116:5608-5618
31. Elias D, Gilly F, Boutitie F et al (2010) Peritoneal colorectal carcinomatosis treated with surgery and perioperative intraperitoneal chemotherapy: retrospective analysis of 523 patients from a multicentric French study. J Clin Oncol 28:63-68
32. Yan TD, Deraco M, Baratti D et al (2009) Cytoreductive surgery and hyperthermic intraperitoneal chemotherapy for malignant peritoneal mesotelioma: multi-institutional experience. J Clin Oncol 27:6237-6242
33. Chua TC, Moran BJ, Sugarbaker PH et al (2012) Early- and long-term outcome data of patients with pseudomixoma peritonei from appendiceal origin treated by a strategy of cytoreductive surgery and hyperthermic intraperitoneal chemotherapy. J Clin Oncol 30:2449-2456
34. Glehen O, Gilly FN, Boutitie F et al (2010) Toward curative treatment of peritoneal carcinomatosis from nonovarian origin by cytoreductive surgery combined with perioperative intraperitoneal chemotherapy: a multi-institutional study of 1290 patients. Cancer 116:5608-5618
35. Deraco M, Kusamura S, Virzì S et al (2011) Cytoreductive surgery and hyperthermic intraperitoneal chemotherapy as upfront therapy for advanced epithelial ovarian cancer: multi-institutional phase II trial. Gynaecol Oncol 122:215-220

Part III

Results of Integrated Treatment

16 Pseudomyxoma Peritonei

Marco Vaira, Manuela Robella, Alfredo Mellano,
and Michele De Simone

16.1 Introduction

Pseudomyxoma peritonei (PMP) is a rare, low-grade, peritoneal malignancy predominated by mucus, with an estimated incidence of two to three cases per million people per year [1]. Werth, in 1884, first described PMP as a rare, unusual reaction of the peritoneum to a jelly-like substance, looking like a myxoma, in relation to an ovarian neoplasm [2]. In 1901, Frankel described PMP associated with an appendiceal cyst [3], but the first description of a benign mucocele of the appendix was reported by Rokitansky in 1842 [4].

PMP is thought to originate in most cases from the rupture of an appendiceal mucinous neoplasm. It is characterized by the slow and progressive extracellular accumulation of mucin and epithelial mucin-secreting cells in the peritoneal cavity; over time, this syndrome results in massive symptomatic distension and associated mechanical and functional gastrointestinal obstruction [5]. Experimental studies by Cheng et al. illustrate that obstruction of the appendix by tumor is necessary for PMP development. The authors created appendiceal mucoceles in rabbits by ligation only, with sterile perforation, and the rabbits did not develop PMP [6, 7].

The pathogenesis of PMP has long been debated: mucinous adenocarcinoma originating from large bowel, ovary, or other intra-abdominal sites may mimic PMP [8]. Synchronous ovarian metastases are not uncommon, and PMP of appendiceal origin can be confused with primary ovarian cancer [9]. Immunohistochemical [10], genetic [11] and pathological [12] studies now provide substantial evidence that in the vast majority of cases, the appendix

M. Robella (✉)
Oncology Surgery Unit,
Candiolo Cancer Instutute, Candiolo (TO), Italy
e-mail: manuela.robella@hotmail.it

A. Di Giorgio, E. Pinto (Eds), *Treatment of Peritoneal Surface Malignancies*,
Updates in Surgery
DOI: 10.1007/978-88-470-5711-1_16,

can be identified as the origin [11, 13]. Immunohistochemical markers creatinine kinases CK7, 18, and 20 may be useful to distinguish primary ovarian neoplasms from metastases by determining their intestinal origin: in PMP, immunoreactivity is particularly positive for CK18 and 20, whereas CK7 is mostly negative [14–17]. CK20, caudal type homebox trascription factor – 2 (CDx-2), and MUC-2 expression seems to be correlated to prognosis [18]. True PMP of ovarian origin has been associated with mature cystic teratomas and is often associated with CK7-positive reaction [19, 20].

16.2 Definition

In 1996, Sugarbaker strictly defined PMP as a grade 1 mucinous adenocarcinoma arising from an adenoma of the appendix [5, 21]. However, within the pathology literature, there was early recognition that the clinicopathologic entity of PMP could be classified into subtypes with different clinical outcomes and histopathologic findings. Ronnet and colleagues proposed a classification distinguishing disseminated peritoneal adenomucinosis (DPAM), arising from a primitive adenoma of the appendix, from peritoneal mucinous carcinomatosis (PMCA), arising from an appendicular adenocarcinoma of the appendix. DPAM represents the classic PMP, with paucicellular mucinous ascites and an indolent clinical course; PMCA has a higher percentage of overtly malignant cells and poorer prognosis. A refined system, in which PMCA was further divided into PMCA and PMCA-I (intermediate), subclassified carcinomas into lesions that would behave more like traditional colorectal cancer (PMCA) and those more likely to have a progressive indolent course (PMCA-I) [12]. However, Ronnett's classification is to date the most frequently used and is reported in the majority of papers in the literature. Most recent purposed classifications are, at least, simplified models: Misdraji et al. classified appendiceal mucinous tumors into low-grade appendiceal mucinous neoplasms (LAMN) and high-grade mucinous adenocarcinomas (MACA) [22]. In 2009, Renehan et al. purposed a classification for precursor lesions of disseminated PMP, the so-called LAMN, subcategorized into LAMN-I (disease confined in the appendiceal lumen), and LAMN-II (Fig. 16.1) (disease in the appendiceal wall or periappendiceal tissue) [23]. In 2010, the American Joint Committee on Cancer (AJCC) and the World Health Organization (WHO) divided PMP into high-grade or low-grade MACA on the basis of the grade of the epithelial cells within the peritoneal mucin [24, 25]. Two particular subsets of disease are represented by signet-ring-cell tumor and goblet-cell carcinoids of the appendix. Those two entities are, in the majority of cases, considered to behave similarly to high-grade tumors, and aggressive treatment is usually recommended [22, 26, 27].

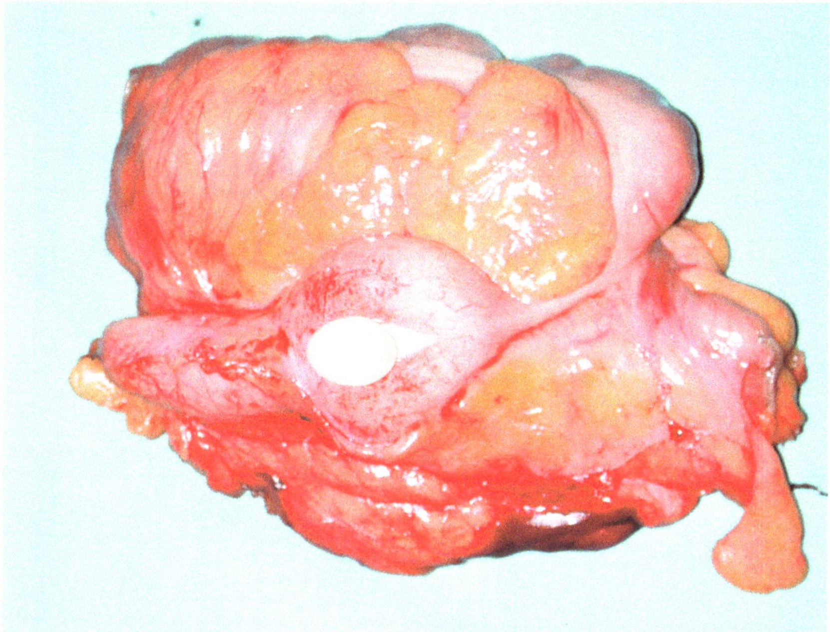

Fig. 16.1 Perforated appendiceal tumor [low-grade appendiceal mucinous neoplasms (LAMN II)]

16.3 Clinical Features

PMP usually manifests with the characteristic jelly belly (Fig. 16.2) appearance, represented by the advanced stage of disease, when most of the abdomen is filled with mucinous ascites and tumor. In fact, cancer cells deposit throughout the entire peritoneal cavity, in contrast to nonmucinous colorectal cancer, where the first metastases are often found near the primary tumor [28]. This kind of presentation can be explained by the so-called redistribution phenomenon consisting of a dissemination pattern associated with intraperitoneal fluid current and gravity. The mobility of the small bowel probably explains why mucus and tumor cells adhere significantly less frequently at these sites, in contrast to more fixed parts, such as antrum, ileocecal region, and rectosigmoid, which are usually massively surrounded by mucus. Usually, patients at this stage present abdominal distension and pain related to obstruction due to the excessive amount of mucinous material. PMP can also manifest with localizing symptoms mimicking acute appendicitis. In female patients, the initial symptoms may be pelvic pressure and palpable ovarian masses. In some cases, mucinous aggregates are discovered incidentally in surgical specimens, such as hernia sacs, thus necessitating the search for the primary neoplasms [29]. Hematogenic or lymphatic dissemination of PMP tumor cells is rare [5, 30–36]

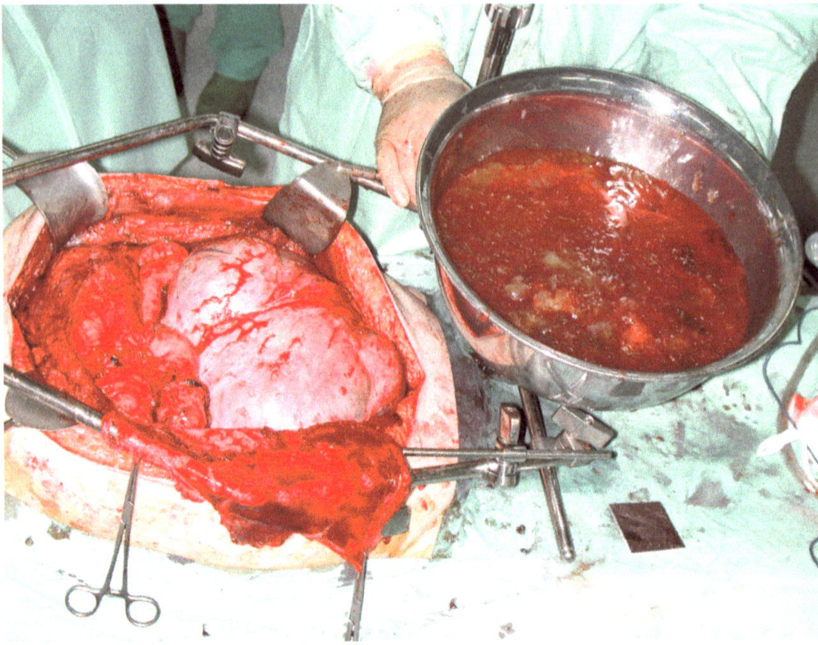

Fig. 16.2 Disseminated peritoneal adenomucinosis [DPAM (jelly belly)]

16.4 Diagnosis

Most patients will have increases in serum tumor markers carbohydrate antigen (CA) 19.9, and carcinoembryonic antigen (CEA), which are useful for both diagnosis and, above all, managing treatment efficacy and recurrence following therapy [37]. Many studies report that preoperative CEA and CA-19.9 levels are useful in predicting disease extent (peritoneal cancer index [PCI]) and surgical success, as well as progression-free (PFS) and overall survival (OS) in patients treated with cytoreductive surgery and hyperthermic intraperitoneal chemotherapy (HIPEC) [38–40] CA-125 is not widely used as a tumor marker for PMP, as it is known to be elevated in a range of benign and inflammatory diseases, thus influencing its specificity. The diagnostic sensitivity of CA-125 for PMP has been examined and approached 60% [41]; the elevated value of this tumor marker seems to be predictive of completeness of cytoreduction and disease-free survival (DFS) [18, 40, 42]. Imaging by ultrasound (US) can be misleading, because the paucicellular mucinous ascites resemble free intraperitoneal fluid [37]; in this case, computed tomography (CT) may be more helpful in preoperative planning by demonstrating the extent of disease. Magnetic resonance imaging (MRI) is scarcely described [43]. Positron emission tomography (PET) in combination with CT might be useful for predicting peritoneal metastasis of high-grade cases [44].

Explorative laparoscopy is an important tool in the diagnosis process: it provides a wide view of the entire abdominal cavity without a large laparotomy, and it may be helpful for definitive histological diagnosis of PMP in patients in whom a primary disease site is not identified. Moreover, laparoscopy allows detection of peritoneal dissemination and establishing ileus involvement from carcinomatosis, which may contraindicate a further laparotomy with curative intent.

16.5 Treatment

Although tumor masses of PMP are often not locally invasive, the mucin is locally destructive. PMP was once treated by iterative debulking operations, which attained unsatisfactory results. Relapses occurred in most cases, and repeated surgeries were more challenging when the disease progressed and scarring, adhesions and distortion of the anatomy developed [45]. A recent study reported the outcome differences between debulking surgery and CRS, both followed by HIPEC, in patients with PMP: CRS and HIPEC were the most efficient treatment modalities, even though associated with a higher morbidity [46].

A serial debulking protocol in patients with limited low-grade appendiceal PMP resulted in a 10-year overall survival of 21–32% [47–49]. Patients with adenocarcinoma who underwent debulking surgery were reported to have a 5-year survival rate of 6% [50] associated with a 30-day postoperative mortality rate of 2.7% [47].

As a result of pioneering work by Sugarbaker, CRS associated with HIPEC have become the mainstays of treatment for PMP [51]. The aim of surgery is complete cytoreduction, as described by Sugarbaker [52], which involves up to six different peritonectomies in combination with visceral resections to remove all macroscopic tumor or, if this is not possible, to leave tumor deposits <2.5 mm [53]. HIPEC attempts to eliminate microscopic residual disease; complete cytoreduction is attempted, especially at the first operation, as intraperitoneal chemotherapy is used selectively in patients who are able to undergo complete or near-complete surgical cytoreduction.

Chemotherapeutic agents, dosage, temperature, and duration of intraperitoneal chemotherapy have not been subject to randomized trials but have been chosen according to knowledge regarding agents' intraperitoneal pharmacokinetics. The commonly used intraoperative agents are mitomycin C (MMC), cisplatin, 5-fluorouracil (5-FU), or a combination of these, usually administered for 30–120 min [54]. For early postoperative intraperitoneal chemotherapy (EPIC), 5-FU, and cyclophosphamide are used for up to 6 days [53].

The cornerstone of successful PMP treatment is represented by correct diagnosis and appropriate treatment. Repeated debulking surgery in misdiagnosed disease, often associated with systemic chemotherapy and especially when performed for low-grade malignancies, leads to progressive decrease in intention-to-treat cytoreductive surgery plus HIPEC. Thus, it is mandatory to refer suspect or certain PMP to a trained center. In fact, despite this treatment strategy, the disease, especially if arising from high-grade primary tumors, may recur: early detection of relapse may provide the opportunity for a further complete CRS plus HIPEC, which may prolong survival [55].

16.5.1 Hyperthermic Intraperitoneal Chemotherapy (HIPEC)

There are two main procedures by which to deliver HIPEC: the open-abdomen technique described by Sugarbaker (coliseum technique) and the closed abdomen technique [56]. No significant differences in terms of results between the two techniques are reported in the literature.

Originally, we perform a semiclosed HIPEC technique (using the computer-assisted perfusion system PERFORMER HT, Rand), which avoids exposing surgical personnel to chemotherapeutic drugs and could reduce the dissipation that occurs with the coliseum technique, allowing the surgeon to mix the perfusate solution and visually check the peritoneal cavity [57]. The protocols we use are based on administering cisplatinum (CDDP) 100 mg/m^2 plus MMC 16 mg/m^2 at a temperature of 41.5° C, or MMC as single drug at 35mg/m^2 for 60 min at a temperature of 40.5°C, according to the Netherland protocol [58].

16.6 Results

16.6.1 Literature Analysis

Recent evidence suggests that optimal surgical resection (complete cytoreduction if possible) combined with HIPEC is the most fundamentally based strategy for treating PMP. Although this treatment is still associated with a major risk of morbidity, the increase in survival may be acceptable when proposing an alternative to debulking procedures alone. As presented in a recent meta-analysis on the improved survival rate of patients with PMP receiving cytoreductive surgery and HIPEC, the mean mortality rate was 3.75 (median 2.45). The mean and median morbidity reported were 35.75 and 40.0, respectively. Mean 3-, 5-, and 10-year survival rates were 77.18%, 76.63%, and 57.3%, respectively. Median 3-, 5-, and 10-year survival rates were 77.85%, 79.5%, and 55.9%, respectively [59]. In Tables 16.1 and 16.2, the most recent and significant studies and related results in terms of outcome and postoperative complications are reported.

16.7 Our Experience

In our Institution, from 1995 to December 2013, ~800 operations for peritoneal carcinomatosis were performed, and in 350 cases, surgical cytoreduction asso-

Table 16.1 Cytoreductive surgery combined with perioperative intraperitoneal chemotherapy for pseudomyxoma peritonei

Study [Reference]	Median FU (months)	Size (*n*)	Median OS (months)	5-year OS (%)	10-year OS (%)	Median DFS (months)	5-year DFS (%)	10-year DFS (%)
Robella et al. (De Simone) 2013 [60]	35	80	144	89	78.5	88	82	68
Arjona-Sanchez et al. 2013 [61]	36	38	36	58.7		36		
Chua et al. 2012 [62] (multicentric)	36	2,298	196	74	63	98		
Sorensen et al. 2012 [63]		93	NR	79	69		58	47
Chua et al. 2011 [64]	34	113	104	79	47	48	47	
Youssef et al. 2011 [65]		456		69	57			
Elias et al. 2010 [66] (multicentric)	88	301	NR	72.6	54.8	78	56	
Alves et al. 2010 [67]		49						
Baratti et al. 2009 [18]	45	102		84.4	79		48.3	
Vaira et al. 2009 [68]		53		94	84		80	70
Elias et al. 2008 [69]	48	105		80.2		97	68.5	
Smeenk et al. 2007 [70]	51.5	103		59.5		25.6	37.4	
Bradley et al. 2006 [26]	101			57				
Gonzalez-Moreno et al. 2006 [71]	48	501	156	71.9	54.5			
Sugarbaker et al. 2006 [72]	35	356						
Smeenk et al. 2006 [73]	35	103						
Deraco et al. 2003 [74] (multicentric)		70		91			54	

FU, follow-up; *OS*, overall survival; *DFS*, disease-free survival; *NR*, not reported

Table 16.2 Morbidity and mortality of cytoreductive surgery combined with perioperative intraperitoneal chemotherapy for pseudomyxoma peritonei

Study [Reference]	Procedure	Morbidity (%)	Mortality (%)
Robella et al. (De Simone) 2013 [60]	HIPEC	52.5	0
Arjona-Sanchez et al. 2013 [61]	HIPEC	18.4	0
Chua et al. 2012 [62] (multicentric)	HIPEC	24	2
Sorensen et al. 2012 [63]	HIPEC-EPIC	24	
Chua et al. 2011 [64]	HIPEC-EPIC	44	1
Youssef et al. 2011 [65]	HIPEC-EPIC	7	1,6
Elias et al. 2010 [66] (multicentric)	HIPEC-EPIC	40	4.4
Alves et al. 2010 [67]	HIPEC-EPIC	9	2
Baratti et al. 2009 [18]	HIPEC		0.98
Vaira et al. 2009 [68]	HIPEC	45	0
Elias et al. 2008 [69]	HIPEC	67.6	7.6
Smeenk et al. 2007 [70]	HIPEC	54	2.9
Bradley et al. 2006 [26]	HIPEC		
Gonzalez-Moreno et al. 2006 [71]	HIPEC-EPIC		
Sugarbaker et al. 2006 [72]	HIPEC-EPIC	40	2
Smeenk et al. 2006 [73]	HIPEC	54	3
Deraco et al. 2003 [74] (multicentric)	HIPEC	14	1.4

EPIC, early postoperative intraperitoneal chemotherapy; *HIPEC*, hyperthermic intraperitoneal chemotherapy

ciated with HIPEC were carried out. We operated about 200 patients presenting PMP; 107 of those underwent CRS plus HIPEC. Inclusion criteria for the procedure were the following:

- Presence of tumor confirmed by histology or cytology;
- Patients aged between 18 and 72 years;
- Performance status (PS) <2 according to the Eastern Cooperative Oncology Group (ECOG);
- No evidence of extraperitoneal disease;
- Absence of concomitant uncompensated cardiopulmonary, hepatic, renal, and metabolic disease;
- No prior abdominal radiotherapy for carcinomatosis or over a wide abdominal area.

Preoperative evaluation always included thoracic and abdominal CT scan to stage peritoneal disease and exclude distant metastases; upper digestive endoscopy and colonoscopy generally completed tumor staging. A careful preoperative evaluation of the patient's general conditions was always performed and included complete blood tests, electrocardiogram, cardiac US, and spirometry.

Follow-up data are available for 95 CRS plus HIPEC performed in 86 patients (11 patients were excluded because follow-up was too short or they were lost). With a median follow-up of 41.6 months (range 3–167 months), we reported a 5-

and 10-year OS of 81.6% and 67.9%, respectively. Median OS was not reached at 10 years. Five- and 10-year DFS were 61.5% and 45.8%, respectively, with a median of 72 months. Morbidity was 37.9% (36/95), with a major complications rate of 22.1% (21/95). Reoperations were required in 13.7% of cases (13/95), with no perioperative deaths. Our results in terms of OS, DFS, morbidity, and mortality rates are comparable with those reported in the literature.

Twenty-eight patients recurred (20 PMCA and 8 DPAM). Most patients relapsed within 2 years (median 23.7 months). A reiterative CRS was performed in 50% of cases, whereas eight patients were treated with a second CRS plus HIPEC; one patient underwent a third procedure.

Tumor histology (p=0.02), PCI >20 (p=0.074), and previous systemic chemotherapy (p=0.038) were identified in the univariate analysis as independent predictors for a poorer long-term OS. Preoperative systemic chemotherapy (p=0.008) and PCI >20 (p=0.001) have a strong negative impact on DFS. In our study, contrary to what is reported in the literature, complete cytoreduction (CC-0 vs CC-1) had a nonstatistically significant impact on outcome. This result may be due to our selection policy, as we do not perform HIPEC if a CC-2 or CC-3 surgical cytoreduction is obtained. In our casuistry, only 13 patients were CC-1; as a consequence, we did not report a statistically significant impact on OS and DFS regarding this factor.

The main prognostic factors influencing OS and DFS reported in the literature are:

- PCI
- Treatment center
- Pathology grade (PMCA vs DPAM)
- Gender
- Use of HIPEC
- Prior systemic chemotherapy
- Major postoperative complications [62, 66].

16.8 Challenging Problems

16.8.1 Recurrence, Treatment, and Repeated CRS plus HIPEC

Despite a much-improved understanding in terms of biology and immunohistochemistry of the disease, the impact of therapy is still incompletely understood; relapses are not uncommon, even if complete surgical cytoreduction is performed, and multiple operations are sometimes required. In the literature, iterative cytoreductive surgery associated or not with HIPEC, presents encouraging results associated with a complications rate comparable with the first procedure. In our experience, disease recurrence occurs within 2 years of CRS plus HIPEC (23.7 months). Histology PMCA is related to relapse in most cases (71.4%). We reported a morbidity rate of 50% (4/8); in one case, reoperation was required for bleeding, but no perioperative mortality was recorded. We detected a 3- and 5-year OS of 77.5% and 34%, respectively (the abrupt decrease is due to the death of two patients from other causes).

A comparable trend is described in the literature, and a long-term DFS is distinctly uncommon, whereas a long-term OS is frequently reported. Some authors reported that most patients recur within 2 years, but a further treatment (CRS, associated or not with HIPEC; or systemic chemotherapy) is feasible, with acceptable morbidity and mortality rates and encouraging outcome results [59]. A paper by Chua [64] who enrolled 113 patients with low-grade PMP, reported a recurrence rate of 41% associated with poor outcome results in early recurrence (<12 months). It is remarkable that patients have been submitted to CRS without repeated HIPEC.

16.8.2 Radiotherapy Treatment for Local Multiple Recurrence

In our experience, 4/28 patients who relapsed presented a repeated, single-site, local recurrence. They were submitted twice to radical surgical removal of relapse, but the disease recurred a third time, and they were treated with radiotherapy at the relapse site. At a median follow-up of 9 months (range 3-13), all four patients were alive without disease progression. In the literature, an interesting paper reported using whole abdominopelvic radiotherapy in palliative treatment for intestinal bowel obstruction caused by recurrent PMP, with resolution of clinical symptoms for 24 months [75].

16.8.3 Treating Appendiceal Mucoceles

The so-called LAMN, divided into LAMN-I and LAMN-II, are often a challenging problem for general surgeons [23]. It appears reasonable, in our experience—and we found a validation in literature reports—to treat LAMN-I disease by appendectomy, associated with multiple peritoneal biopsies and peritoneal washing for cytological examination, histological examination of appendiceal lymph nodes, and margins of resection. We must emphasize that either laparotomic or laparoscopic appendectomy must be performed safely in order to maintain appendiceal-wall integrity. In case of negative biopsies, resection margins, cytology, and lymph nodes, appendectomy is to be considered curative.

LAMN-II must be considered a precursor lesion of PMP syndrome: in the literature, an incidence of progression ranging from 22.2% [76] to 16.6% [77] is reported. In order to avoid inappropriate treatment, those patients, if not managed in emergency, must be treated in specialized centers. In fact, in these cases, it is generally recommended to combine HIPEC and surgery. An increasing aggressiveness in operative procedures is required, shifting from a LAMN-

II tumor with negative lymph nodes, resection margins, and cytology that requires appendectomy + HIPEC, to a perforated tumor with positive cytology, resection margins, and lymph nodes, which requires right colectomy associated with a peritonectomy procedure and HIPEC [76, 78–80].

16.9 Trial Reports

No randomized trials report significant evidence regarding the real effectiveness of cytoreductive surgery vs. HIPEC. A single meta-analysis on the outcome of PMP treated with CRS plus HIPEC only reported on some single-center and three multicenter studies; there were no data regarding independent factors influencing results in terms of morbidity and long-term survival rates [59]. A phase-II study evaluating the role of MMC and capecitabine in patients with advanced, unresectable PMP enrolled 40 patients and showed stabilization or reduction of mucinous disease in half of the patients; 89% reported improvement in their global health status [81].

16.10 Conclusions and Future Perspectives

From the reported data, some key points may be summarized:

1. Treating PMP with CRS plus HIPEC is more than a promising option and may be considered the gold standard for treating this rare and complex disease;
2. Repeated surgical debulking of disease or systemic chemotherapy in misdiagnosed PMP or in DPAM disease decreases, at the least, the intention-to-treat using CRS plus HIPEC;
3. Treating LAMN-II, and the particular features and rarity of PMP, strongly suggest addressing suspected or diagnosed PMP patients to a specialized referral center in order to ensure the optimal diagnostic and therapeutic course to the patients and to collect data for statistical analysis and treatment improvement;
4. Multicentric studies and randomized trials based on relevant clinical endpoints and appropriate control groups are necessary in order to achieve a better understanding of the role of surgery in PMP; in consideration of the rarity of this disease, collecting large series of patients treated in specialized centers is necessary to provide useful information for further treatment improvement, focusing not only on first-presentation disease but also on the optimal management of recurrent disease;
5. Some case reports in the literature explore alternative or experimental treatment options in peculiar situations:
   a. Possible new role of adjuvant systemic chemotherapy (FOLFOX4) in the treatment of PMP [82];
   b. Potential applicability of ascorbic acid and hydrogen peroxide for

mucolysis on compact mucin secreted in PMP [83];

c. Possible benefit of bevacizumab-based combination therapy in advanced cases in order to achieve disease stabilization and clinical improvement [84];
d. Recent studies highlight the possible role of bacteria in PMP disease: these data may support the hypothesis that adding antimicrobials to the standard PMP treatment could improve patient survival [85];
e. Potential application of anti-inflammatory drugs that seem to inhibit extracellular mucin production in PMP, decreasing compressive symptoms and increasing the disease-free interval [86].

In conclusion, immunohistochemical, genetic, and pharmacological studies may help our understanding and improve outcomes of a particular subset of or recurrent PMP. Also, it seems appropriate that when recognized and diagnosed, patients with this rare disease be referred to specialized centers to undergo state of the art treatment.

References

1. Smeenk RM, van Velthuysen ML, Verwaal VJ et al (2008) Appendiceal neoplasms and pseudomyxoma peritonei: a population based study. Eur J Surg Oncol 34:196–201
2. Werth R (1884) Klinische und anatomische untersuchungen zur lehre von den bauchgeschwuelsten und der laparotomie. Arch Gynaecol Obstet 24:100-118
3. Fraenkel E (1901) Ueber das sogennante pseudomyxoma peritonei. Munch Med Wochenschr 48:965-971
4. Weaver CH (1937) Mucocele of the appendix with pseudomucinous degeneration. Am J Surg 36:523
5. Sugarbaker PH, Ronnett BM, Archer A et al (1996) Pseudomyxoma peritonei syndrome. Adv Surg 30:233-280
6. Cheng KK (1949) An experimental study of mucocele of the appendix and pseudomyxoma peritonei. J Pathol Bacteriol 61:217-225
7. Grodinsky M, Rubnitz AS (1941) Mucocele of the appendix and pseudomyxoma peritonei: a clinical review and experimental study, with case report. Surg Gynecol Obstet 73:345-354
8. Baratti D, Kusamura S, Nonaka D et al (2008) Pseudomyxoma peritonei: clinical pathological and biological prognostic factors in patients treated with cytoreductive surgery and hyperthermic intraperitoneal chemotherapy (HIPEC). Ann Surg Oncol 15:526–534
9. Jarvinen P, Lepisto A (2010) Clinical presentation of pseudomyxoma peritonei. Scand J Surg 99:213-216
10. Carr NJ, Emory TS, Sobin LH (2002) Epithelial neoplasms of the appendix and colorectum: an analysis of cell proliferation, apaptosis and expression of p53, CD44, bcl-2. Arch Pathol Lab Med 126:837–841
11. Szych C, Staebler A, Connolly DC et al (1999) Molecular genetic evidence supporting the clonality and appendiceal origin of pseudomyxoma peritonei in women. Am J Pathol 154:1849–1855
12. Ronnett BM, Zahn CM, Kurman RJ et al (1995) Disseminated peritoneal adenomucinosis and peritoneal mucinous carcinomatosis: a clinicopathologic analysis of 109 cases with emphasis on distinguishing pathologic features, site of origin, prognosis and relationship to "pseudomyxoma peritonei". Am J Surg Pathol 19:1390–1408
13. Mukherjee A, Parvaiz A, Cecil TD et al (2004) Pseudomyxoma peritonei usually originates from the appendix: a review of the evidence. Eur J Gynaecol Oncol 25:411-414
14. Young RH, Gilks CB, Scully RE (1991) Mucinous tumors of the appendix associated with

mucinous tumors of the ovary and pseudomyxoma peritonei. A clinicopathological analysis of 22 cases supporting an origin in the appendix. Am J Surg Pathol 15:415-429
15. Prayson RA, Hart WR, Petras RE (1994) Pseudomyxoma peritonei. A clinicopathologic study of 19 cases with emphasis on site of origin and nature of associated ovarian tumors. Am J Surg Pathol 18:591-603
16. Ronnett BM, Shmookler BM, Diener-West M et al (1997) Immunohistochemical evidence supporting the appendiceal origin of pseudomyxoma peritonei in women. Int J Gynecol Pathol 16:1-9
17. Guerrieri C, Franlund B, Fristedt S et al (1997) Mucinous tumors of the vermiform appendix and ovary, and pseudomyxoma peritonei: histogenetic implications of cytokeratin 7 expression. Hum Pathol 28:1039-1045
18. Baratti D, Kusamura S, Nonaka D et al (2009) Pseudomyxoma Peritonei: Biological Features Are the Dominant Prognostic Determinants After Complete Cytoreduction and HyperthermicIntraperitoneal Chemotherapy. Ann Surg 249:243-249
19. Ronnett BM, Seidman JD (2003) Mucinous tumors arising in ovarian mature cystic teratomas: relationship to the clinical syndrome of pseudomyxoma peritonei. Am J Surg Pathol 27:650-657
20. McKenney JK, Soslow RA, Longacre TA (2008) Ovarian mature teratomas with mucinous epithelial neoplasms: morphologic heterogeneity and association with pseudomyxoma peritonei. Am J Surg Pathol 32:645-655
21. Sugarbaker PH (1996) Pseudomyxoma peritonei. Cancer Treat Res 81:105-119
22. Misdraji J, Yantiss RK, Graeme-Cook FM et al (2003) Appendiceal mucinous neoplasms: a clinicopathologic analysis of 107 cases. Am J Surg Pathol 27:1089-1103
23. Renehan A, O'Dwyer S, Stern P (2009) Pseudomyxoma peritonei. In: Schwab M (ed) Cancer encyclopedia. Springer, London, pp 2134-2138
24. Panarelli NC, Yantiss RK (2011) Mucinous neoplasms of the appendix and peritoneum. Arch Pathol Lab Med 135:1261-1268
25. Bosman FT, Carneiro F, Hruban RH et al (2010) Classification of tumours of the digestive system. 4th ed. Lyon, France: IARC:112-125
26. Bradley RF, Stewart JH, Russell GB et al (2006) Pseudomyxoma peritonei of appendiceal origin: a clinicopathologic analysis of 101 patients uniformly treated at a single institution, with literature review. Am J Surg Pathol 30:551-559
27. Van ES, Offerhaus GJ, Hart AA et al (2007) Goblet cell carcinoid of the appendix: a specific type of carcinoma. Histopathology 51:763-773
28. Sugarbaker PH (1994) Pseudomyxoma peritonei. A cancer whose biology is characterized by a redistribution phenomenon. Ann Surg 219:109-111
29. Young RH (2004) Pseudomyxoma peritonei and selected other aspects of the spread of appendiceal neoplasms. Semin Diagn Pathol 21:134-150
30. Lee BY, Kim HS, Lee SH et al (2004) Pseudomyxoma peritonei: extraperitoneal spread to the pleural cavity and lung. J Thorac Imaging 19:123-126
31. Mortman KD, Sugarbaker PA, Shmookler BM et al (1997) Pulmonary metastases in pseudomyxoma peritonei syndrome. Ann Thorac Surg 64:1434-1436
32. Geisinger KR, Levine EA, Shen P et al (2007) Pleuropulmonary involvement in pseudomyxoma peritonei: morphologic assessment and literature review. Am J Clin Pathol 127:135-143
33. Peek DF, Beets GL (1999) Pseudomyxoma peritonei in the pleural cavity: report of a case. Dis Colon Rectum 42:113-115
34. Yoshida R, Yoshioka K, Yoshitaka H et al (2002) Pseudomyxoma peritonei of appendiceal cancer with metastasis to the stomach: report of a case. Surg Today 32:547-550
35. Smeenk RM, Verwaal VJ, Antonini N et al (2007) Progression of pseudomyxoma peritonei after combined modality treatment: management and outcome. Ann Surg Oncol 14:493-499
36. Mets T, Van Hove W, Louis H (1977) Pseudomyxoma peritonei. Report of a case with extraperitoneal metastasis and invasion of the spleen. Chest 72:792-794
37. Smeenk RM, Verwaal VJ, Zoetmulder FA (2007) Pseudomyxoma peritonei. Cancer Treat Rev 33:138-145

38. Kusamura S, Hutanu I, Baratti D et al (2013) Circulating tumor markers: predictors of incomplete cytoreduction and powerful determinants of outcome in pseudomyxoma peritonei. J Surg Oncol 108:1-8
39. Koh JL, Liauw W, Chua T et al (2013) Carbohydrate antigen 19-9 (CA 19-9) is an independent prognostic indicator in pseudomyxoma peritonei post cytoreductive surgery and perioperative intraperitoneal chemotherapy. J Gastrointest Oncol 4:173-181
40. Taflampas P, Dayal S, Chandrakumaran K et al (2014) Pre-operative tumour marker status predicts recurrence and survival after complete cytoreduction and hyperthermic intraperitoneal chemotherapy for appendiceal Pseudomyxoma Peritonei: Analysis of 519 patients. Eur J Surg Oncol http://dx.doi.org/10.1016/j.ejso.2013.12.021.
41. Baratti D, Kusamura S, Martinetti A, et al (2007) Prognostic value of circulating tumor markers in patients with pseudomyxoma peritonei treated with cytoreductive surgery and hyperthermic intraperitoneal chemotherapy. Ann Surg Oncol 14:2300-2308
42. Alexander-Sefre F, Chandrakumaran K, Banerjee S et al (2005) Elevated tumour markers prior to complete tumour removal in patients with pseudomyxoma peritonei predict early recurrence. Colorectal Dis 7:382-386
43. Gollub MJ, DeCorato D, Schwartz LH (2000) MR enteroclysis: evaluation of small-bowel obstruction in a patient with pseudomyxoma peritonei. Am J Roentgenol 174:688-690.
44. Passot G, Glehen O, Pellet O (2010) Pseudomyxoma peritonei: role of 18F-FDG PET in preoperative evaluation of pathological grade and potential for complete cytoreduction. Eur J Surg Oncol 36:315-323
45. Jarvinen P, Ristimaki A, Kantonen J et al (2013) Feasibility of radical cytoreductive surgery and hyperthermic intraperitoneal chemotherapy for pseudomyxoma peritonei of appendiceal origin. Scand J Surg 102:145-151
46. Andreasson H, Graf W, Nygren P et al (2012) Outcome differences between debulking surgery and cytoreductive surgery in patients with pseudomyxoma peritonei. Eur J Surg Oncol 38:962-968
47. Jarvinen P, Jarvinen HJ, Lepisto A (2010) Survival of patients with pseudomyxoma peritonei treated by serial debulking. Colorectal Dis 12:868-872
48. Gough DB, Bonohue JH, Schutt AJ et al (1994) Pseudomyxoma peritonei. Long-term patient survival with an aggressive regional approach. Ann Surg 219:112-119
49. Miner TJ, Shia J, Jaques DP et al (2005) Long-term survival following treatment of pseudomyxoma peritonei: an analysis of surgical therapy. Ann Surg 241:300-308
50. Nitecki SS, Wolff BG, Schlinkert R et al (1994) The natural history of surgically treated primary adenocarcinoma of the appendix. Ann Surg 219:51-57
51. Sugarbaker PH (2001) Cytoreductive surgery and perioperative intraperitoneal chemotherapy as a curative approach to pseudomyxoma peritonei syndrome. Eur J Surg Oncol 27:239-243
52. Sugarbaker PH (2006) New standard of care for appendiceal epithelial neoplasms and pseudomyxoma peritonei syndrome? Lancet Oncol 7:69-76
53. Moran B, Baratti D, Yan TD et al (2008) Consensus statement on the loco-regional treatment of appendiceal mucinous neoplasms with peritoneal dissemination (Pseudomyxoma peritonei). J Surg Oncol 98:277-282
54. Yan TD, Black D, Savady R et al (2006) A systematic review on the efficacy of cytoreductive surgery and perioperative intraperitoneal chemotherapy for pseudomyxoma peritonei. Ann Surg Oncol 14:484–492
55. Esquivel J, Sugarbaker PH (2001) Second-look surgery in patients with peritoneal dissemination from appendiceal malignancy: analysis of prognostic factors in 98 patients. Ann Surg 234(2):198–205
56. Sugarbaker PH (1999) Management of peritoneal-surface malignancy: the surgeon's role. Langenbecks Arch Surg 384:576–587
57. De Simone M, Barone R, Vaira M et al (2003) Semi-closed hyperthermic –antiblastic peritoneal perfusion (HAPP) in the treatment of peritoneal carcinosis. J Surg Oncol 82:138-140
58. Glehen O, Sugarbaker PH, Elias D et al (2004) Cytoreductive surgery combined with peri-

operative intraperitoneal chemotherapy for the management of peritoneal carcinomatosis from colorectal cancer. A multi-institutional study of 506 patients. J Clin Oncol 22:3284-3292
59. McBride K, McFadden D, Osler T (2013) Improved survival of patients with pseudomyxoma peritonei receiving intraperitoneal chemotherapy with cytoreductive surgery: a systematic review and meta-analysis. J Surg Res 183:246-252
60. Robella M, Vaira M, Marsanic P et al (2013) Treatment of pseudomyxoma peritonei with cytoreductive surgery and hyperthermic intraperitoneal chemotherapy (HIPEC): a single center experience. Minerva Chir 68:569-577
61. Arjona-Sanchez A, Munoz-Casares FC, Casado-Adam A et al (2013) Outcome of patients with aggressive pseudomyxoma peritonei treated by cytoreductive surgery and intraperitoneal chemotherapy. World J Surg 37:1263-1270
62. Chua TC, Moran BJ, Sugarbaker PH et al (2012) Early- and Long-Term Outcome Data of Patients With Pseudomyxoma Peritonei From Appendiceal Origin Treated by a Strategy of Cytoreductive Surgery and Hyperthermic Intraperitoneal Chemotherapy. J Clin Oncol 30:2449-2456
63. Sorensen O, Flatmark K, Reed W et al (2012) Evaluation of complete cytoreductive surgery and two intraperitoneal chemotherapy techniques in pseudomyxoma peritonei. Eur J Surg Oncol 38:969-976
64. Chua TC, Liauw W, Morris DL (2011) Early recurrence of pseudomyxoma peritonei following treatment failure of cytoreductive surgery and perioperative intraperitoneal chemotherapy is indicative of a poor survival outcome. Int J Colorectal Dis 27:381-389
65. Youssef H, Newman C, Chandrakumaran K et al (2011) Operative findings, early complications, and long-term survival in 456 patients with pseudomyxoma peritonei syndrome of appendiceal origin. Dis Colon Rectum 54:293-299
66. Elias D, Gilly F, Quenet F et al (2010) Pseudomyxoma peritonei: A French multicentric study of 301 patients treated with cytoreductive surgery and intraperitoneal chemotherapy. Eur J Surg Oncol 36:456-462
67. Alves S, Mohamed F, Yadegarfar G et al (2010) Prospective longitudinal study of quality of life following cytoreductive surgery and intraperitoneal chemotherapy for pseudomyxoma peritonei. Eur J Surg Oncol 36:1156-1161
68. Vaira M, Cioppa T, De Marco G et al (2009) Management of pseudomyxoma peritonei by cytoreduction + HIPEC (Hyperthermic Intraperitoneal Chemotherapy): results analysis of a twelve-year experience. In Vivo 23:639-644
69. Elias D, Honore´ C, Ciuchende R et al (2008) Peritoneal pseudomyxoma: results of systematic policy of complete cytoreductive surgery and hyperthermic intraperitoneal chemotherapy. Br J Surg 95:1164-1171
70. Smeenk RM, Verwaal VJ, Antonini N et al (2007) Survival analysis of pseudomyxoma peritonei patients treated by cytoreductive surgery and hyperthermic intraperitoneal chemotherapy. Ann Surg 245:104-109
71. Gonzalez-Moreno S, Sugarbaker PH (2004) Right hemicolectomy does not confer a survival advantage in patients with mucinous carcinoma of the appendix and peritoneal seeding. Br J Surg 91:304–311
72. Sugarbaker PH, Alderman R, Edwards G et al (2006) Prospective morbidity and mortality assessment of cytoreductive surgery plus perioperative intraperitoneal chemotherapy to treat peritoneal dissemination of appendiceal mucinous malignancy. Ann Surg Oncol 13:1–11
73. Smeenk RM, Verwaal VJ, Zoetmulder FAN (2006) Toxicity and mortality of cytoreduction and intraoperative hyperthermic intraperitoneal chemotherapy in pseudomyxoma peritonei—a report of 103 procedures. Eur J Surg Oncol 32:186–190
74. Deraco M, De Simone M, Rossi CR et al (2003) An Italian multicentric phase II study on peritonectomy and intra-peritoneal hyperthermic perfusion (IPHP) to treat patients with pseudomyxoma peritonei. J Exp Clin Cancer Res 22:35-39
75. Berkovic P, van de Voorde L, De Meerleer G et al (2014) Whole abdominopelvic radiotherapy in the palliative treatment of pseudomyxoma peritonei. Strahlenther Onkol 190:223-228
76. Pai Rk, Beck AH, Norton JA et al (2009) Appendiceal mucinous neoplasms: clinicopatholog-

ic study of 116 cases with analysis of factors predicting recurrence. Am J Surg Pathol 33:1425-1439
77. Smeenk RM, van Velthuysen ML, Verwaal VJ et al (2008) Appendiceal neoplasms and pseudomyxoma peritonei: a population based study. Eur J Surg Oncol 34:196-201
78. McDonald JR, O'Dwyer ST, Rout S et al (2012) Classification of cytoreductive surgery for low grade appendiceal mucinous neoplasms. Br J Surg 99:987-992
79. Fish R, Selvasekar C, Crichton P et al (2014) Risk-reducing laparoscopic cytoreductive surgery and hyperthermic intraperitoneal chemotherapy for low-grade appendiceal mucinous neoplasm: early outcomes and technique. Surg Endosc 25:341-345
80. Dhage-Ivatury S, Shugarbaker PH (2006) Update on the surgical approach to mucocele of the appendix. J Am Coll Surg 202:680-684
81. Farquharson AL, Pranesh N, Witham G et al (2008) A phase II study evaluating the use of concurrent mitomycin C and capecitabine in patients with advanced unresectable pseudomyxome peritonei. Br J Cancer 99:591-596
82. Chen CF, Huang CJ, Kang WI et al (2008) Experience with adjuvant chemotherapy for pseudomyxoma peritonei secondary to mucinous adenocarcinoma of the appendix with oxaliplatin/fliotouracil/leucovorin (FOLFOX4). World J Surg Oncol 6:118
83. Pillai K, Akhter J, Chua TC (2012) Mucolysis by ascorbic acid and hydrogen peroxide on compact mucin secreted in pseudomyxoma peritonei. J Surg Res 174:e69-73
84. Sun WL, Hutarew G, Gradl J et al (2009) Successfu antiangiogenic combination therapy for pseudomyxoma peritonei with bevacizumab and capecitabine. Cancer Biol Ther 8:1459-1462
85. Gilbreath JJ, Semino-Mora C, Friedline CJ et al (2013) A core microbiome associated with the peritoneal tumors of pseudomyxoma peritonei. Orphanet J Rare Dis 8:105
86. Choudry HA, Mavanur A, O'Malley ME et al (2012) Chronic anti-inflammatory drug therapy inhibits gel-forming mucin production in a murine xenograft model of human pseudomyxoma peritonei. Ann Surg Oncol 19:1402-1409

Peritoneal Mesothelioma

17

Marcello Deraco, Dario Baratti, Shigeki Kusamura, Antonello D. Cabras, Federica Perrone, and Nadia Zaffaroni

17.1 Introduction

Diffuse malignant peritoneal mesothelioma (DMPM) is an exceedingly uncommon tumor arising from mesothelial cells. Macroscopically, the disease is characterized by thousands of small tumor nodules that grow to form plaques, masses, or layers covering all peritoneal surfaces. DMPM has been considered a pathological entity without effective treatment options until the 1990s, when initial surgical experiences integrating cytoreductive surgery (CRS) with hyperthermic intraperitoneal chemotherapy (HIPEC) showed a significant impact on patient prognosis [1–3]. These encouraging results prompted clinical and basic science researchers to intensify their efforts in an attempt to identify new prognostic factors and therapeutic targets to optimize patient selection for treatment and therapeutic strategies. The translation of these advancements into clinical practice will be the challenge for the coming years [4, 5]. Treatment guidelines and investigational perspectives concerning DMPM were defined by the Consensus Conference, Milan (4–6 December 2006) [6].

17.2 Epidemiology

Epidemiological, biological, and clinical behaviors of DMPM are different from its better know and more frequent pleural counterpart. From the Surveillance, Epidemiology, and End Results (SEER) program and European Cancer Incidence and Mortality (EUROCIM) data [7, 8], age-standardized incidence

M. Deraco (✉)
Department of Surgery, National Cancer Institute,
Milan, Italy
e-mail: marcello.deraco@istitutotumori.mi.it

A. Di Giorgio, E. Pinto (Eds), *Treatment of Peritoneal Surface Malignancies*,
Updates in Surgery
DOI: 10.1007/978-88-470-5711-1_17,

rates among men range from 0.5 to approximately three cases per million population. About 2,500 new cases of mesothelioma are registered each year in the USA. Higher rates are reported in smaller areas with widespread past use of asbestos, such as the harbor city of Genoa, Italy (age-standardized incidence in men in 1995 was 5.5/1,000,000) [9]. According to recent epidemiological data, a 5–10 % increase in annual disease-related mortality will be observed worldwide until 2020. The disease has likely reached its incidence peak in the USA, but in Europe and Australia, the peak is expected during this decade [10].

17.3 Etiology

The role of asbestos exposure in DMPM origin is not clear, as in pleural forms. It was estimate that 58 % of men and only 20 % of women with DMPM had past asbestos exposure [11]. Therefore, it has been suggested that disease etiology may differ between sexes [12]. Since no asbestos exposure is documented in about 20–40 % of patients with DMPM, it has been suggested that other factors, such as Simian virus 40 (SV40), may be implicated as possible cofactors in mesothelioma oncogenesis. Furthermore, observations gathered in Cappadocia, Turkey, resulted in the hypothesis of a genetic susceptibility with an autosomal dominant pattern [13, 14]

17.4 Diagnosis

17.4.1 Clinical Presentation

DMPM growth is characterized by peritoneal seeding, eventually leading to death because of intractable ascites, bowel encasement, and bowel obstruction. Patients are usually diagnosed at an advanced disease stage. In an Italian series of 81 DMPM patients, the most frequent symptoms leading to diagnosis were ascites, abdominal pain, and asthenia. Weight loss, anorexia, abdominal mass, fever, diarrhea, and vomiting were less common; presentation with abdominal hernia occurred in 13 % of patients and thrombocytosis with anemia in 73 %. In about 25 % of female patients, diagnosis was triggered by nonspecific gynecological symptoms [15].

Cytological examination of ascitic fluid is mostly nondiagnostic. In the Washington Cancer Institute series, diagnosis of DMPM was made by fluid sampling in none of 68 patients. In 44 % of patients, diagnosis was obtained by laparotomy, in 52 % by laparoscopy, and in 4 % by ultrasound/computed tomography (US/CT)-guided biopsy [12]. CT-scan is the preferred radiological tool for disease staging and patient selection for treatment [16].

17.4.2 Histology, Immunohistochemistry, and Staging

According to the 2012 update of the Guidelines for Pathologic Diagnosis of Malignant Peritoneal Mesothelioma of the Consensus Statement from the International Mesothelioma Interest Group (iMIG), DMPM can be classified into epithelial, sarcomatoid, and biphasic variants, analogously to the pleural form. Histological subtypes are outlined in Table 17.1 [17]. Epithelial DMPM is further classified by its predominant patterns: tubulopapillary, solid, deciduoid, storiform-like, fascicular-like, papillary, microcystic, and granular. Tubulopapillary areas are sometimes difficult to distinguish from well-differentiated mesothelioma. There is usually some degree of nuclear pleomorphism. [17, 18].

Sarcomatoid DMPM can show the histologic patterns produced by any soft-tissue tumor. A mixture of sarcomatoid and epithelial components gives rise to biphasic or mixed variants (Fig. 17.1), which are usually aggressive tumors. Occasionally, sarcomatous areas may be markedly hypocellular, resulting in small biopsy specimens being misinterpreted as reactive fibrosis [17, 18].

It must be emphasized that conventional pathological techniques have low sensitivity and specificity in the diagnosis of DMPM. Thus, misdiagnosis between neoplasms originating from other abdominal organs is relatively common. Therefore, immunohistochemical studies play an important role in the diagnostic workup. In particular, DMPM must be distinguished from benign reactive lesions and metastatic carcinoma. At present, a specific marker for mesothelioma is not available, and diagnosis relies on the combination of positive [calretinin, cytokeratin (CK)-5/6, monoclonal antibody (MAb) D2-40, podoplanin, mesothelin, and Wilms tumor-1 (WT1)] and negative [claudin-4, carcinoembryonic antigen (CEA), MAbs MOC-31 and B72.3, and antihuman epithelial antigen (Ber-EP4) markers [17].

Table 17.1 Diffuse malignant peritoneal mesothelioma (DMPM) types and subtypes

Types	Subtypes	Percentage
Malignant	Epithelial	75
	Tubulopapillary nonglandular (solid)	13
	Sarcomatous	6
	Biphasic (mixed)	6
	Undifferentiated	Very rare
	Desmoplastic	Very rare
	Lymphohistiocytic	Very rare
	Small cell	Very rare
	Deciduoid	Very rare
Borderline/low malignant	Well-differentiated papillary	Rare
	Multicystic	Rare

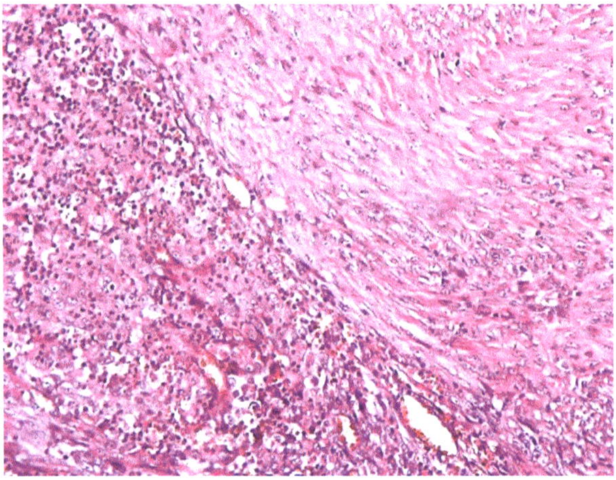

Fig. 17.1 Biphasic diffuse malignant peritoneal mesothelioma (DMPM) histology: combination of an epithelial and a sarcomatoid cells

Thyroid transcription factor 1 (TTF-1) can assist in distinguishing DMPM from lung carcinoma, homeobox protein CDX-2 from colon carcinoma, and cytokeratin (CK)-7 and paired-box (PAX)-8 from ovarian carcinoma or serous papillary peritoneal carcinoma. Renal cell carcinoma marker (RCC-Ma) may be helpful in establishing renal origin [19, 20].

Gathering data from eight international centers, a new tumor/node/metastasis (TNM) staging system for DMPM was recently proposed. Peritoneal cancer index (PCI) was categorized into T1 (PCI 1–10), T2 (PCI 11–20), T3 (PCI 21–30), and T4 (PCI 30–39). T1 N0 M0 was defined as stage I, T2/T3 N0 M0 as stage II, and T4 and/or N1 and/or M1 as stage III. The 5-year survival associated with stage I, II, and III disease was 87 %, 53 %, and 29 %, respectively [21].

17.4.3 Serum Tumor Markers

Although mesothelin and osteopontin showed their potential usefulness in diagnosing and assessing prognosis of pleura mesothelioma patients, no information is available for DMPM [22]. The clinical role of serum markers was studied in 60 patients with DMPM treated at the Istituto Nazionale Tumori (INT) in Milan, Italy. Baseline diagnostic sensitivity was 53.3 % for cancer antigen (CA)125, 0 for CEA, 3.8 % for CA19.9, and 48.5 % for CA15.3 [23]. These data may help in the initial evaluation of peritoneal tumors from unknown site of origin. When therapy response was assessed, CA125 normalized after adequate CRS plus HIPEC in 21/22 patients with elevated baseline levels. CA125 remained high in all patients with persistent macroscopic disease after surgery. Also, CA125 became positive in 12/12 patients with elevated baseline levels, developing disease progression after adequate CRS plus HIPEC. A borderline prognostic significance for baseline CA125 levels was observed only in individuals not previously treated with systemic chemotherapy (sCHT).

17.5 Treatment Results

17.5.1 Systemic Chemotherapy

In our institution, we investigated the role of sCHT in 116 DMPM patients treated with CRS plus HIPEC. No significant survival difference was seen among three subsets of patients: (1) those treated by sCHT before CRS plus HIPEC ($n = 60$), (2) patients who had sCHT after CRS plus HIPEC ($n = 30$), and (3) the group receiving no sCHT ($n = 26$). However, administration of platinum compounds plus pemetrexed was related with a statistically significant borderline survival advantage ($p = 0.09$) [24]. Even looking at other centers' experiences, no high-quality clinical data to define the role of sCHT in DMPM management is available.

DMPM is a poorly chemoresponsive tumor. A systematic meta-analysis of all prospective clinical trials published up to 2001 involving pleural or peritoneal mesothelioma demonstrated that cisplatin was the most active single agent and that cisplatin with doxorubicin was the most active combination in terms of treatment response [25]. However, these results should be interpreted with caution, as comparisons were not made in a randomized framework.

In a German series and the pemetrexed expanded access program, DMPM response rates were comparable with those observed for pleural disease [26, 27]. Other agents showing activity in DMPM are vinorelbine and gemcitabine, either alone or combined with platinum compounds. In historical case series, standard therapy with palliative surgery and systemic/intraperitoneally administered chemotherapy (IP-CHT) was associated with a median survival of ~ 1 year [4]. However, the hypothesis that chemotherapeutic drugs have limited efficacy seems to be confirmed by the poor median survival, ranging from 9 to 15 months, observed in individuals affected by DMPM who receive sCHT alone [2].

17.5.2 Cytoreductive Surgery plus Hyperthermic Intraperitoneal Chemotherapy

The 2006 Milan Consensus Conference on Peritoneal Surface Malignancies concluded that the standard treatment of DMPM is based on the integration of CRS-HIPEC and sCHT [6].

The aim of CRS is complete removal of all neoplastic implants from the abdominal cavity, which is possible only by peritonectomy (PRT) procedures and multivisceral resections. The pattern of DMPM dissemination implies complete distribution on peritoneal surfaces, and most cases are diagnosed with widespread tumor (Fig. 17.2). Also, microscopic disease is frequently identified at pathological examination, even when no evidence of disease is noted at macroscopic intraoperative examination. Therefore, we recommend complete

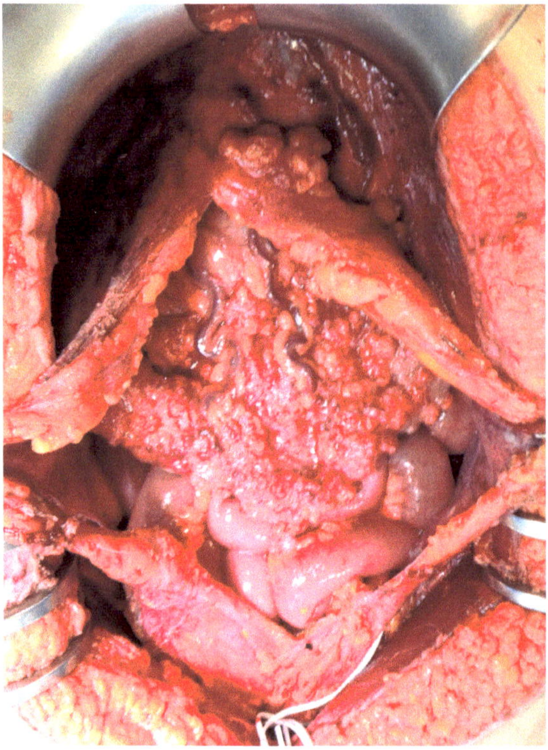

Fig. 17.2 Intraoperative high Peritoneal Cancer Index (PCI) in diffuse malignant peritoneal mesothelioma (DMPM): typical omental cake, peritoneal thickening, abdominal mass, and mesenterial thickening

parietal PRT for this disease [28]. Conversely, organ resections are indicated only in case of their massive involvement.

With the aim of consolidating macroscopic CRS, locoregional treatment allowing high peritoneal (and low systemic) drug concentration is used. This procedure, HIPEC, combines the pharmacological advantage with moderate hyperthermia. CRS is performed according to the technique originally described by Sugarbaker, with minor variations [29, 30] (Fig. 17.3) HIPEC is performed according to the closed-abdomen technique with cisplatin (45 mg/L perfusate) and doxorubicin (15 mg/L perfusate) for 90 min at a temperature of 42.5 C, based on a recent dose-finding study [31]. Perfusate volume is 4–6 L, and mean flow is 700 ml/min. The extracorporeal circulation device, Performer LRT® (RAND, Medolla, Italy), is used.

Analysis of published data allows us to conclude that median survival grew from 12 months with sCHT to 53 months with CRS plus HIPEC plus sCHT [32–34]. In our institutional experience, postoperative quality of life (QoL) was satisfactory, related morbidity and mortality acceptable, and financial cost-effectiveness reasonable [35, 36].

According to our most recent study, median overall (OS) and progression-free

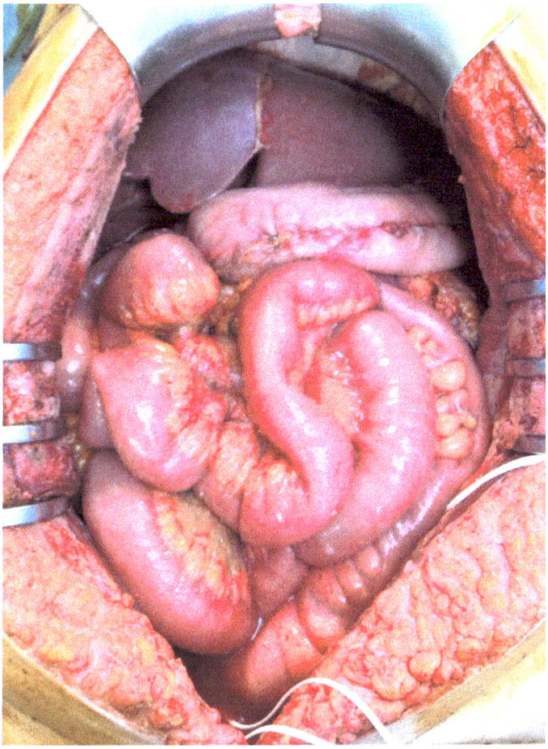

Fig. 17.3 High Peritoneal Cancer Index (PCI) diffuse malignant peritoneal mesothelioma (DMPM): result after mesenteric peritonectomy

(PFS) survival were 63.2 and 25.1 months in 108 patients undergoing complete CRS plus HIPEC (residual tumor < 2.5 mm). The survival curve reached a plateau after 7 years, suggesting that patients surviving > 7 years may be cured. Actual cure rate was 19/39 patients with potential follow-up of 7 years (43.6 %) [37].

17.6 Prognostic Factors

In a large collaborative study, the most significant prognostic factors were epithelial subtype, no node metastases, completeness of cytoreduction (CC), and administration of HIPEC [33]. In pattern-of-failure analysis, the small bowel was the site most commonly involved at recurrence; residual tumor > 2.5 mm was the only independent risk factor for recurrence [38]. CC has consistently been one of the most predominant prognostic factors. It is related to the extent of peritoneal involvement and surgeon skill to remove all peritoneal disease [1–3, 32–34]. Lymph node metastases are rare in DMPM but correlate with poor outcome. This supports the necessity that any suspicious node be systematically removed during the CRS procedure [32, 33].

Biphasic and sarcomatoid histological variants are correlated with poor prognosis, although their clinical utility as prognostic factors is limited by their rarity [1]. Other pathological prognostic variables are nuclear/nucleolar size, depth of tumor invasion, and mitotic count.

In the above-mentioned series, a Ki67-positive cell rate < 10 % correlated at multivariate analysis with better OS and PFS [37]. The role of proliferative index for prognostic stratification was confirmed in an exhaustive clinicopathological analysis by Deraco et al. (personal communication) using the technology of tissue microarray (TMA), results of which were presented at the Ninth International Symposium on Locoregional Cancer Therapies, Steamboat Springs, CO, USA, 15–17 February 2014.

17.7 Molecular Biology

In DMPM, molecular and cellular mechanisms underlying the proliferative potential and resistance to therapy are still poorly understood. The biology of this disease has been thoroughly investigated by clinical and basic science researchers at Milan INT during the last decade. It has been demonstrated that p16 expression is frequently absent or reduced in patients with DMPM and that EGFR overexpression is more common in peritoneal than in pleural forms. However, no correlation with prognosis of overexpression of EGFR and matrix metalloproteases (MMP)-2 and -9 was found in patients treated in our institution [39].

Telomerase activity (TA) is expressed in the majority of DMPM and negatively impacts prognosis [40]. In DMPM specimens from 38 patients undergoing various therapies; we assessed TA using the telomeric repeat amplification protocol. The alternative lengthening of telomeres (ALT) mechanisms were studied by assaying ALT-associated promyelocytic leukemia nuclear bodies. ALT or TA alone was found in 18.2 % and 63.6 % of cases, respectively; both ALT and TA were positive in two cases. In the overall series, TA expression was significantly associated with disease relapse (p = 0.018) and cancer-related death (p =0.045); ALT was not associated with outcome. In a subset analysis, the prognostic relevance of TA was confirmed in patients uniformly treated by CRS plus HIPEC.

Overexpression of cytoprotective factors, including survivin and members of the inhibitors of apoptosis protein (IAP) family, were demonstrated by Zaffaroni et al. [5]. Those authors analyzed DMPM proliferative and apoptotic features and tested a survivin knockdown approach in a human DMPM cell line. DMPM cells were transfected with small-interfering RNA (siRNA) targeting survivin messenger RNA (mRNA). Survivin expression, growth rate, and ability to undergo spontaneous and drug-induced apoptosis was measured, showing low proliferation rates and poor apoptotic activity in DMPM cells. Survivin was expressed in 91 % of cases and the other IAPs in 69–100 %. Transfection of

DMPM cells with survivin siRNA resulted in a survivin inhibition, a time-dependent cell-growth decrease, and an enhancement of spontaneous and drug-induced apoptosis. These results suggest that survivin may be a potential target for biological treatments in DMPM.

We demonstrated by in vitro experiments that nortopsentin heteroanalogs inhibit cyclin-dependent kinase (CDK)-1 activity, reduce cell growth, induce a concentration-dependent cell cycle arrest in the gap 2/mitosis (G2/M) phase, increase apoptotic rate, and downregulate survivin in a DMPM cell line. Additionally, the combined administration of nortopsentin heteroanalogs and paclitaxel further increased the cytotoxic effect.

In surgical samples from 20 DMPM patients undergoing CRS plus HIPEC at our center, Perrone et al. studied the expression of tyrosin kinase receptors (TKR) and the status of TKR downstream pathways, with mTOR and its effectors S6 ribosomal protein (S6), and 4E binding protein 1 (4EBP1), through biochemical and mutational analysis and fluorescent in situ hybridization (FISH). By immunoprecipitation/Western blot, activation/phosphorylation was shown in 90 % of cases for EGFR, 75 % for PDGFRβ, and 45 % of cases for PDGFRα. In 100 % of cases, no EGFR, PDGFRα, or PDGFRβ mutation or gene amplification was demonstrated. Primarily, AKT, extracellular signal-regulated kinase (ERK) 1/2, mTOR, S6, and 4EBP1 were highly expressed and activated. No mutations in *PI3KCA*, *PTEN*, *KRAS*, and *BRAF* genes were seen. The ligand- and heterodimerization-dependent activation/expression of EGFR and PDGFRβ was demonstrated. Taken together, these findings strongly suggest the potential of TKR and their downstream effectors as targets for molecularly tailored treatments. Based on the concurrent activation of TKR and their downstream effectors, we designed a clinicobiological study to test the combination TKR and mTOR inhibitors. In a further analysis, we evaluated the EGFR inhibitor gefitinib, the mTOR inhibitor everolimus (RAD001), and the multiple TKR inhibitor, sorafenib, in a DMPM cell line: gefitinib and RAD001 alone showed poor cytotoxic activity; sorafenib had a stronger effect on cellular proliferation, and sequential treatment with RAD001 followed by sorafenib induced a marked synergistic effect in DMPM cells [41].

17.8 Multicystic and Well-differentiated Papillary Peritoneal Mesothelioma

Multicystic (MPM) and well-differentiated papillary (WDPPM) PM are exceedingly rare tumors with uncertain malignant potential. At Milan NCI, MPM and WDPPM have been treated with CRS plus HIPEC because of their propensity to recur locoregionally and to evolve into truly malignant neoplasms. We treated four women with MPM and eight with WDPPM; one patient underwent a second procedure due to MPM peritoneal recurrence. Seven patients had recurrent disease after prior debulking. Due to the low aggressiveness of these diseases, uterus and ovaries were spared in four young women. Optimal CRS with microscopic or minimal (≤ 2.5 mm) residual disease was achieved in 12/13 procedures.

After a median follow-up of 27 (range 6–94) months, disease progression developed in two patients and tumor-related death in one. At the time of this writing, the first patient was disease free after the repeated procedure. In the second patient, we documented a transition of typical WDPPM to biphasic DMPM; this woman died of disease progression after incomplete CRS followed by HIPEC. Five-year OS and PFS were 90 % and 79 %, respectively. The difference in PFS after 11 debulking operations carried out in seven patients before referral to the Milan NCI was statistically significant in favor of CRS plus HIPEC ($p = 0.016$). According to these data, definitive tumor eradication by CRS plus HIPEC is recommended as the standard option to prevent disease recurrence or transition into malignant conditions [42].

17.9 Future Perspectives

During the last two decades, CRS plus HIPEC has become the standard treatment for DMPM. Several studies have addressed DMPM biology and natural history, identifying new biological prognostic factors and therapeutic targets. However, there is still a critical need for effective systemic therapies for these patients. Several research lines are currently active at the Milan NCI:

- A prospective study, supported by the Health Ministry, aims to evaluate the potential efficacy of integrating CRS plus HIPEC and systemic treatment into an individualized, comprehensive approach based on molecular characterization of the disease.
- Further investigations on microRNA and other biological markers using the TMA technique aim to identify new prognostic factors and therapeutic targets.
- New efforts should be taken to validate prospectively the proposed TNM staging system.

Acknowledgement
Contents are partially based on Deraco M, Baratti D, Kusumara S (2012) Diffuse malignant peritoneal mesothelioma. In Sugarbaker et al. Cytoreductive Surgery and Perioperative Chemotherapy for Peritoneal Surface Malignancy: Textbook and Video Atlas, Cine-Med, Incorporated, pp 115-126.

References

1. Feldman AL, Libutti SK, Pingpank JF et al (2003) Analysis of factors associated with outcome in patients with malignant peritoneal mesothelioma undergoing surgical debulking and intraperitoneal chemotherapy. J Clin Oncol 21:4560-4567

2. Sugarbaker PH, Yan TD, Stuart OA, Yoo D (2006) Comprehensive management of diffuse malignant peritoneal mesothelioma. Eur J Surg Oncol 32:686-691
3. Deraco M, Nonaka D, Baratti D et al (2006) Prognostic analysis of clinicopathologic factors in 49 patients with diffuse malignant peritoneal mesothelioma treated with cytoreductive surgery and intraperitoneal hyperthermic perfusion. Ann Surg Oncol 13:229-237
4. Deraco M, Baratti D, Zaffaroni N et al (2007) Advances in clinical research and management of diffuse peritoneal mesothelioma. Recent Results Cancer Res 169:137-155
5. Zaffaroni N, Costa A, Pennati M et al (2007) Survivin is highly expressed and promotes cell survival in malignant peritoneal mesothelioma. Cell Oncol 29:453-466
6. Deraco M, Bartlett D, Kusamura S, Baratti D (2008) Consensus statement on peritoneal mesothelioma. J Surg Oncol 98:268-272
7. European Network of Cancer Registries. Eurocim Version 4.0. European Incidence Database V2.3, CI5 Dictionary (2001). Lyon, France: IARC
8. Surveillance, Epidemiology, and End Results (SEER) Program. http://www.seer.cancer.gov
9. Boffetta P (2007) Epidemiology of peritoneal mesothelioma: a review. Annals of Oncology 18:985-990
10. Peto J, Decarli A, La Vecchia C et al (1999) The European mesothelioma epidemic. Br J Cancer 79:666-672
11. Spirtas R, Heineman EF, Bernstein L et al (1994) Malignant mesothelioma: attributable risk of asbestos exposure. Occup Environ Med 51:804-811
12. Sugarbaker PH, Welch LS, Mohamed F, Glehen O (2003) A review of peritoneal mesothelioma at the Washington Cancer Institute. Surg Oncol Clin North Am 12:605-621
13. Gazdar AF, Carbone M (2003) Molecular pathogenesis of mesotheliom and its relationship to Simian virus 40. Clin Lung Cancer 5:177-181
14. Roushdy-Hammady I, Siegel J, Emri S et al (2001) Genetic-susceptibility factor and malignant mesothelioma in the Cappadocian region of Turkey. Lancet 357:444-445
15. de Pangher V, Recchia L, Cafferata M et al (2010) Malignant peritoneal mesothelioma: a multicenter study on 81 cases. Ann Oncol 21:348-353
16. Yan TD, Haveric N, Carmignani CP et al (2005) Abdominal Computed Tomography Scans in the Selection of Patients with Malignant Peritoneal Mesothelioma for Comprehensive Treatment with Cytoreductive Surgery and Perioperative Intraperitoneal Chemotherapy. Cancer 103:839-849
17. Husain AN, Colby T, Ordonez N et al (2013) Guidelines for pathologic diagnosis of malignant mesothelioma: 2012 update of the consensus statement from the International Mesothelioma Interest Group. Arch Pathol Lab Med 137:647-667
18. Weiss SW (1994) World health Organization International Histological Classification of Tumors: Histological typing of soft tissue tumors. Springer-Verlag, Berlin
19. King J, Thatcher N, Pickering C, Hasleton P (2006) Sensitivity and specificity of immunohistochemical antibodies used to distinguish between benign and malignant pleural disease: a systematic review of published reports. Histopathology 49:561-568
20. Deraco M, Baratti D, Cabras AD et al (2010) Experience with peritoneal mesothelioma at the Milan National Cancer Institute. World J Gastrointest Oncol 2:76-84
21. Yan TD, Deraco M, Elias D et al (2011) A novel tumor-node-metastasis (TNM) staging system of diffuse malignant peritoneal mesothelioma using outcome analysis of a multi-institutional database. Cancer 117:1856-63
22. Robinson BWS, Creaney J, Lake R et al (2003) Mesothelin-family proteins and diagnosis of mesothelioma. Lancet 362:1612-6
23. Baratti D, Kusamura S, Martinetti A et al (2007) Circulating CA125 in patients with peritoneal mesothelioma treated with cytoreductive surgery and intraperitoneal hyperthermic perfusion. Ann Surg Oncol 14:500-508
24. Deraco M, Baratti D, Hutanu I et al (2013)The role of perioperative systemic chemotherapy in diffuse malignant peritoneal mesothelioma patients treated with cytoreductive surgery and hyperthermic intraperitoneal chemotherapy. Ann Surg Oncol 20:1093-1100
25. Berghmans T, Paesmans M, Lalami Y et al (2002) Activity of chemotherapy and immunother-

apy on malignant mesothelioma: a systematic review of the literature with meta-analysis. Lung Cancer 38:111-121
26. Jänne PA, Wozniak AJ, Belani CP et al (2005) Open-label study of pemetrexed alone or in combination with cisplatin for the treatment of patients with peritoneal mesothelioma: outcomes of an expanded access program. Clin Lung Cancer 7:40-46
27. Carteni G, Manegold C, Martin Garcia G et al (2009) Malignant peritoneal mesothelioma. Results from the International Expanded Access Program using pemetrexed alone or in combination with a platinum agent: Lung Cancer 64:211-218
28. Baratti D, Kusamura S, Cabras AD, Deraco M (2012) Cytoreductive surgery with selective versus complete parietal peritonectomy followed by hyperthermic intraperitoneal chemotherapy in patients with diffuse malignant peritoneal mesothelioma: a controlled study. Ann Surg Oncol 19:1416-1424
29. Sugarbaker PH (1995) Peritonectomy Procedures. Ann Surg 221:29-42
30. Deraco M, Baratti D, Kusamura S et al (2009) Surgical technique of parietal and visceral peritonectomy for peritoneal surface malignancies. J Surg Oncol 100:321-328
31. Rossi CR, Foletto M, Mocellin S et al (2002) Hyperthermic intraoperative intraperitoneal chemotherapy with cisplatin and doxorubicin in patients who undergo cytoreductive surgery for peritoneal carcinomatosis and sarcomatosis: phase I study. Cancer 94:492-499
32. Baratti D, Kusamura S, Cabras AD et al (2010) Lymph node metastases in diffuse malignant peritoneal mesothelioma. Ann Surg Oncol 17:45-53
33. Yan TD, Deraco M, Baratti D et al (2009) Cytoreductive surgery and hyperthermic intraperitoneal chemotherapy for malignant peritoneal mesothelioma: multi-institutional experience. J Clin Oncol 27:6237-6242
34. Deraco M, Casali P, Inglese MG et al (2003) Peritoneal mesothelioma treated by induction chemotherapy, cytoreductive surgery, and intraperitoneal hyperthermic perfusion. J Surg Oncol 83:147-153
35. Deraco M, Baratti D, Kusamura S (2007) Morbidity and quality of life following cytoreduction and HIPEC. Cancer Treat Res 134:403-418
36. Baratti D, Scivales A, Balestra MR et al (2010) Cost analysis of the combined procedure of cytoreductive surgery and hyperthermic intraperitoneal chemotherapy (HIPEC). Eur J Surg Oncol 36:463-469
37. Baratti D, Kusamura S, Cabras AD et al (2013) Diffuse malignant peritoneal mesothelioma: long-term survival with complete cytoreductive surgery followed by hyperthermic intraperitoneal chemotherapy (HIPEC). Eur J Cancer 49:3140-148
38. Baratti D, Kusamura S, Cabras AD et al (2009) Diffuse malignant peritoneal mesothelioma: Failure analysis following cytoreduction and hyperthermic intraperitoneal chemotherapy (HIPEC). Ann Surg Oncol 16:463-472
39. Nonaka D, Kusamura S, Baratti D et al (2005) Diffuse malignant mesothelioma of the peritoneum: a clinicopathological study of 35 patients treated locoregionally at a single institution. Cancer 104:2181-2188
40. Villa R, Daidone MG, Motta R et al (2008) Multiple mechanisms of telomere maintenance exist and differentially affect clinical outcome in diffuse malignant peritoneal mesothelioma. Clin Cancer Res 14:4134-4140
41. Perrone F, Jocollè G, Pennati M et al (2010) Receptor tyrosine kinase and downstream signalling analysis in diffuse malignant peritoneal mesothelioma. Eur J Cancer 46:2837-2848
42. Baratti D, Vaira M, Kusamura S et al (2010) Multicystic peritoneal mesothelioma: outcomes and patho-biological features in a multi-institutional series treated by cytoreductive surgery and Hyperthermic Intraperitoneal Chemotherapy (HIPEC). Eur J Surg Oncol 36:1047-1053

Peritoneal Carcinomatosis from Gastric Cancer

18

Franco Roviello, Tommaso Cioppa, Daniele Marrelli,
Stefano Caruso, and Enrico Pinto

18.1 Introduction

Gastric cancer (GC) is the fourth most common cancer worldwide and the second leading cause of cancer-related mortality [1, 2]. In addition to hematogenous spread, GC may disseminate along the inside surface of the peritoneal cavity, leading to a condition of peritoneal carcinomatosis (PC). In patients undergoing a potentially curative resection of GC, PC may occur in 5–20% [3]. PC of gastric origin has an extremely poor prognosis, with a median survival estimated to be 1–3 months. Systemic chemotherapy has limited effects on this condition, with a median survival of 7–10 months [4–9]. Since 1990, cytoreductive surgery (CRS) combined with hyperthermic intraperitoneal chemotherapy (HIPEC) has been used to treat PC from gastrointestinal and ovarian malignancies [10, 11]. CRS is used primarily to treat gross and macroscopic disease, as experimental studies suggest that local chemotherapy may penetrate to a maximal depth of 3 mm [12]. Additionally, CRS also removes intra-abdominal adhesions, allowing greater distribution of cytotoxic agents [13]. The ultimate intent of CRS plus HIPEC is to excise all macroscopic disease and, upon completion, treat the residual tumor or microscopic disease of the peritoneal cavity with chemotherapy agents delivered directly to the site of disease. This higher local concentration of cytotoxic chemotherapy reaches residual microscopic tumor cells [12], and the combination of hyperthermia and chemotherapy has a synergistic effect, thus augmenting the cytotoxicity of chemotherapeutics [13]. Another advantage of localizing chemotherapy within the peritoneum is that it minimizes undesirable systemic effects [12]. The addition of hyperthermia has

F. Roviello (✉)
Department of Medical, Surgical, and Neurological Sciences, General and Oncologic Surgery Unit, University of Siena, Siena, Italy
e-mail: franco.roviello@unisi.it

A. Di Giorgio, E. Pinto (Eds), *Treatment of Peritoneal Surface Malignancies*,
Updates in Surgery
DOI: 10.1007/978-88-470-5711-1_18,

two potential benefits: First, it may induce apoptosis, denature proteins, and impair DNA repair [14]. Second, it allows greater drug accumulation within tumor nodules [15-17]. HIPEC can be performed with a closed, semiclosed, or open technique; the most common chemotherapeutic agents used are cisplatin and mitomycin, with the induction of intra-abdominal temperatures typically between 40 °C and 44.8 °C. Treatment duration normally ranges between 30 and 120 min. Despite the paucity of evidence to support systemic chemotherapy for treating PC, it is often used for patients with PC from GC. The lack of its effectiveness for PC is related to the presence of a peritoneal barrier [18]; however, the use of neoadjuvant chemotherapy is reported to reduce the burden of macroscopic PC [19, 20].

An important consideration for PC from GC is the timing of PC, specifically the presence of synchronous PC during the initial diagnosis versus metachronous development of PC following initial treatment for GC. It may be speculated that metachronous PC represents disease progression; however, this speculation remains controversial. Because PC is usually not visible on standard imaging techniques (i.e., computed tomography), diagnosing metachronous disease while it is still considered resectable may be difficult. For this reason, some surgeons may consider synchronous PC more treatable than metachronous PC.

PC of GC origin treated with CRS plus HIPEC demonstrated improved survival when complete cytoreduction (CC) is attained. In 1988, Fujimoto et al. [21] were the first to report the application of HIPEC in 15 patients with PC secondary to advanced GC, with a low postoperative morbidity rate (13%) and a mean survival of 7.2 months. This new treatment modality gradually gained acceptance in many countries, and a number of groups have reported their experiences with it in recent yers (Table 18.1) [22-26]. Elias et al. [14] report the highest median survival (MS) for patients with Completeness of Cytoreduction score (CC-0) to be 60 months; however, these results have not been repeated in a randomized controlled trial.

In the world literature, nine studies reported a total of 24 treatment-related deaths from a total of 467 patients, an overall mortality rate of 5.1% and morbidity of 21.5% (Table 18.2) [23, 27-34]. A recent review of CRS plus HIPEC for treating PC of any origin reported a mean mortality rate of 2.9%, with tertiary centers reporting a mortality rate ranging from 0.9% to 5.8% [35]. Combined morbidity was reported to be 28.8 %; the most common complications following CRS plus HIPEC were abscesses, fistulas, and anastomotic leaks [36]. CRS plus HIPEC for PC from GC has comparatively similar mortality and morbidity rates as for PC of other organ origins.

Since PC from GC is essentially a fatal disease with conventional treatment options, these mortality and morbidity rates may be acceptable to patients. The importance of achieving CC is emphasized in the literature, with a twofold increase in MS with a CC score of 0 or 1. This suggests that CRS plus HIPEC for PC from GC should only be considered in select patients if the surgeon is very confident that a CC-0 is possible. The overall morbidity rate was reported

Table 18.1 Outcome rates after CRC plus HIPEC in the last 10 years in patients with PC from GC

Study [Reference]	Year	Patients	Drug	Temperature (°C)	Duration	Mortality	Morbility	Survival
Yan et al. [22]	2007	34	CDDP 120 mg + MMC 30 mg	42.5–43.5	60–90	–	14.7%	3 yrs 5.9% (CC, 0–1, 12 mo)
Glehen et al. [23]	2010	159	MMC 30–50 mg/m^2 + CDDP or LOHP 340–460 mg/m^2 + Irinotecan 100–200 mg/m^2	41–43	30–120	6.5%	27.8%	5 yrs 5.9% (CC, 23%)
Yang et al. [24]	2010	28	CDDP 120 mg or HCPT 20 mg + MMC 30 mg	42.5–43.5	90–120	0%	14.3%	2 yrs 42.8% (CC0, 43.4 mo)
Yonemura et al. [25]	2005	107	CDDP 300 mg Etoposide 150 mg MMC 30 mg	42–43	60	2.8%	21.5%	5 yrs 6.7% (CC0, 13% CC> 0, 2%)
Glehen et al. [26]	2004	49	MMC 10 mg/L	45–48	90	4%	27%	5 yrs 16% (CC0–1, 29.4%)

CRS, cytoreductive surgery; HIPEC, hyperthermic intraperitoneal chemotherapy; *PC*, peritoneal carcinomatosis; *GC*, gastric cancer; *MMC*, mitomycin-C; *CDDP*, cisplatin; *LOHP*, oxaliplatin; *HCPT*, hydroxycamptothecin; *CC*, Completeness of Cytoreduction score

Table 18.2 Mortality rates of CRS plus HIPEC

Study [Reference]	Treatment-related deaths	Mortality (%)	Cause of death
Glehen et al. [23]	11	6.5	2 MOFs , 2 septic shocks, 1 fistula, 1 PE, 1 CVA, 1 toxicity
Yang et al. [27]	3	10.7	2 ileus, 1 ARDS, 1 pneumonia
Scaringi et al. [28]	1	11	Septic shock
Roviello et al. [29]	1	1.6	MOF
Farma et al. [30]	1	5.6	CVA
Yonemura et al. [31]	3	7	1 ARF, 1 A-leak, 1 bleeding
Mussa et al. [32]	1	14.3	
Fujimura et al. [33]	0	0	
Beaujard et al. [34]	3	3.6	1 PE, 1 MOF, 1 septic shock
Total; median	24	5.1	

CRS, cytoreductive surgery; HIPEC, hyperthermic intraperitoneal chemotherapy; *ARDS,* adult respiratory distress syndrome; *MOF,* multiple organ failure; *CVA,* cerebrovascular accident; *ARF,* acute renal failure; *A-leak,* anastomosis leak; *PE,* pulmonary embolism

by eight authors to be 21.5% (Table 18.3) [27-31, 33, 34]. CRS plus HIPEC may improve survival in select patients with with PC from GC: MS is increased to 15 months in patients with CC-0 compared with 3 months with only basic supportive therapy.

18.2 Role of Systemic Chemotherapy in Peritoneal Carcinomatosis from Gastric Cancer

PC from GC is typically treated with systemic chemotherapy; however, its efficacy is difficult to determine based on the literature. Three clinical trials found that systemic chemotherapy improved MS in metastatic GC to 7–10 months; however, patient populations were heterogeneous and inconsistently randomized, with the majority having no PC [5–7]. Similarly, Preusser et al. [37] reported decreased response rates to systemic chemotherapy in patients with PC. No clinical trials have directly compared CRS plus HIPEC vs. systemic chemotherapy in patients with PC from GC.

18.3 Role of HIPEC in Peritoneal Carcinomatosis from Gastric Cancer

Tumor extent in the gastric serosa and lymphatic spread are the two most important factors affecting prognosis in patients with GC [38-40]: when the gastric

Table 18.3 Morbidity and complications of CRS plus HIPEC for PC from GC

Study [Reference]	Overall morbidity (%)	Reoperation (%)	Sepsis	Fistula	Abscess	Hematologic toxicity	Ileus	Anastomotic leak
Yang et al. [27]	14.3		1		1		2	1
Scaringi et al. [28]	27			9	5	2		
Roviello et al. [29]	27.9	8.2		5	2	5	1	
Farma et al. [30]	55.6				1	3		
Yonemura et al. [31]	21.5			1	6			6
Fujimura et al. [33]	50	33.3			2			
Beaujard et al. [34]	9.6	4.8				3	2	1
Median	21.5							

CRS, cytoreductive surgery; HIPEC, hyperthermic intraperitoneal chemotherapy; *PC*, peritoneal carcinomatosis; *GC*, gastric cancer

serosa is infiltrated, PC occurs frequently [41] (Fig. 18.1). In this condition, ~ 50% of patients with advanced GC (AGC) will develop PC despite undergoing radical surgery. PC is also common in GC, being already present in 5–20% of patients explored for potentially curative surgery.

The presence of free peritoneal tumor cells (FPTC) in washing specimens were identified in up to 24 % of patients with GC stage Ib and up to 40 % in stages II and III [41]; in 10–38% of cases, the peritoneum was the only site of recurrence [42-46] (Fig. 18.2).

The 5-year survival rate in patients with PC from GC is < 3% [47], with an overall mean and MS of 6.5 and 3.1 months, respectively [34]. Saito et al. [48] reported a 5-year survival rate of patients with advanced GC with FPTC of 15.3 %, similar to that of patients having macroscopical peritoneal metastasis (14.8 %).

Systemic chemotherapy may improve MS up to 12 months in advanced/metastatic GC, but a similar survival benefit has not been reported in macroscopic PC. Yonemura et al. [49] affirmed that the use of adjuvant systemic chemotherapy after radical resection in patients with FPTC showed a survival benefit. Patients treated with adjuvant chemotherapy survived significantly longer than patients in the control group: the 1- and 2-year respective survival rates were 88 % and 44 % in the adjuvant group and 53 % and 9 % in the adjuvant group and the control group. Neoadjuvant chemotherapy (NACT) has been described to decrease the load of macroscopic PC from GC [50]. Yano et al. [51] reported a small series of four of 26 patients (15.4 %) affected by PC from GC

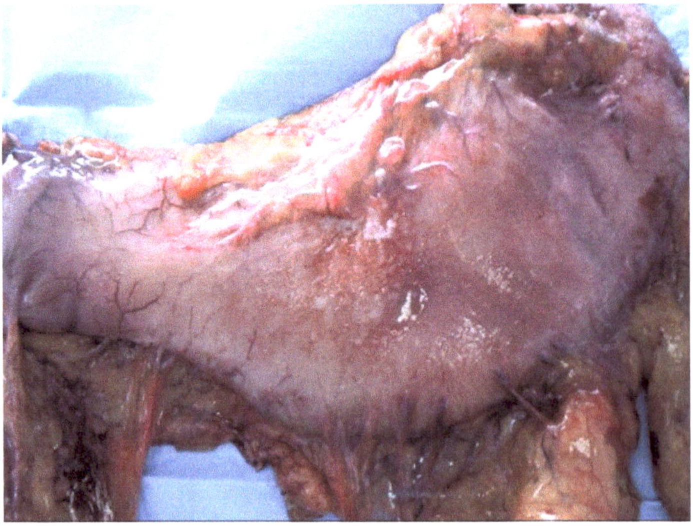

Fig. 18.1 Gastric cancer with serosal invasion

who attained complete remission of peritoneal metastasis after NACT. All these patients subsequently underwent curative resection. Inokuchi et al. [52] reported a partial response in nine of 13 patients (69 %). However, a further study suggested that after NACT, detecting FPTC can change from positive to negative and vice versa: ten of 42 patients (24 %) with negative peritoneal cytology shifted to positive for FPTC during NACT, whereas seven of 19 (37 %) with FPTC-positive cytology at staging laparoscopy turned negative.

GC peritoneal spread remains a major problem, and some authors finally suggest that there is no role for surgery in these instances.

As with other types of PC, in PC from GC, HIPEC after CRS is performed to eliminate FPTC and prevent or delay PC [53]. A number of studies have been conducted with the aim of demonstrating a significant reduction in the rate of subsequent PC and an increase in survival of patients with AGC when radical surgery was combined with HIPEC [22, 54–57]. Yonemura et al. [58] demonstrated that HIPEC could significantly improve the MS from 15 to 48 months and the 5-year survival rate from 12 % to 42 % in patients with FPTC. However results of CRS plus HIPEC treatment of PC from GC seem to be less encouraging in terms of survival, morbidity, and mortality when compared with PC from other tumor types [59–61]. In a French retrospective multicenter study, the PC from GC group showed the worst outcome, with 3- and 5-year survival rates of 18 % and 13 %, respectively. In 2010, Li et al. [62] reported a series of 128 patients with PC from GC: the MS in the unresected group was 6 months, compared with 11.8 months for resected patients. Moreover, the authors observed a significantly improved survival in patients treated with surgery plus HIPEC compared with those treated with surgery alone, but postoperative complications were more frequent in HIPEC cases than in patients with resection alone (20.0 % vs. 13.2 %,

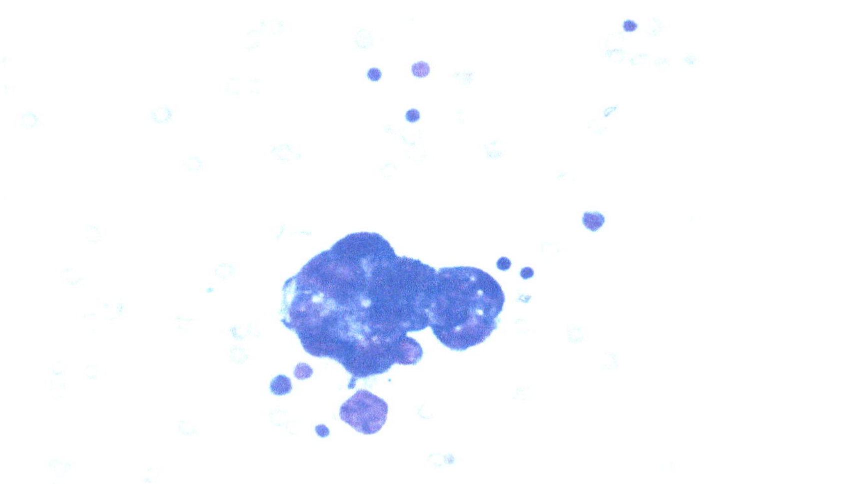

Fig. 18.2 Free peritoneal tumor cells (FPTC) in washing specimen

$P = 0.34$). Yang et al. [27] published the final results of a phase III randomized trial to evaluate efficacy and safety of CRS plus HIPEC for treating PC from GC. Median overall survival (OS) was 6.5 months in the CRS-alone group and 11 months in the CRS plus HIPEC group ($P = 0.046$). This outcome was even more significant in patients with synchronous PC from GC ($n = 51$): median OS was 12 months in the CRS plus HIPEC group ($n = 24$) and 6.5 months in the CRS group ($n = 27$, $P = 0.029$). The 1-, 2-, and 3-year survival rates were, respectively, 29.4 %, 5.9 %, and 0 % for CRS group and 41.2 %, 14.7 %, and 5.9 % for the CRS plus HIPEC group.

CC score has been demonstrated to influence survival, but HIPEC obtained a significant advantage in patients with CC 0–1 compared with those with CC 2–3. Multivariate analysis recognized CRS plus HIPEC, synchronous PC, CC 0–1, systemic chemotherapy, and no serious adverse events as major independent predictors for better survival. HIPEC was ~ 2.6 times more likely to increase survival. In a systematic review, Gill et al. [36] analyzed survival, mortality, and morbidity in the treatment of PC from GC with CRS plus HIPEC: overall MS was 7.9 months. In the subgroup of patients with residual nodules after CRS < 0.25 cm in diameter, MS rose to 15 months. The 1- and 5-year survival rates were 43 % and 13 %, respectively. The treatment-related mortality rate was 4.8 % and morbidity 21.5 %.

In conclusion, in PC from GC, CRS plus HIPEC proved, with good evidence, to improve survival, with acceptable morbidity and mortality rates. It is extremely important to obtain the diagnosis and the diffusion grade of PC from GC before CRS plus HIPEC with the use of staging laparoscopy. The role of surgery is fundamental; CC was strictly related to improved survival. In patients with PC from GC, multimodal treatment is mandatory, with the pivotal role being HIPEC after CRS.

18.4 Surgical Cytoreduction and Hyperthermic Intraperitoneal Chemotherapy

Two recent studies reported MS times > 15 months in patients with PC from GC treated with CRS plus HIPEC [24]. Importantly, both studies also reported CC score as an independent prognostic factor for survival. The experience of institutions and surgeons performing CRS plus HIPEC shows that CC seems to be associated not only with survival but with both mortality and morbidity. The multi-institutional study by Glehen et al. [23], which comprised 159 patients from 15 institutions, reported that the institution at which CRS plus HIPEC was performed was an independent prognostic factor of postoperative complications. CRS plus HIPEC are considered technically challenging procedures with steep learning curves. Smeenk et al. [63] performed CRS plus HIPEC for PC over a 10-year period and analyzed the rate of CC and postoperative morbidity over three consecutive treatment periods. They reported a significantly increased CC rate from 35.6 % to 65.1 % and a subsequent decreased postoperative morbidity from 71.2 % to 34.1 %. Furthermore, they reported that the peak of the learning curve was reached after 130 procedures. Yan et al. [64] compared morbidity rates following CRS plus HIPEC for peritoneal surface malignancies (PSM) in 140 consecutive patients. They reported that severe morbidity rates decreased from 30 % to 10 % when comparing the last 70 cases with the first 70 cases. Controversy remains regarding the treatment of patients with PC from GC: systematic review demonstrates similar mortality and morbidity rates for CRS plus HIPEC for PC from GC compared with PC from other organs. Survival improved in these patients compared with basic supportive therapy; however, systemic chemotherapy data specifically for this population is scarce.

A recent trial comparing gastrectomy, metastasectomy, plus systemic therapy versus systemic therapy alone (GYMSSA trial) was recently conducted in patients with GC [65]. As a prospective phase III randomized trial, GYMSSA has the potential to clarify whether an aggressive surgical approach combined with HIPEC and systemic chemotherapy may benefit GC patients. However the trial included patients with limited metastatic disease, including lung and liver metastases, while HIPEC focused on PC from GC without evidence of distant metastases.

18.5 Adjuvant Role of Hyperthermic Intraperitoneal Chemotherapy

Peritoneal metastasis is the most common type of recurrence and cause of death after surgery in patients with GC [66], developing in ~ 20–50 % of patients who undergo a curative gastrectomy and increasing to 80 % for those with positive peritoneal cytology [67–69]. Tumour-positive cytology has been clearly correlated with intraperitoneal (IP) recurrence and is significantly associated with decreased disease-free (DFS) and OS rates [54, 55, 70] Intravenously administered chemotherapy plus radiotherapy showed no significant survival advantage as adjuvant treatment for patients with a high risk of PC from GC.

Several studies [29, 71–73], including a number of randomized clinical trials (RCTs), have been performed to investigate the usefulness of HIPEC in a prophylactic setting or as adjuvant treatment after potentially curative GC resection. The RCTs conducted by Koga et al. [74] reported a considerably higher 3-year survival rate of patients in the HIPEC plus surgery group (83.0 %) compared with those in the control group (67.3 %), although this was not statistically significant. Similar results were obtained from RCTs reported by Hamazoe et al. [75], with a lower incidence of peritoneal recurrence and a higher 5-year survival rate of patients in the HIPEC group compared with the control group (64.2 % vs. 52.5 %), although the survival benefit did not achieve a statistically significant difference. The RCT conducted by Fujimoto et al. [76] was the first to demonstrate significantly improved peritoneal recurrence and long-term survival rates in the surgery plus HIPEC group compared with surgery alone after curative resection: in addition, peritoneal recurrence rate in the HIPEC group was significantly lower ($p < 0.0001$) compared with that of the control group. In their randomized trials, Fujimura et al. [33] and Yonemura et al. [77] showed a significantly higher rate of survival after adjuvant HIPEC combined with surgery compared with surgery alone: their results showed the independent and synergistic effect of hyperthermia, along with chemotherapeutic agents, against cancer cells, which seems to increase greatly at temperatures of 42.5 °C–43 °C. Yonemura et al. [31] more recently confirmed similar results in an RCT involving normothermic intraperitoneal chemotherapy (NIPEC) procedures: the 5-year survival rate of patients treated with the combination of HIPEC and surgery was significantly higher, at 61 %, than those of the other two groups (NIPEC plus surgery and surgery alone).

Overall, randomized clinical trials on adjuvant HIPEC procedures demonstrate that the peritoneal recurrence rate decreased and survival improved with this treatment modality in patients with advanced GC.

Xu et al. [78] reviewed all available randomized trials investigating the use of HIPEC after radical, potentially curative, resection for locally advanced GC: the authors found seven RCTs comparing surgery plus HIPEC with surgery alone. Based on their results, HIPEC benefitted the patient after curative resection versus resection alone, and in particular, the combination of HIPEC or activated carbon particles was superior to other forms of HIPEC. Similarly, Yan et al. [79] reviewed all clinical trials studying the adjuvant role of perioperative IPEC in resectable GC: based on the meta-analysis of the pooled data from 1,648 patients, a significant improvement in survival was noted with HIPEC alone or HIPEC plus EPIC. A trend toward survival improvement with normothermic IPEC (NIPEC) was also shown, whereas there was no significant trend with either EPIC alone or HIPEC.

18.6 Discussion

The combination of CRS plus HIPEC is to date the only therapeutic strategy with a hope of long-term survival at 5-years in patients with PC of GC. HIPEC could be performed with the aim of minimizing the rate of peritoneal recurrences (adjuvant intent), but several RCTs confirm the survival advantage and the potential adjuvant role of HIPEC in preventing PC in advanced GC.

Patients with serosa-invasive tumors or positive peritoneal cytology are the high-risk groups that show a significant risk of PC and very poor survival prospects: these groups can reasonably be considered for HIPEC and may particularly benefit from this treatment for preventing peritoneal recurrence.

The most recent TNM classification includes IP free cancer cell detection as part of the staging process, denoting M1 when positive, but the incorporation of peritoneal cytology into the algorithm of GC treatment is not universally accepted. Advanced techniques, (immunoassays, immunohistochemistry, and reverse transcriptase polymerase chain reaction) have better sensitivity in detecting IP free cancer cells with better correlation to peritoneal recurrence compared with the traditionally conventional cytological evaluation of peritoneal fluid. Thus, IP free cancer cell detection should be a useful tool for clinical decision making in both neoadjuvant and adjuvant settings, directing more or less aggressive strategies, including chemoperfusion techniques.

The therapeutic approach may also be orientated based on whether patients in whom IP cytology was or was not converted from positive to negative following neoadjuvant therapy.

In conclusion, HIPEC is useful to improve survival in selected patients with advanced GC by reducing the risk of peritoneal recurrence (adjuvant intent) and in patients with peritoneal disease when CC can be achieved (curative intent); patients with unresectable PC it should excluded from such treatment.

At this time, the new frontier is to evaluate the combination treatment with both targeted locoregional and systemic therapies in these patients. The European Union Network of Excellence (EUNE) for Gastric Cancer consequently drafted the following study protocol: patients with gastric cancer infiltrating the serosa (T3-T4), lymph node metastasis (N1), or positive peritoneal cytology will be included. All patients will receive three cycles of platinum-based therapy as defined by the MAGIC protocol [80], followed by D2. Patients will then be randomized to undergo surgery with HIPEC using oxaliplatin or surgery alone (GASTRICHIP, unpublished).

At the same time, new bidirectional chemotherapy, called neoadjuvant intraperitoneal and systemic chemotherapy (NIPS), has been proposed to attack PC from both sides of the peritoneum: in fact, after diagnosis of PC, the patient receives simultaneously chemotherapy IP and intravenously (IV) and . In terms of response rate and progression-free survival (PFS) in patients with advanced GC, bidirectional therapy with HIPEC (cisplatin) plus chemotherapy IV (docetaxel, 5-fluorouracil, and leucovorin) shows a significant advantage compared with chemotherapy IV only.

After NIPS, the disappearance of peritoneal free cancer cells has been reported, and the incidence of CC has increased accordingly. Although severe complications post-NIPS were reported in four of 79 patients, this strategy achieved a change in washing cytology from positive to negative in 41 of 79 patients (63 %). Following NIPS, a surgical phase is accomplished by CRS plus HIPEC to enable CC. After surgery, EPIC is performed on postoperative days 1–5, and systemic chemotherapy is performed on postoperative days 30–40. This protocol is the example of maximum application of all combined therapies that at this time are available to treat this disease [81].

In the past decade, a new drug for IP treatment of GC was developed in Germany. Catumaxomab (trade name Removab®) is a rat–mouse hybrid monoclonal antibody (MAb) composed of one "half" (one heavy chain and one light chain) of an antiepithelial cell adhesion molecule (EpCAM) antibody and one half of an anti-CD3 antibody, thus finally binding both EpCAM and CD3. EpCAM is an epithelial differentiation antigen that is expressed on normal epithelial cells and on almost all carcinomas (especially gastrointestinal and ovarian carcinomas) and functions as a cell adhesion molecule [82]. In addition, the Fc region can bind to an Fc receptor on accessory cells, such as other antibodies, which has led to the drug being called a trifunctional antibody. Actually, catumaxomab is used to treat malignant ascites, as in a phase III randomized trial, IP application of this anti-EpCAM antibody showed significant benefits in puncture-free survival (survival without repeated paracentesis) for patients with malignant ascites [83]. The study demonstrated no statistically significant increases in median OS for other cancers, whereas in patients with GC, a small survival increase was associated with the use of catumaxomab.

18.7 Conclusions and Remarks

Based on current evidence, we can only conclude that CRS plus HIPEC may be an efficacious treatment in patients with PC from GC when CC is achievable. The correct patient selection, the use of new antidrug agents, and increasing experience in specialized centers may contribute to a better result for select patients presenting with GC and PC, and CRS plus HIPEC may eventually become an accepted treatment strategy for these patients. Patients who show a significant risk of PC and very poor survival prognosis can reasonably be considered for HIPEC and may particularly benefit from this treatment in order to prevent peritoneal recurrence. The standardization of surgical procedures and HIPEC techniques, integrated with new anticancer drugs and new bidirectional chemotherapy protocols using NIPS is the goal to improve further the results of this promising treatment strategy.

References

1. Bertuccio P, Chatenoud L, Levi F et al (2009) Recent patterns in gastric cancer: A global overview. Int J Cancer 125:666–673
2. Parkin DM, Bray F, Ferlay J et al (2005) Global cancer statistics, 2002. CA Cancer J Clin 55:74–108
3. Ikeguchi M, Oka A, Tsujitani S et al (1994) Relationship between area of serosal invasion and intraperitoneal free cancer cells in patients with gastric cancer. Anticancer Res 14:2131–2134
4. Sadeghi B, Arvieux C, Glehen O et al (2000) Peritoneal carcinomatosis from non-gynecologic malignancies: Results of the EVOCAPE 1 multicentric prospective study. Cancer 88:358–363
5. Pyrhonen S, Kuitunen T, Nyandoto P et al (1995) Randomized comparison of fluorouracil, epidoxorubicin and methotrexate (FEMTX) plus supportive care with supportive care alone in patients with non-resectable gastric cancer. Br J Cancer 71:587–591
6. Murad AM, Santiago FF, Petroianu A et al (1993) Modified therapy with 5-fluorouracil, doxorubicin, and methotrexate in advanced gastric cancer. Cancer 72:37–41
7. Scheithauer W, Kornek G, Zeh G et al (1995) Palliative chemotherapy versus supportive care in patients with metastatic gastric cancer: A randomized trial. 68 Second International Conference on Biology, Prevention, Treatment of GI Malignancy. Koln, Germany [AQ8]
8. Hanazaki K, Mochizuki Y, Machida T et al (1999) Post-operative chemotherapy in non-curative gastrectomy for advanced gastric cancer. Hepatogastroenterology 46:1238–1243
9. Chu DZ, Lang NP, Thompson C et al (1989) Peritoneal carcinomatosis in non gynecologic malignancy. A prospective study of prognostic factors. Cancer 63:364–367
10. Sugarbaker PH (1995) Peritonectomy procedures. Ann Surg 221:29–42
11. Sugarbaker PH, Jablonski KA (1995) Prognostic features of 51 colorectal and 130 appendiceal cancer patients with peritoneal carcinomatosis treated by cytoreductive surgery and intraperitoneal chemotherapy. Ann Surg 221:124–132
12. van Ruth S, Verwaal VJ, Zoetmulder FA (2003) Pharmacokinetics of intraperitoneal mitomycin C. Surg Oncol Clin N Am 12: 771–780
13. van de Vaart PJ, van der Vange N, Zoetmulder FA et al (1998) Intraperitoneal cisplatin with regional hyperthermia in advanced ovarian cancer: Pharmacokinetics and cisplatin-DNA adduct formation in patients and ovarian cancer cell lines. Eur J Cancer 34:148–154
14. Elias D, Antoun S, Goharin A et al (2000) Research on the best chemohyperthermia technique of treatment of peritoneal carcinomatosis after complete resection. Int J Surg Investig 1:431–439
15. Christophi C, Winkworth A, Muralihdaran V et al (1998) The treatment of malignancy by hyperthermia. Surg Oncol 7:83–90
16. Jacquet P, Averbach A, Stuart OA et al (1998) Hyperthermic intraperitoneal doxorubicin: Pharmacokinetics, metabolism, and tissue distribution in a rat model. Cancer Chemother Pharmacol 41:147–154
17. Storm FK (1989) Clinical hyperthermia and chemotherapy. Radiol Clin North Am 27:621–627
18. Van Cutsem E, Moiseyenko VM, Tjulandin S et al (2006) Phase III study of docetaxel and cisplatin plus fluorouracil compared with cisplatin and fluorouracil as first-line therapy for advanced gastric cancer: A report of the V325 Study Group. J Clin Oncol 24:4991–4997
19. Koichi M, Fujii M, Kanamori N et al (2006) Neoadjuvant chemotherapy with S-q and CD-DP in advanced gastric cancer. J Cancer Res Clin Oncol 132:781–785
20. Yano M, Shiozaki H, Inoue M et al (2002) Neoadjuvant chemotherapy followed by salvage surgery: Effect of survival of patients with primary noncurative gastric cancer. World J Surg 26:1155–1159
21. Fujimoto S, Sherestha RD, Kokubun M et al (1988) Intraperitoneal Hyperthermic perfusion combined with surgery for gastric cancer patients with peritoneal seeding. Ann Surg 208:36-41
22. Yan TD, Black D, Sugarbaker PH et al (2007) A systematic review and meta-analysis of the randomized controlled trials on adjuvant intraperitoneal chemotherapy for resectable gastric cancer. Ann Surg Oncol 14:2702-2713

23. Glehen O, Gilly FN, Arvieux C et al (2010) Association Francaise de Chirurgie. Peritoneal carcinomatosis from gastric cancer: a multi-institutional study of 159 patients treated by cytoreductive surgery combined with perioperative intraperitoneal chemotherapy. Ann Surg Oncol 17:2370–2377
24. Yang XJ, Li Y, Yonemura Y (2010) Cytoreductive surgery plus hyperthermic intraperitoneal chemotherapy to treat gastric cancer with ascites and/or peritoneal carcinomatosis: Results from a Chinese center. J Surg Oncol 101:457-464
25. Yonemura Y, Kawamura T, Bandou E et al (2005) Treatment of peritoneal dissemination from gastric cancer by peritonectomy and chemohyperthermic peritoneal perfusion. Br J Surg 92:370–375
26. Glehen O, Schreiber V, Cotte E et al (2004) Cytoreductive surgery and intraperitoneal chemohyperthermia for peritoneal carcinomatosis arising from gastric cancer. Arch Surg 139:20–26
27. Yang XJ, Huang CQ, Suo T et al (2011) Cytoreductive surgery and hyperthermic intraperitoneal chemotherapy improves survival of patients with peritoneal carcinomatosis from gastric cancer: final results of a phase III randomized clinical trial. Ann Surg Oncol 18:1575-1581
28. Scaringi S, Kianmanesh R, Sabate JM et al (2008) Advanced gastric cancer with or without peritoneal carcitomatosis treated with hyperthermic intraperitoneal chemotherapy: a single western center experience. Eur J Surg Oncol 34:1246-1252
29. Roviello F, Marrelli D, Neri A et al (2006) Treatment of peritoneal carcinomatosis by cytoreductive surgery and intraperitoneal hyperthermic chemoperfusion (IHCP): postoperative outcome and risk factors for morbidity. World J Surg 30:2033–2040
30. Farma JM, Pingpank JF, Lubutti SK et al (2005) Limited survival in patients with carcinomatosis from foregut malignancies after citoreduction and continuos hyperthermic peritoneal perfusion. J Gastroint Surg 9:1346-1353
31. Yonemura Y, de Aretxabala X, Fujimura T et al (2001) Intraoperative chemohyperthermic peritoneal perfusion as an adjuvant to gastric cancer: final results of a randomized controlled study. Hepatogastroenterology 48:1776–1782
32. MussaA, Sandrucci S, Zanon C (2001) Intraoperative chemohyperthermia for advanced gastric: a new procedure with closed abdomen and previously constructed anastomosis. Tumori 87:18-20
33. Fujimura T, Yonemura Y, Muraoka K et al (1994) Continuous hyperthermic peritoneal perfusion for the prevention of peritoneal recurrence of gastric cancer: randomized controlled study. World J Surg 18:150–155
34. Beaujard AC, Glehen O, Caillot JL et al (2000) Intraperitoneal chemohyperthermia with mitomicin C for digestive tract cancer patients with peritoneal carcinomatosis. Cancer 88:2512-2519
35. Chua TC, Yan TD, Saxena A et al (2009) Should the treatment of peritoneal carcinomatosis by cytoreductive surgery and hyperthermic intraperitoneal chemotherapy still be regared as a highly morbid procedure? A systematic review of morbidity and mortality. Ann Surg 249:900–907
36. Gill RS, Al-Adra DP, Nagendran J et al (2011) Treatment of gastric cancer with peritoneal carcinomatosis by cytoreductive surgery and HIPEC: a systematic review of survival, mortality, and morbidity. J Surg Oncol 104: 692-698
37. Preusser P, Wilke H, Achterrath W et al (1989) Phase II study with the combination etoposide, doxorubicin, and cisplatin in advanced measurable gastric cancer. J Clin Oncol 7:1310–1317
38. Nakamura K, Ueyama T, Yao T et al (1992) Pathology and prognosis of gastric carcinoma. Findings in 10,000 patients who underwent primary gastrectomy. Cancer 70:1030-1037
39. Takahashi T, Hagiwara A, Sawai K et al (1991) Intensive intraoperative local chemotherapy for lymph node and peritoneal metastases in gastric cancer. Onkologie 14:152-157
40. Yu CC, Levison DA, Dunn JA et al (1995) Pathological prognostic factors in the second British-Stomach Cancer Group trial of adjuvant therapy in resectable gastric cancer. Br J Cancer 71:1106-1110

41. Ikeguchi M, Oka A, Tsujitani S et al (1994) Relationship between area of serosal invasion and intraperitoneal free cancer cells in patients with gastric cancer. Anticancer Res 14:2131-213
42. D'Angelica M, Gonen M, Brennan MF et al (2004) Patterns of initial recurrence in completely resected gastric adenocarcinoma. Ann Surg 240:808-816
43. Siewert JR, Lordick F, Ott K et al (2006) Curative vs palliative strategies in locoregional recurrence of gastrointestinal malignancies. Chirurg 77:227-235
44. Ott K, Lordick F, Blank S, Büchler M (2011) Gastric cancer: surgery in 2011. Langenbecks Arch Surg 396:743-758
45. Wu B, Wu D, Wang M, Wang G (2008) Recurrence in patients following curative resection of early gastric carcinoma. J Surg Oncol 98: 411-414
46. Yonemura Y (1996) Contemporary approaches towards cure of gastric cancer. Kanazawa: Maeda Shoten Co., p. 115
47. Sadeghi B, Arvieux C, Glehen O et al (2000) Peritoneal carcinomatosis from non-gynecologic malignancies: results of the EVOCAPE 1 multicentric prospective study. Cancer 88:358-363
48. Saito H, Kihara K, Kuroda H et al (2011) Surgical outcomes for gastric cancer patients with intraperitoneal free cancer cell, but no macroscopic peritoneal metastasis. J Surg Oncol 104:534-537
49. Yonemura Y, Endou Y, Bando E et al (2006) The usefulness of oral TS-1 treatment for potentially curable gastric cancer patients with intraperitoneal free cancer cells. Cancer Ther 4:135-142
50. Kochi M, Fujii M, Kanamori N et al (2006) Neoadjuvant chemotherapy with S-1 and CDDP in advanced gastric cancer. J Cancer Res Clin Oncol 132:781-785
51. Yano M, Shiozaki H, Inoue M et al (2002) Neoadjuvant chemotherapy followed by salvage surgery: effect on survival of patients with primary noncurative gastric cancer. World J Surg 26:1155-1159
52. Inokuchi M, Yamashita T, Yamada H et al (2006) Phase I/II study of S-1 combined with irinotecan for metastatic advanced gastric cancer. Br J Cancer 94:1130-1135
53. Averbach AM, Jacquet P (1996) Strategies to decrease the incidence of intra-abdominal recurrence in resectable gastric cancer. Br J Surg 83:726-733
54. Yonemura Y, Ninomiya I, Kaji M (1995) Prophylaxis with intraoperative chemohyperthermia against peritoneal recurrence of serosal invasion-positive gastric cancer. World J Surg 19:450-454
55. Xu DZ, Zhan YQ, Sun XW et al (2004) Meta-analysis of intraperitoneal chemotherapy for gastric cancer. World J Gastroenterol 10:2727-2730
56. Fujimoto S, Takahashi M, Mutou T et al (1999) Successful intraperitoneal hyperthermic chemoperfusion for the prevention of postoperative peritoneal recurrence in patients with advanced gastric carcinoma. Cancer 85:529-534
57. Yonemura Y, de Aretxabala X, Fujimura T (2001) Intraoperative chemohyperthermic peritoneal perfusion as an adjuvant to gastric cancer: final results of a randomized controlled study. Hepatogastroenterology 48:1776-1782
58. Yonemura Y, Bando E, Kawamura T et al (2007) Cytoreduction and intraperitoneal chemotherapy for carcinomatosis from gastric cancer. Cancer Treat Res 134:357-373
59. Hall JJ, Loggie BW, Shen P et al (2004) Cytoreductive surgery with intraperitoneal hyperthermic chemotherapy for advanced gastric cancer. J Gastrointest Surg 8:454-463
60. Samel S, Singal A, Becker H, Post S (2000) Problems with intraoperative hyperthermic peritoneal chemotherapy for advanced gastric cancer. Eur J Surg Oncol 26:222-226
61. Glehen O, Gilly FN, Boutitie F et al (2010) Toward curative treatment of peritoneal carcinomatosis from nonovarian origin by cytoreductive surgery combined with perioperative intraperitoneal chemotherapy: a multi-institutional study of 1,290 patients. Cancer 116:5608-5618
62. Li C, Yan M, Chen J et al (2010) Surgical resection with hyperthermic intraperitoneal chemotherapy for gastric cancer patients with peritoneal dissemination. J Surg Oncol 102:361-365
63. Smeenk RM, Verwall VJ, Zoetmulder FAN (2007) Learning curve of combined modality treatment in peritoneal surface disease. Br J Surg 94:1408-1414

64. Yan TD, Links M, Fransi S et al (2007) Learning curve for cytoreductive surgery and perioperative intraperitoneal chemotherapy for peritoneal surface malignancy—A journey to becoming a nationally funded peritonectomy center. Ann Surg Oncol 14:2270–2280
65. Kerkar SP, Kemp CD, Duffy A et al (2009) The GYMSSA trial: A prospective randomized trial comparing gastrectomy, metastasectomy plus systemic therapy versus systemic therapy alone. Trials 10:121
66. Maekawa S, Saku M, Maehara Y et al (1996) Surgical treatment for advanced gastric cancer. Hepatogastroenterology 43:178–186
67. Fujimoto S, Takahashi M, Mutou T et al (1999) Successful intraperitoneal hyperthermic chemoperfusion for the prevention of postoperative peritoneal recurrence in patients with advanced gastric carcinoma. Cancer 85:529–534
68. Bando E, Yonemura Y, Takeshita Y et al (1999) Intraoperative lavage for cytological examination in 1,297 patients with gastric carcinoma. Am J Surg 178:256–262
69. Boku T, Nakane Y, Minoura T et al (1990) Prognostic significance of serosal invasion and free intraperitoneal cancer cells in gastric cancer. Br J Surg 77:436–439
70. Bonenkamp JJ, Songun I, Hermans J, van de Velde CJ (1996) Prognostic value of positive cytology findings from abdominal washings in patients with gastric cancer. Br J Surg 83:672–674
71. Glehen O, Schreiber V, Cotte E et al (2004) Cytoreductive surgery and intraperitoneal chemohyperthermia for peritoneal carcinomatosis arising from gastric cancer. Arch Surg 139:20–26
72. Glehen O, Mohamed F, Gilly FN (2004) Peritoneal carcinomatosis from digestive tract cancer: new management by cytoreductive surgery and intraperitoneal chemohyperthermia. Lancet Oncol 5:219–28
73. Ikeguchi M, Kondou A, Oka A (1995) Effects of continuous hyperthermic peritoneal perfusion on prognosis of gastric cancer with serosal invasion. Eur J Surg 161:581–586
74. Koga S, Hamazoe R, Maeta M et al (1988) Prophylactic therapy for peritoneal recurrence of gastric cancer by continuous hyperthermic peritoneal perfusion with Mitomycin C. Cancer 61:232–237
75. Hamazoe R, Maeta M, Kaibara N (1994) Intraperitoneal thermochemotherapy for prevention of peritoneal recurrence of gastric cancer. Final results of a randomized controlled study. Cancer 73:2048–2052
76. Fujimoto S, Takahashi M, Mutou T et al (1999) Successful intraperitoneal hyperthermic chemoperfusion for the prevention of postoperative peritoneal recurrence in patients with advanced gastric carcinoma. Cancer 85:529–534
77. Yonemura Y, Ninomiya I, Kaji M et al (1995) Prophylaxis with intraoperative chemohyperthermia against peritoneal recurrence of serosal invasion-positive gastric cancer. World J Surg 19:450–454
78. Xu DZ, Zhan et al (2004) Meta-analysis of intraperitoneal chemotherapy for gastric cancer. World J Gastroenterol 10: YQ, Sun XW 2727–2730
79. Yan TD, Black D, Sugarbaker PH et al (2007) A systematic review and meta-analysis of the randomized controlled trials on adjuvant intraperitoneal chemotherapy for resectable gastric cancer. Ann Surg Oncol 14:2702–1342
80. Cunningham D, Allum WH, Stenning SP et al (2006) MAGIC Trial Participants. Perioperative chemotherapy versus surgery alone for resectable gastro-oesophageal cancer. N Engl J Med 355:11–20
81. Yonemura Y, Elnemr A, Endou Y et al (2010) Multidisciplinary therapy for treatment of patients with peritoneal carcinomatosis from gastric cancer. World J Gastrointest Oncol 2:85–97
82. Heiss MM, Murawa P, Koralewski P et al (2010) The trifunctional antibody catumaxomab for the treatment of malignant ascites due to epithelial cancer: Results of a prospective randomized phase II/III trial. Int J Cancer 127:2209-2221
83. Ströhlein MA, Lordick F, Rüttinger D et al (2011) Immunotherapy of peritoneal carcinomatosis with the antibody catumaxomab in colon, gastric, or pancreatic cancer: an open-label, multicenter, phase I/II trial. Onkologie 34:101-108

19 Peritoneal Carcinomatosis from Colorectal Cancer

Antonio Sommariva and Carlo Riccardo Rossi

19.1 Introduction

In 2012, 447,000 new cases of colorectal cancer (CRC) were reported in Europe [1]. In two large population-based studies, peritoneal carcinomatosis (PC) was present in 4.8–8.3 % of all CRC patients [2, 3]. Incidence rates may vary among study populations, as the incidence of PC is slightly higher (> 10%) in hospital-based studies [4, 5], most likely related to selection bias. In general, PC incidence is probably underestimated, as it is well known that radiological imaging has a low sensibility for detecting peritoneal cancer nodules with respect to other common metastatic sites (liver, lung, lymph nodes), and not all patients undergo a surgical procedure for PC confirmation. PC is reported as being isolated in 42–77 % of cases [2, 4, 6, 7] and is more often associated with colon than with rectal cancer, with an approximate proportion of 1:5 [3]. Colorectal PC can be distinguished as two different clinical entities: synchronous (at the time of primary presentation) or metachronous (after primary treatment). In more than half of the cases, PC presents as synchronous (49–61%) [4, 5, 6, 7].

Substantially, CRC gives rise to the occurrence of PC in two ways: intraperitoneal (IP) spread may occur before surgery as a transmural invasion cancer, or after potential curative surgery, when tumoral cells fall into the abdominal cavity directly from the tumor, from the bowel cavity, or from dissected lymphatics and vessels [8]. Data from two large study populations affected with CRC identified several risk factors (epidemiological, clinical,

A. Sommariva (✉)
Melanoma and Sarcoma Unit,
Veneto Institute of Oncology IOV,
Padova, Italy
e-mail: antonio.sommariva@ioveneto.it

A. Di Giorgio, E. Pinto (Eds), *Treatment of Peritoneal Surface Malignancies*,
Updates in Surgery
DOI: 10.1007/978-88-470-5711-1_19, © Springer-Verlag Italia 2015

Table 19.1 Risk factors for peritoneal dissemination in colorectal cancer

T stage of primary (T4)
Lymph-node status (N1–2)
Mucinous/signet-ring-cell histology
Right-sided tumors
Positive peritoneal cytology
Emergency/nonradical surgery
Perforated/ruptured primary
Ovarian metastases
Previously resected peritoneal nodules
Young age

histological) for PC [2, 3, ,9]. Serosal involvement of the primary (T4 tumors) is frequently associated with synchronous PC [2] and represents an established risk factor for subsequent metachronous PC [3, 5, 9] (Table 19.1). Exfoliation and subsequent seeding of malignant cells throughout the peritoneal cavity is a logical explanation of this phenomenon, which can also be considered for perforated/occlusive primary tumors (spontaneous or iatrogenic) [3, 10]. Right-sided colon tumors are also significantly associated with synchronous PC [2] and represent an independent predictor for metachronous PC [3]. Lymph node status (N1/N2) is another significant predictor of peritoneal failure [3]. Younger patients seem to be at higher risk for PC (at presentation of the primary or during follow-up) [2, 3, 5]. The reasons are unknown but may in part be explained by the fact that older patients less frequently undergo a surgical procedure for PC diagnosis or treatment; thus underestimation in this population may explain this difference. Primary CRC with mucinous histology seems more frequently associated with PC at presentation [2]. Preliminary data on the identification of gene-expression profiling of CRC at risk of PC would have the benefit of better defining therapeutic strategy and follow-up of each individual patient [11, 12].

19.2 Role of Systemic Chemotherapy

Systemic chemotherapy has been considered for many years the only therapeutic option for CRC patients with PC. In the era of 5-fluorouracil (5-FU)-based therapy, the results of systemic chemotherapy for CRC PC were discouraging [4, 6]. Considering a multivariate analysis on predictors of outcome in patients with CRC stage IV disease treated with 5-FU, PC is associated with the worst outcome (median survival 7.7 months) with respect to patients (median survival 11.6 months) with other site of metastases (liver, lung, lymph nodes) [13]. Significant progress has been made in the medical management of metastatic

CRC. The introduction of oxaliplatin and irinotecan to 5-FU-based regimens, coupled more recently with targeted biological therapy (bevacizumab and cetuximab) has improved outcomes for PC patients, leading to a median survival > 20 months [14–19]. The more adverse outcome of PC with respect to other sites of metastatic disease was also confirmed within modern chemotherapy combination treatments, with an estimated 30 % reduction in overall survival (OS) for patients with PC with respect to other unresectable metastatic sites [15]. A possible explanation can be that only patients with more advanced disease were included in those trials, as "no measurable disease" by imaging techniques is a frequent ineligibility criterion for randomized controlled trials (RCT). A part from these considerations, median survival of patients with PC without other sites of metastasis (isolated PC) ranges from 21.8 to 23.9 months [14, 18], suggesting that metastatic CRC confined in the abdominal cavity represents a distinct biological entity with a more favorable prognosis. Although these retrospective and uncontrolled data indicate that modern systemic chemotherapy has led to a better outcome for patients with PC, prospective studies investigating its effect on the subset of patients with isolated PC are still lacking, as are data on the most efficient treatment combination for this clinical entity.

19.3 Role of Surgery

Results of surgical resection for stage IV CRC in recent decades has led to the change in indications for radical surgery of metastases, which are no longer being considered an absolute contraindication. In selected patients with colorectal liver metastasis, though in the absence of prospective randomized clinical trials, radical resection is now considered the standard of care, as a survival benefit has been clearly deduced from historical controls since the late 1990s [20]. For extrahepatic metastatic disease (lung, lymph node, peritoneum), a reasonable number of published studies suggest a potential survival benefit in a highly selected group of patients [21, 22]. The use of surgery for colorectal PC was once restricted to complication palliation, such as intestinal obstruction or perforation. A potential beneficial role of radical surgery in a subset of CRC patients with peritoneal implants has been suggested by some retrospective studies [23–26]. Radical removal of limited peritoneal implants (around the primary tumor or on the ovarian surface) is associated with improved prognosis, whereas gross residual disease and tumor load at the completion of surgery are factors negatively affecting survival.

19.4 Role of Surgery plus Intraperitoneal Chemotherapy

Based on the rationale of the "metastatic insufficiency" of some forms of PC from CRC, the combined approach based on maximal CRS and IP-administered chemotherapy (IP-CHT) was proposed by Sugarbaker, who first demonstrated the feasibility of this treatment and identified prognostic factors for patient selection [27]. After this pioneering experience, several studies (single institution and multicenter) have investigated the utility of CRS associated with IP drug delivery for selected patients with CRC peritoneal involvement, in most cases under hyperthermic conditions [hyperthermic intraperitoneal chemotherapy (HIPEC)] [28, 29]. These studies reported longer survival (median range between 12.8 and 60.1 months) for patients undergoing surgery plus HIPEC versus historical controls treated with systemic chemotherapy alone. However, these results should be interpreted with caution. The selection criteria were extremely heterogeneous; in some trials, patients with hematogenous (liver) metastases were also included in the final analysis, whereas in others, more favorable histology (appendix, pseudomyxoma) was present. Moreover, the timing of IP-CHT (intra-/postoperative), HIPEC method (closed vs. open), and drug type and dosage varied widely among studies. Nonetheless, results of these studies appear much better than those reported in historical control patients treated with chemotherapy alone. These encouraging results were confirmed by a randomized controlled trial promoted by The Netherlands Cancer Institute, which compared standard [5-FU/leucovorin (LV) with or without palliative surgery] with experimental (CRS plus HIPEC) treatment [30]. This trial showed a significant advantage in survival (12.6 vs. 22.3 months) in favor of CRS plus HIPEC group and was stopped prematurely for ethical reasons. These results were confirmed by other comparative studies [17–19, 31] (Table 19.2). Level of evidence at present justifies the use of CRS plus HIPEC in selected patients in centers with significant experience in treating peritoneal surface malignancies, preferably in the context of prospective trials. The decision-making process should be based upon defined selection criteria, which should be discussed in a multidisciplinary meeting involving surgeons, oncologists, and radiologists. Different scoring systems have been proposed to identify with good accuracy patients with severe colorectal PC and predicted short survival outcome. However, none of studies was prospectively tested [32, 33]. A full explanation of potential risks and benefits of CRS plus HIPEC should be given to the patients, explaining treatment alternatives and taking into account the individual motivation in undergoing this treatment (Fig. 19.1).

19.5 Selection Criteria

19.5.1 Cytoreduction Completeness

The maximum size of residual disease remaining after surgical cytoreduction has a strong prognostic value for colorectal PC [34]. Median survival of patients with incomplete surgery (i.e., residual disease > 2.5 mm) and IP—CHT is only 8 months. This observation leads to the conclusion that it is necessary to achieve

Table 19.2 Results of modern chemotherapy in colorectal peritoneal carcinomatosis

Study [Reference]	Study type	Study period	Patients (*N*)	Chemotherapy type	Extraperitoneal metastasis	Median overall survival (months)	Median progression-free survival (months)
Elias et al. [18]	Retrospective analysis of institutional multihospital cancer registries	1998–2003	48	Oxaliplatin–irinotecan based ± bevacizumab/cetuximab	No	23.9	NA
Franko et al. [19]	Retrospective analysis of institutional multihospital cancer registries	2001–2007	38	Oxaliplatin–irinotecan based ± bevacizumab/cetuximab	Yes	16.8	NA
Klaver et al. [14]	Eindhoven cancer registry analysis	2006–2009	136	Not reported (national guidelines)	No	21.8	15
Franko et al. [15]	Retrospective analysis of two phase III trials of North Central Treatment Group (N9741-N9841)	1998–2003	364	Oxaliplatin–irinotecan based	Yes	15.7	5.8
Klaver et al. [16]	Retrospective analysis of two phase III trials of the Dutch Colorectal Cancer Group (CAIRO 1 and 2)	2003–2005	81	Oxaliplatin–irinotecan based ± bevacizumab/cetuximab	Yes	15.2	7.2
Chua et al. [17]	Retrospective analysis of multicentre prospective collected databases	1988–2009	32	Oxaliplatin–irinotecan based ± bevacizumab/cetuximab	No	23	NA

NA, not available

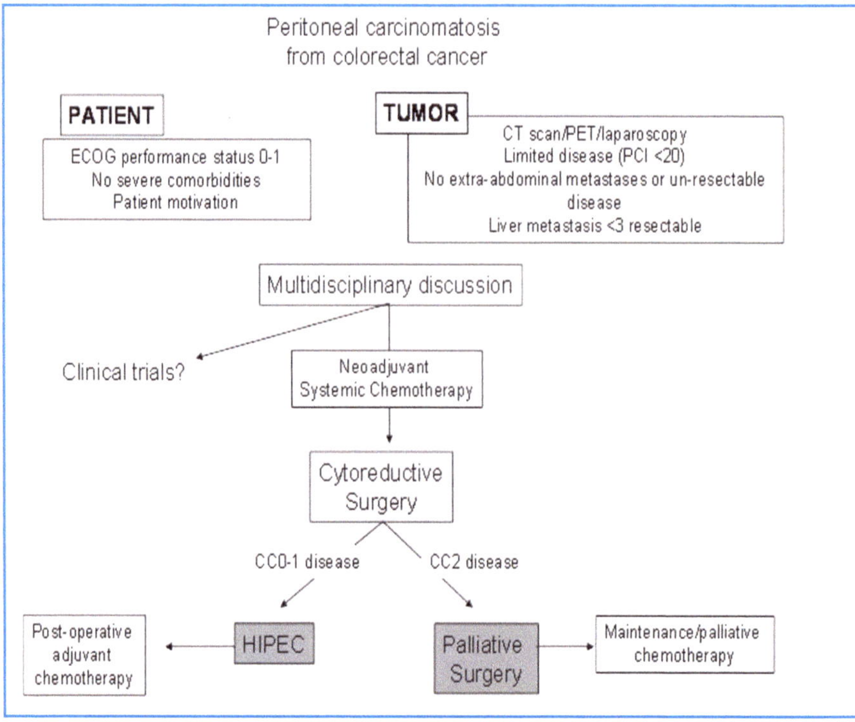

Fig. 19.1 Algorithm for selecting and treating patients with colorectal peritoneal carcinomatosis at Veneto Institute of Oncology. *HIPEC,* hyperthermic intraperitoneal chemotherapy; *ECOG,* Eastern Cooperative Oncology Group; *CT,* computed tomography; *PET,* positron emission tomography; *PCI,* Peritoneal Cancer Index; *CC,* Completeness of Cytoreduction score

complete cytoreduction before treating a patient with HIPEC, as confirmed by a consensus statement built on expert opinion [35]. The possibility of obtaining complete cytoreduction depends on established clinical and radiological criteria valid for all types of peritoneal malignancies selected for HIPEC. Biliary tract, ureteral, and multiple small-bowel obstruction and extensive small-bowel mesentery and gastrohepatic ligament involvement represent situations in which direct penetration beyond the peritoneal barrier into unresectable or marginally resectable structures make a complete or near complete cytoreduction unlikely and are associated with an unacceptable risk of complication [36].

A learning-curve effect on cytoreduction has been demonstrated, with the zenith of the learning curve (graded by the percentage of complete cytoreductions) reached after approximately 130 procedures. [37]. On this basis, the complete cytoreduction rate reflects a center's experience on patient selection and treatment expertise, meaning that all colon cancers with peritoneal dissemination should be referred to an experienced peritoneal-surface malignancy center for accurate clinical, radiological, and—possibly—surgical assessment of carcinomatosis resectability.

19.5.2 Peritoneal Diffusion

Disease extent, calculated as the number of abdominal regions involved and volume of nodules in each region, represents an important prognostic criteria in colorectal PC patients selected for CRS plus HIPEC. Among the different scoring systems, the Peritoneal Cancer Index (PCI) is the most frequently used for staging and was elected the best intraoperative staging system in treating peritoneal surface malignancies [38], although other staging systems are proven to have a prognostic value for colorectal PC [39, 40]. The prognostic cutoff values for PCI were investigated in a large multi-institutional retrospective study of 523 patients treated with CRS and IP-CHT between 1990 and 2007. When PCI is > 20, median survival is 18 months, which is no longer than after systemic chemotherapy alone [34]. For these reasons, PCI > 20 is now considered a relative contraindication to CRS plus HIPEC, a statement confirmed by one international expert consensus [36]. Although computed tomography (CT) and positron emission tomography (PET) technology and expertise in PC could improve in the near future, at present, scores of preoperative radiological PCI formulation before surgical exploration significantly underestimate intraoperative PCI [41]. It has been calculated that 12 % of patients selected for CRS plus HIPEC after CT scan became ineligible for treatment after surgical exploration [42]. Laparoscopic exploration has been proposed as a complementary method for predicting PCI in patients selected for CRS plus HIPEC [43]. Because a clear underestimation of the laparoscopic PCI score compared with open PCI has been shown [44, 45], a more defined clinical and radiological selection process is necessary to understand which patients are eligible for pre-CRS plus HIPEC laparoscopy workup. This would avoid unnecessary laparotomy in a higher percentage of cases and contribute to a more cost-effective treatment and better QoL for these patients.

19.5.3 Primary tumor

Primary tumor site is considered an important prognostic factor. Patients with rectal cancer treated with CRS and peritoneal IP-CHT have a worse survival rate with respect to colon cancer [46, 47]. Moreover, aggressiveness of primary tumor histology (signet-ring-cell histology, grading, lymph node involvement) suggests a worse prognosis [34, 48–50].

19.5.4 Extraperitoneal Disease

CRS plus HIPEC is usually contraindicated in the presence of systemic disease, and colorectal patients with peritoneal carcinomatosis associated with extraperitoneal metastases are usually deemed not suitable for treatment and are referred to an oncologist for systemic chemotherapy. Surgery for limited and stable metastatic disease has sometimes been offered to patients with multiple disease sites (liver, lung, peritoneum), but the issue remains under investigation, and results of the few available studies are influenced by a high selection bias [21]. A single-center experience reported a 28 % 5-year survival rate in patients who underwent an R0 resection of extrahepatic disease simultaneously with hepatectomy for colorectal liver metastasis [51]. Although the reported experience remains limited, an increasing number of studies on this subject have been published [52]. Patients with metastases in the liver and peritoneum who were selected for curative resection and HIPEC showed a trend toward a lower OS when compared with patients with isolated peritoneal disease treated with CRS plus HIPEC. However, patients with liver and peritoneal metastases show a better survival trend after CRS plus HIPEC when compared with modern systemic chemotherapy alone. Hence, there is insufficient evidence to exclude patients with liver and peritoneal disease from a potentially curative treatment. In these patients, the selection process should be more accurate, taking into account the potential added morbidity of liver resection and that only patients with low peritoneal burden (PCI < 10) and liver disease (< 3 metastases) will probably reap benefits from this combined approach [53–55].

19.6 Italian Experience

The Italian experience is collected in a prospective database that includes operative, postoperative, and follow-up data of patients treated in five Italian centers and represents the largest Italian study on multimodal treatment of colorectal PC. A recent update investigating 146 consecutive patients treated during from 1995 to 2007 confirms that the cytoreduction completeness represents the most important prognostic factor, along with the presence of liver metastases resected at any time during the disease, of unfavorable sites such as small intestine, hepatic hilum, diaphragm, and of gross involvement of retroperitoneal lymph nodes [56].

19.7 Open Questions

19.7.1 Need for Treatment Standardization

Among the oncological community, a main criticism regarding benefits of IP administration of drugs for colorectal carcinomatosis is the absolute lack of standardization. There is a high variability in HIPEC modality (open vs. closed), chosen drugs (mitomycin vs. oxaliplatin based), drug dosage, perfusate volume, inflow temperature, and perfusion duration [57]. Both mitomycin C and oxaliplatin are considered for IP administration for their high molecular weight, resulting in a high IP concentration and limited systemic absorption and toxicity. For mitomycin C, a dose-escalation study fixed the maximum tolerated dose as single agent at 35 mg/m^2 [58]. For oxaliplatin, a dosage of 460 mg/m^2 in 2 l/m^2 of 5 % dextrose at 42–44 °C over 30 min was recommended [59]. In that protocol, IV administration of 5-FU (400 mg/m^2) and LV (20 mg/m^2) 1 h before HIPEC was proposed to enhance IP-administered oxaliplatin activity. Combination drug therapies with a mitomycin C and oxaliplatin dose reduction have been studied, some of which have been adopted by centers worldwide, although not always tested in a phase I trial. The combination of mitomycin C (15–20 mg/m^2) and doxorubicin (15 mg/m^2) has been tested in the USA and Germany [60]. In Italy, the preferred drug combination is mitomycin C (3.3 mg/m^2/l) plus cisplatinum (25 mg/m^2/l) for 60–90 min [56]. In a few uncontrolled studies comparing mitomycin C and oxaliplatin-based regimens, no clear difference in toxicity (hematological, renal), postoperative complication rate, disease free and OS were detected when comparing the two HIPEC protocols [60, 61].

In absence of level I evidence, the choice of drugs and technique for HIPEC administration remains mainly based on the tradition of the center rather than on a critical evaluation of toxicity and efficacy. While waiting designed prospective trials to determine the best HIPEC protocol, the first attempt for achieving a consensus on this issue emerged in the fifth international workshop on peritoneal surface malignancies held in Milan in 2006 [62]. In this context, substantial agreement was obtained and published by the American Society of Peritoneal Surface Malignancies (ASPSM) regarding the optimal HIPEC delivery method for colorectal carcinomatosis [63]. The standardization of HIPEC delivery protocols in colorectal PC through consensus documents and multi-institutional registries is the first step toward a clear definition of the optimal treatment regimen in relation to morbidity, mortality, and long-term outcome.

19.7.2 Comparing CRS plus HIPEC and New Systemic CHT

Despite the substantial benefits of CRS plus HIPEC with respect to systemic chemotherapy in colorectal PC demonstrated in a RCT and in several uncontrolled comparative studies, significant scepticism remains with regard to the wide applicability of CRS plus HIPEC in terms of safety and efficacy. Improved response and prolonged OS rates of patients with stage IV CRC obtained after the introduction of modern chemotherapy (median survival > 20 months) raises the question of whether CRS plus HIPEC remains the optimal treatment option for colorectal carcinomatosis. The question appears even more urgent after the introduction of biologic therapy [vascular endothelial growth factor (VEGF) and epithelial growth factor receptor (EGFR) inhibitors], is reported to improve survival outcome compared with standard treatment alone [17, 64]. The role of modern systemic chemotherapy in colorectal PC is poorly investigated, and few data are available regarding patients with isolated peritoneal involvement. A prospective study on systemic chemotherapy restricted to peritoneal carcinomatosis has not yet been done. The question of whether CRS plus HIPEC offers a significant advantage in terms of survival compared with a highly selected and well-matched group of patients with colorectal PC treated with "modern" chemotherapy regimens alone remains unanswered, and some trials attempting to clarify this issue are ongoing at the time of this writing (Table 19.3). CRS plus HIPEC should be matched in the near future with the improved results of systemic chemotherapy, keeping in mind that treatment-related mortality and morbidity, side effects, and QoL play a pivotal role in therapeutic planning in a population with a relatively short life expectancy.

19.7.3 Role of Adjuvant Chemotherapy

Systemic adjuvant chemotherapy in a patient population with carcinomatosis of colonic origin selected for CRS and IP-CHT showed a positive prognostic impact in two large registry studies [34, 48]. Half of the patients with isolated PC treated with CRS plus HIPEC showed systemic recurrence during their life course, and the rationale for treating those patients with systemic chemotherapy was mainly directed at preventing hematogenous metastases (liver, lung, bone). Moreover, neoadjuvant chemotherapy allows for better patient selection for CRS plus HIPEC, excluding those with systemic progression and considering only those with a more favorable tumor biology (better drug responsiveness, lack of metastatic potential). The activity of systemic chemotherapy on colorectal peritoneal nodules is largely unknown. As for rectal cancer and liver metastasis, the radiological and histological response of peritoneal nodules to neoadjuvant chemotherapy can theoretically provide important information on tumor chemosensitivity and suggest the optimal postoperative regimen after surgery (Figs. 19.2 and 19.3). At present, the few available data show that failure to respond to systemic adjuvant treatment before CRS plus HIPEC is not necessarily associated with an unfavorable outcome [65, 66]. For this reason, failure to respond to previous adjuvant systemic treatment should not be considered an exclusion criterion for treatment with CRS plus HIPEC. A possible explanation for the supposed little efficacy of systemically administered drugs could be the poor vascularization of peritoneal nodules, which prevents a therapeutic drug concentration. A pilot study aimed at evaluating the response rate and characteristics of patients with initially unresectable colorectal PC seems to confirm a substantial unresponsiveness to systemically administered chemotherapy [67]. In that study, all patients were evaluated with laparoscopy before and after chemotherapy; and in none of them was systemic administration of chemotherapy able to convert unresectable PC into resectable PC, a condition that would have made those patients potentially suitable candidates for CRS plus HIPEC. At laparoscopy, 78 % of patients showed progressive disease,

Table 19.3 Registered trials on CRS plus HIPEC for peritoneal carcinomatosis from colorectal cancer

Title	ID number	Sponsor	Country	Phase	Primary end point	Study start date	Status
A randomized phase-III study comparing cytoreductive surgery plus intraperitoneal chemotherapy versus modern systemic chemotherapy in colorectal peritoneal carcinomatosis	ClinicalTrials.gov ID:	Uppsala University	Sweden	III	Overall survival	June 2003	Completed
Cytoreductive surgery associated with hyperthermic chemotherapy: intraperitoneal versus systemic chemotherapy in the treatment of resectable colorectal carcinomatosis. IOV-CAR-CRC-1-2012	EudraCT no: 2012-004058-27	Veneto Oncology Institute, Padua	Italy	II	Overall survival	January 2013	Recruiting
Multicentric phase III trial comparing simple follow-up to exploratory laparotomy plus "in principle" HIPEC in colorectal patients initially treated with surgery and adjuvant chemotherapy who have a high risk of developing colorectal peritoneal carcinomatosis. ProphyloCHIP	ClinicalTrials.gov ID: NCT01226394 EudraCT no.: 2009-015598-11	Gustave Roussy, Cancer Campus, Grand Paris	France	III	Disease-free survival	April 2010	Recruiting
Randomized phase II study to evaluate an audit approach: surgical systematically associated with intraperitoneal	EudractCT no. 2012-002739-27	University of Milan, "Luigi Sacco" Hospital	Italy	II	Overall survival	June 2012	Recruiting

(cont.) →

Table 19.3 (*continued*)

chemohyperthermia and possible cytoreductive surgery versus standard follow-up in patients at high risk of developing peritoneal carcinomatosis from colorectal carcinoma							
Prospective randomized trial evaluating mandatory second look surgery with HIPEC and CRS versus standard of care in subjects at high risk of developing colorectal peritoneal metastases	ClinicalTrials.gov ID: NCT01095523	National Cancer Institute (NCI)	USA	II	Overall survival	January 2010	Withdrawn
Multimodality treatment including pre- and postoperative systemic chemotherapy plus cetuximab, cytoreductive surgery (CRS) and hyperthermic intraperitoneal chemotherapy (HIPEC) in patients with peritoneal carcinomatosis arising from wild type *K-ras* colon cancer: a prospective multicenter phase II Study. COMBACT trial	ClinicalTrials.govID: NCT01540344 EudraCT no.: 2009 -014040-11	University of Regensburg	Germany	II	Progression-free survival	October 2010	Recruiting
Neoadjuvant chemotherapy, cytoreductive surgery with hyperthermic intraperitoneal	EudraCT no.: 2010-020787-37	University Medical Center, Groningen	Netherlands	II	Safety of neo-adjuvant chemotherapy	November 2011	Recruiting

(*cont.*)

Table 19.3 (*continued*)

chemotherapy for peritoneal carcinomatosis of colorectal origin (NACHO trial)							
Phase II study comparing normothermic versus hyperthermic intraoperative chemoperfusion with oxaliplatin in patients with peritoneal metastases from appendiceal or colon cancer	ClinicalTrials.govID: NCT01575730	University Hospital, Ghent	Belgium	II	Morbidity/mortality, oxaliplatin pharmacokinetics	June 2012	Recruiting
Phase III study evaluating the use of systemic chemotherapy and chemohyperthermia intraperitoneal preoperatively (CHIP) and after maximum resection of peritoneal carcinomatosis originating with colorectal cance (Prodige 7/ACCORD 15)	ClinicalTrials.gov ID: NCT00769405 EudraCT no: 2006-006175-20	UNICANCER	France/ Spain	III	Overall survival	February 2008	Recruiting
Randomized phase 2 study comparing second-look laparoscopy to standard follow-up in patients with no radiologic evidence of disease at 6 months after complete resection of colorectal mucinous carcinoma	ClinicalTrials.gov ID: NCT01628211	National Cancer Institute, Naples	Italy	II	Overall survival	April 2012	Recruiting

CRS, cytoreductive surgery; *HIPEC*, hyperthermic intraperitoneal chemotherapy
Data source: U.S. National Institutes of Health, National Cancer Institute NCI (*http://clinicaltrials.gov/ct2/home*) and European Clinical Trials Database, EudraCT (*https://eudract.ema.europa.eu/*)

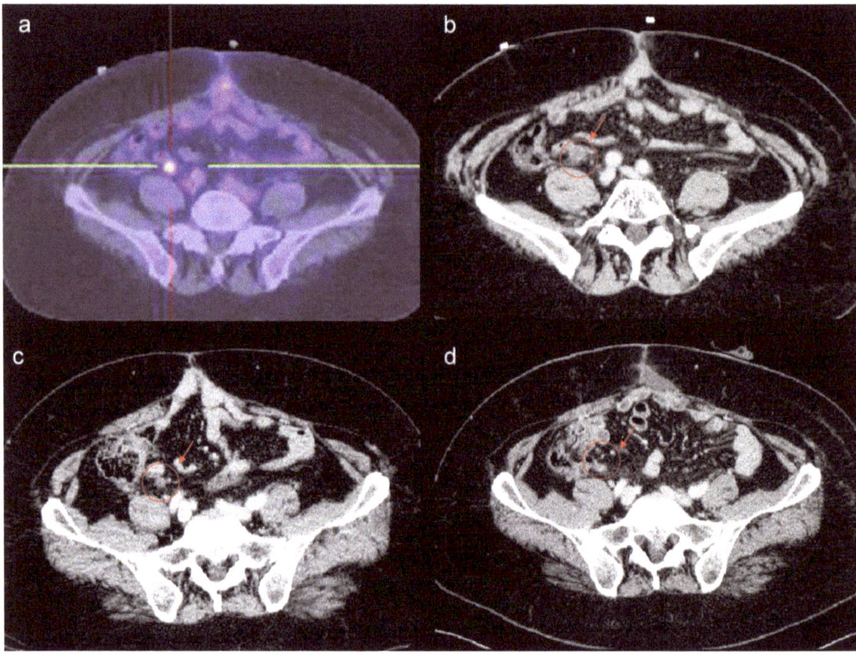

Fig. 19.2 Radiological response to neoadjuvant chemotherapy of peritoneal nodule from mucinous adenocarcinoma. Positron emission tomography/computed tomography (*CT*) (**a**) and *CT* (**b**) before chemotherapy; *CT* scan before cytoreductive surgery (*CRS*) plus hyperthermic intraperitoneal chemotherapy (*HIPEC*) (**c**) and 3 months after surgery (**d**)

and no macroscopic response was documented. Interestingly, laparoscopic evaluation showed an important discrepancy with respect to that obtained with radiological evaluation. These findings suggest a substantial unreliability of disease response assessment based on preoperative imaging alone.

Moreover, the influence of neoadjuvant chemotherapy on surgical complications in patients selected for CRS plus HIPEC remains largely unknown. Administration of bevacizumab before surgery with complete cytoreduction followed by HIPEC for colorectal carcinomatosis is associated with a twofold increase in morbidity rates. Therefore, the safety and efficacy of bevacizumab before HIPEC remains to be evaluated [68]. The potential benefit of neoadjuvant chemotherapy is under study in prospective trials (Table 19.4)

19.7.4 Role of HIPEC

Even though data from animal models confirm the efficacy of IP-CHT on experimentally induced carcinomatosis [69, 70], the additive role of HIPEC in treating colorectal PC has never been exhaustively investigated in clinical studies. Doubts about the effect of IP-CHT also spring from a randomized prospec-

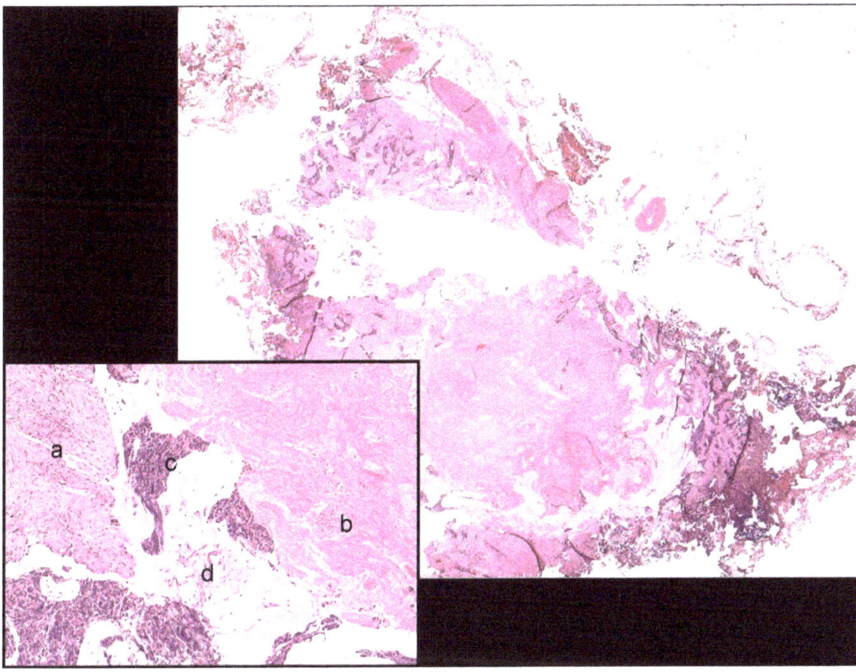

Fig. 19.3 Histological response of mucinous adenocarcinoma to peritoneal implants after neoadjuvant chemotherapy before cytoreductive surgery (*CRS*) plus hyperthermic intraperitoneal chemotherapy (*HIPEC*) (same patient as in Fig. 19.2; hematoxylin and eosin × 10). Fibrosis (**a**); necrosis (**b**) exists with tumoral tissue (**c**); mucinous lakes (**d**)

tive study that compared radical surgery of colorectal carcinomatosis associated with IP-CHT or not [71]. The study, interrupted due to poor enrollment, confirms the validity of complete surgical cytoreduction, whereas the therapeutic impact of IP-CHT does not appear to be significant. This single observation also supports the impression that the results of combined CRS and IP-CHT seem not to be influenced by the type of perfusion technique used or by the drugs employed [61]. This point remains controversial, as in the context of a CRS protocol, HIPEC appears superior to normothermic IP-CHT, with improved outcome and no significant increase in mortality or morbidity rates [72]. In another nonrandomized trial, HIPEC confers a significant survival advantage with respect to a control group (surgery only), even in patients in whom the tumor was not optimally debulked [Completeness of Cytoreduction (CC) scores 2–3) [73]. In addition to the question regarding the real therapeutic value of HIPEC in CRS for colorectal carcinomatosis, another issue yet to be clarified is its possible role in favoring postsurgical complications, estimated to be in the order of 12–52 % [74]. HIPEC determines a different incidence of systemic toxicity (especially hematological and renal) depending on the drug type and dosage. Its true role in the event of postsurgical complications (fistulas and abscesses) is quite difficult to determine and therefore remains inade-

Table 19.4 Comparative studies on cytoreduction surgery (CRS) plus intraperitoneally administered chemotherapy vs. systemically administered chemotherapy for colorectal peritoneal carcinomatosis

Study [Reference]	Study period	Study Type	Level of evidence	No.	Therapy	Median survival	Log-rank test
Verwaal et al. [30]	1998–2001	Randomized CT	Ib	54	CRS plus HIPEC (mitomycin C IP)	22.3	P =0.03
				51	Systemic chemotherapy (5-FU IV plus LV ± irinotecan IV) ± palliative surgery	12.6	
Mahteme et al. [31]	1991–1999	Case control study	IIb	18	CRS plus EPIC (5-FU IP)	32	P=0.01
				18	Systemic chemotherapy (5-FU IV plus LV/methotrexate plus 5-FU IV plus LV)	24	
Elias et al. [18]	1998–2003	Case control study	IIb	48	CRS plus HIPEC (oxaliplatin IP plus single-bolus 5-FU IV) plus systemic chemotherapy (5-FU IV plus LV plus oxaliplatin/irinotecan)	62.7	P<0.05
				48	Systemic chemotherapy (5-FU IV plus LV plus oxaliplatin/irinotecan) ± palliative surgery	23.9	
Franko et al. [19]	2001–2007	Case control study	IIb	67	CRS plus HIPEC (mitomycin C IP) plus systemic chemotherapy (5-FU IV plus LV ± oxaliplatin/irinotecan ± biological agents)	34.7	P<.001
				38	Systemic Chemotherapy (5-FU IV plus LV ± oxaliplatin/irinotecan ± biological agents)	16.8	
Chua et al. [17]	1998–2009	Case control study	IIb	110	CRS plus chemotherapy IP (not specified) plus systemic chemotherapy (5-FU IV plus LV ± oxaliplatin/irinotecan ± biological agents)	38.0	P =0.01
				184	Best supportive care or systemic chemotherapy (5-FU IV plus LV ± oxaliplatin/irinotecan ± biological agents) ± palliative surgery	9.0	

LV, leucovorin; *IV*, intravenously; *IP*, intraperitoneally

quately investigated. Only one study reports a rate of surgical complications significantly correlated with chemotherapeutic drug dosage [75]. At this writing, a randomized multicenter trial was ongoing in France (Prodige 7) aimed at evaluating whether the therapeutic advantage of multimodal treatment (CRS plus HIPEC) in PC of colorectal origin is related to the synergistic effect of IP-CHT with oxaliplatin [76].

19.7.5 Prophylactic HIPEC

The application of IP-CHT as prophylactic treatment in CRC patients at high risk of peritoneal seeding represents an appealing strategy supported by increasing evidence of the clinical and pathological risk factors for PC (Table 19.1) [2, 3, 9]. One review identified a high risk of peritoneal failure in the presence of synchronous PC, synchronous isolated ovarian metastases, and perforated primary tumor [10]. At lower risk are patients with tumors with serosal or adjacent organ invasion, mucinous/signet-ring-cell carcinomas, and positive cytology. Prophylactic IP-CHT has been tested both in a postoperative setting (normothermic) and for intraoperative (HIPEC) therapy (Table 19.5).

The outcome of prophylactic postoperative normothermic IP-CHT appears controversial. A significant improvement in survival [77, 78] and locoregional recurrence was noted in two RCTs comparing adjuvant IP-administered 5-FU with IV-administered chemotherapy alone, although results were not confirmed by two successive RCT with a similar design [79, 80]. The lack of confirmed efficacy regarding prophylactic IP-CHT may be related to the normothermic drug-delivery method and the use of 5-FU, which is not considered the best option for treating peritoneal implants. The necessity of narrower selection criteria, which only includes patients with primary CRC at higher risk of PC, was also investigated. An Italian case–control study investigated the role of prophylactic HIPEC in a selected group of patients with colon cancer (T3/4 and mucinous/signet-ring-cell histology) [81]. The experimental group underwent resection of the primary together with omentum, ovaries, cecal appendix, and hepatic round ligament, followed by oxaliplatin-based HIPEC. A significantly lower rate of peritoneal recurrence and longer DFS were detected in the prophylactic group with respect to retrospective selection of patients who fulfilled the same inclusion criteria (4 % vs. 22 %; 36.8 vs. 21.8 months, respectively). The comparative study was nonrandomized, and no difference in OS was observed. In another uncontrolled study, a group of CRC patients with positive cytology at the time of primary resection were selected for postoperative IP administration of mitomycin C. In a multivariate analysis, IP-CHT was the only significant prognostic factor for peritoneal recurrence survival, even though OS was not affected by the locoregional treatment [82]. These studies show that an aggressive prophylactic surgical approach associated with IP-CHT may positively modify the natural course of peritoneal disease and be of benefit in selected

Table 19.5 Published studies on prophylactic intraperitoneally administered chemotherapy in "high-risk" CRC patients

Study [Reference]	Type	Study period	Patients (*N*)	Indication	Experimental protocol	Results
Scheithauer et al. [77]	RCT	1991–1995	241	Stage III/T4	5-FU/LV IV vs 5-FU/LV IV + IP	Reduced locoregional recurrence (local ± peritoneal) in stage III
Vaillant et al. [79]	RCT	1986–1991	267	Stage II/III	5-FU IV vs 5-FU IP	No benefit on peritoneal recurrence, DS and OS
Nordlinger et al. [80]	RCT	1993–1998	1,857	Stage II/III	5-FU/LV/folate IV vs 5-FU/LV/folate plus IP/5-FU intraportally	No survival benefit
Sammartino et al. [81]	Case–control study	2006–2008	75	Mucinous/signet-ring cell histology, T3/4	FOLFOX IV vs FOLFOX IV plus extended surgery plus oxaliplatin HIPEC	Lower peritoneal recurrence, no survival benefit
Noura et al. [82]	Case–control study	1985–2006	52	Positive cytology	Postoperative mitomycin C IP	Better peritoneal RFS and CSS

CRC, colorectal cancer; *RCT*, randomized controlled trial; *IV*, intravenously; *IP*, intraperitoneally; *5-FU*, 5-fluorouracil; *LV*, leucovorin; *FOLFOX*, folinic acid (leucovorin); 5-FU, oxaliplatin; *HIPEC*, hyperthermic intraperitoneal chemotherapy; *RFS*, recurrence-free survival; *CSS*, cancer-specific survival

CRC patients at the moment of primary treatment, but this strategy should be further investigated in RCT.

19.7.6 Second-look plus HIPEC

According to a similar rationale, a prophylactic HIPEC as completion of second-look surgery has been proposed in the setting of patients at high risk of peritoneal recurrence. A study on systematic second look surgery plus HIPEC has been performed in a group of CRC patients at high risk of peritoneal recurrence (minimal peritoneal carcinomatosis resected with the primary, spontaneous tumor perforation or inadvertent rupture of the tumor, ovarian metastasis) [83]. After six months of systemic chemotherapy and no clinical or radiological evidence of disease, second-look surgery followed by CRS (if peritoneal carcinomatosis was present) and systematic HIPEC was performed. This protocol revealed early carcinomatosis in 56% of patients with a mean PCI ranging between 5 and 9. After a median follow-up of 30 months, the 5-year disease-free survival (DFS) and OS rate were 44 % and 90 %, respectively. Peritoneal recurrences occurred in 17 % of cases, mostly in patients with macroscopic PC discovered during the second-look procedure. Three randomized control trials are ongoing in the USA [84] and Europe attempting to answer several questions about what issues must be addressed: the real impact on outcome (survival and morbidity) of this aggressive strategy with respect to simple follow-up, the timing of second-look surgery, and patients best suited to undergo the regimen (Table 19.3).

References

1. Ferlay J, Steliarova-Foucher E, Lortet-Tieulent J et al (2013) Cancer incidence and mortality patterns in Europe: estimates for 40 countries in 2012. Eur J Cancer 49:1374-1403
2. Lemmens VE, Klaver YL, Verwaal VJ et al (2011) Predictors and survival of synchronous peritoneal carcinomatosis of colorectal origin: a population-based study. Int J Cancer 128:2717-2725
3. Segelman J, Granath F, Holm T et al (2012) Incidence, prevalence and risk factors for peritoneal carcinomatosis from cancer. Br J Surg 99:699-705
4. Jayne DG, Fook S, Loi C, Seow-Choen F (2002) Peritoneal carcinomatosis from colorectal cancer. Br J Surg 89:1545-1550
5. Kerscher AG, Chua TC, Gasser M et al (2013) Impact of peritoneal carcinomatosis in the disease history of colorectal cancer management: a longitudinal experience of 2406 patients over two decades. Br J Cancer 108:1432-1439
6. Chu DZ, Lang NP, Thompson C et al (1989) Peritoneal carcinomatosis in nongynecologic malignancy. A prospective study of prognostic factors. Cancer 63:364-367
7. Sadeghi B, Arvieux C, Glehen O et al (2000) Peritoneal carcinomatosis from non-gynecologic malignancies: results of the EVOCAPE 1 multicentric prospective study. Cancer 88:358-363
8. Koppe MJ, Boerman OC, Oyen WJ, Bleichrodt RP (2006) Peritoneal carcinomatosis of col-

orectal origin: incidence and current treatment strategies. Ann Surg 243:212-222
9. Hompes D, Tiek J, Wolthuis A et al (2012) HIPEC in T4a colon cancer: a defendable treatment to improve oncologic outcome? Ann Oncol 23:3123-3129
10. Honore C, Goere D, Souadka A et al (2013) Definition of patients presenting a high risk of developing peritoneal carcinomatosis after curative surgery for colorectal cancer: a systematic review. Ann Surg Oncol 20:183-192
11. Levine EA, Blazer DG, 3rd, Kim MK et al (2012) Gene expression profiling of peritoneal metastases from appendiceal and colon cancer demonstrates unique biologic signatures and predicts patient outcomes. J Am Coll Surg 214:599-606; discussion 606-597
12. de Cuba EM, Kwakman R, van Egmond M et al (2012) Understanding molecular mechanisms in peritoneal dissemination of colorectal cancer : future possibilities for personalised treatment by use of biomarkers. Virchows Arch 461:231-243
13. Kohne CH, Cunningham D, Di Costanzo F (2002) Clinical determinants of survival in patients with 5-fluorouracil-based treatment for metastatic colorectal cancer: results of a multivariate analysis of 3825 patients. Ann Oncol 13:308-317
14. Klaver YL, Lemmens VE, Creemers GJ et al (2011) Population-based survival of patients with peritoneal carcinomatosis from colorectal origin in the era of increasing use of palliative chemotherapy. Ann Oncol 22:2250-2256
15. Franko J, Shi Q, Goldman CD et al (2012) Treatment of colorectal peritoneal carcinomatosis with systemic chemotherapy: a pooled analysis of north central cancer treatment group phase III trials N9741 and N9841. J Clin Oncol 30:263-267
16. Klaver YL, Simkens LH, Lemmens VE (2012) Outcomes of colorectal cancer patients with peritoneal carcinomatosis treated with chemotherapy with and without targeted therapy. Eur J Surg Oncol 38:617-623
17. Chua TC, Morris DL, Saxena A et al (2011) Influence of modern systemic therapies as adjunct to cytoreduction and perioperative intraperitoneal chemotherapy for patients with colorectal peritoneal carcinomatosis: a multicenter study. Ann Surg Oncol 18:1560-1567
18. Elias D, Lefevre JH, Chevalier J et al (2009) Complete cytoreductive surgery plus intraperitoneal chemohyperthermia with oxaliplatin for peritoneal carcinomatosis of colorectal origin. J Clin Oncol 27:681-685
19. Franko J, Ibrahim Z, Gusani NJ et al (2010) Cytoreductive surgery and hyperthermic intraperitoneal chemoperfusion versus systemic chemotherapy alone for colorectal peritoneal carcinomatosis. Cancer 116:3756-3762
20. Tomlinson JS, Jarnagin WR, DeMatteo RP et al (2007) Actual 10-year survival after resection of colorectal liver metastases defines cure. J Clin Oncol 25:4575-4580
21. Carpizo DR, D'Angelica M (2009) Liver resection for metastatic colorectal cancer in the presence of extrahepatic disease. Lancet Oncol 10:801-809
22. Ashley AC, Deschamps C, Alberts SR (2006) Impact of prognostic factors on clinical outcome after resection of colorectal pulmonary metastases. Clin Colorectal Cancer 6:32-37
23. Marcus EA, Weber TK, Rodriguez-Bigas MA et al (1999) Prognostic factors affecting survival in patients with colorectal carcinomatosis. Cancer Invest 17:249-252
24. Bloemendaal AL, Verwaal VJ, van Ruth S, Boot H, Zoetmulder FA (2005) Conventional surgery and systemic chemotherapy for peritoneal carcinomatosis of colorectal origin: a prospective study. Eur J Surg Oncol 31:1145-1151
25. Elias D, Ouellet JF, Bellon N (2003) Extrahepatic disease does not contraindicate hepatectomy for colorectal liver metastases. Br J Surg 90:567-574
26. Kobayashi H, Kotake K, Sugihara K (2014) Outcomes of surgery without HIPEC for synchronous peritoneal metastasis from colorectal cancer: data from a multi-center registry. Int J Clin Oncol 19:98-105
27. Sugarbaker PH, Jablonski KA (1995) Prognostic features of 51 colorectal and 130 appendiceal cancer patients with peritoneal carcinomatosis treated by cytoreductive surgery and intraperitoneal chemotherapy. Ann Surg 221:124-132
28. Cao C, Yan TD, Black D, Morris DL (2009) A systematic review and meta-analysis of cytoreductive surgery with perioperative intraperitoneal chemotherapy for peritoneal carcino-

matosis of colorectal origin. Ann Surg Oncol 16:2152-2165
29. Yan TD, Black D, Savady R, Sugarbaker PH (2006) Systematic review on the efficacy of cytoreductive surgery combined with perioperative intraperitoneal chemotherapy for peritoneal carcinomatosis from colorectal carcinoma. J Clin Oncol 24:4011-4019
30. Verwaal VJ, van Ruth S, de Bree E et al (2003) Randomized trial of cytoreduction and hyperthermic intraperitoneal chemotherapy versus systemic chemotherapy and palliative surgery in patients with peritoneal carcinomatosis of colorectal cancer. J Clin Oncol 21:3737-3743
31. Mahteme H, Hansson J, Berglund A et al (2004) Improved survival in patients with peritoneal metastases from colorectal cancer: a preliminary study. Br J Cancer 90:403-407
32. Cashin PH, Graf W, Nygren P, Mahteme H (2012) Patient selection for cytoreductive surgery in colorectal peritoneal carcinomatosis using serum tumor markers: an observational cohort study. Ann Surg 256:1078-1083
33. Cashin PH, Graf W, Nygren P, Mahteme H (2013) Comparison of prognostic scores for patients with colorectal cancer peritoneal metastases treated with cytoreductive surgery and hyperthermic intraperitoneal chemotherapy. Ann Surg Oncol 20:4183-4189
34. Elias D, Gilly F, Boutitie F, Quenet F et al (2010) Peritoneal colorectal carcinomatosis treated with surgery and perioperative intraperitoneal chemotherapy: retrospective analysis of 523 patients from a multicentric French study. J Clin Oncol 28:63-68
35. Esquivel J, Sticca R, Sugarbaker P et al (2007) Cytoreductive surgery and hyperthermic intraperitoneal chemotherapy in the management of peritoneal surface malignancies of colonic origin: a consensus statement. Society of Surgical Oncology. Ann Surg Oncol 14:128-133
36. Esquivel J, Elias D, Baratti D et al (2008) Consensus statement on the loco regional treatment of colorectal cancer with peritoneal dissemination. J Surg Oncol 98:263-267
37. Smeenk RM, Verwaal VJ, Zoetmulder FA (2007) Learning curve of combined modality treatment in peritoneal surface disease. Br J Surg 94:1408-1414
38. Portilla AG, Shigeki K, Dario B, Marcello D (2008) The intraoperative staging systems in the management of peritoneal surface malignancy. J Surg Oncol 98:228-231
39. Witkamp AJ, de Bree E, Kaag MM et al (2001) Extensive cytoreductive surgery followed by intra-operative hyperthermic intraperitoneal chemotherapy with mitomycin-C in patients with peritoneal carcinomatosis of colorectal origin. Eur J Cancer 37:979-984
40. Gilly FN, Carry PY, Sayag AC et al (1994) Regional chemotherapy (with mitomycin C) and intra-operative hyperthermia for digestive cancers with peritoneal carcinomatosis. Hepatogastroenterology 41:124-129
41. Koh JL, Yan TD, Glenn D, Morris DL (2009) Evaluation of preoperative computed tomography in estimating peritoneal cancer index in colorectal peritoneal carcinomatosis. Ann Surg Oncol 16:327-333
42. Esquivel J, Chua TC (2009) CT versus intraoperative peritoneal cancer index in colorectal cancer peritoneal carcinomatosis: importance of the difference between statistical significance and clinical relevance. Ann Surg Oncol 16:2662-2663; author reply 2264
43. Sommariva A, Zagonel V, Rossi CR (2012) The role of laparoscopy in peritoneal surface malignancies selected for hyperthermic intraperitoneal chemotherapy (HIPEC). Ann Surg Oncol 19:3737-3744
44. Pomel C, Appleyard TL, Gouy S et al (2005) The role of laparoscopy to evaluate candidates for complete cytoreduction of peritoneal carcinomatosis and hyperthermic intraperitoneal chemotherapy. Eur J Surg Oncol 31:540-543
45. Iversen LH, Rasmussen PC, Laurberg S (2013) Value of laparoscopy before cytoreductive surgery and hyperthermic intraperitoneal chemotherapy for peritoneal carcinomatosis. Br J Surg 100:285-292
46. Gomes da Silva R, Cabanas J, Sugarbaker PH (2005) Limited survival in the treatment of carcinomatosis from rectal cancer. Dis Colon Rectum 48:2258-2263
47. Verwaal VJ, van Tinteren H, van Ruth S, Zoetmulder FA (2004) Predicting the survival of patients with peritoneal carcinomatosis of colorectal origin treated by aggressive cytoreduction and hyperthermic intraperitoneal chemotherapy. Br J Surg 91:739-746
48. Glehen O, Kwiatkowski F, Sugarbaker PH et al (2004) Cytoreductive surgery combined with

perioperative intraperitoneal chemotherapy for the management of peritoneal carcinomatosis from colorectal cancer: a multi-institutional study. J Clin Oncol 22:3284-3292
49. Pelz JO, Stojadinovic A, Nissan A et al (2009) Evaluation of a peritoneal surface disease severity score in patients with colon cancer with peritoneal carcinomatosis. J Surg Oncol 99:915
50. Yonemura Y, Canbay E, Ishibashi H (2013) Prognostic factors of peritoneal metastases from colorectal cancer following cytoreductive surgery and perioperative chemotherapy. ScientificWorldJournal 2013:978394
51. Elias D, Sideris L, Pocard M et al (2004) Results of R0 resection for colorectal liver metastases associated with extrahepatic disease. Ann Surg Oncol 11:274-280
52. de Cuba EM, Kwakman R, Knol DL et al (2013) Cytoreductive surgery and HIPEC for peritoneal metastases combined with curative treatment of colorectal liver metastases: Systematic review of all literature and meta-analysis of observational studies. Cancer Treat Rev 39:321-327
53. Elias D, Benizri E, Pocard M et al (2006) Treatment of synchronous peritoneal carcinomatosis and liver metastases from colorectal cancer. Eur J Surg Oncol 32:632-636
54. Glockzin G, Renner P, Popp FC et al (2011) Hepatobiliary procedures in patients undergoing cytoreductive surgery and hyperthermic intraperitoneal chemotherapy. Ann Surg Oncol 18:1052-1059
55. Elias D, Faron M, Goere D et al (2014) A Simple Tumor Load-Based Nomogram for Surgery in Patients with Colorectal Liver and Peritoneal Metastases. Ann Surg Oncol doi:10.1245/s10434-014-3506-z
56. Cavaliere F, De Simone M, Virzi S et al (2011) Prognostic factors and oncologic outcome in 146 patients with colorectal peritoneal carcinomatosis treated with cytoreductive surgery combined with hyperthermic intraperitoneal chemotherapy: Italian multicenter study S.I.T.I.L.O. Eur J Surg Oncol 37:148-154
57. Esquivel J (2009) Technology of hyperthermic intraperitoneal chemotherapy in the United States, Europe, China, Japan, and Korea. Cancer J 15:249-254
58. Zoetmulder FA, van der Vange N, Witkamp AJ et al (1999) Hyperthermic intra-peritoneal chemotherapy (HIPEC) in patients with peritoneal pseudomyxoma or peritoneal metastases of colorectal carcinoma; good preliminary results from the Netherlands Cancer Institute. Ned Tijdschr Geneeskd 143:1863-1868
59. Elias D, Bonnay M, Puizillou JM (2002) Heated intra-operative intraperitoneal oxaliplatin after complete resection of peritoneal carcinomatosis: pharmacokinetics and tissue distribution. Ann Oncol 13:267-272
60. Glockzin G, von Breitenbuch P, Schlitt HJ, Piso P (2013) Treatment-related morbidity and toxicity of CRS and oxaliplatin-based HIPEC compared to a mitomycin and doxorubicin-based HIPEC protocol in patients with peritoneal carcinomatosis: a matched-pair analysis. J Surg Oncol 107:574-578
61. Hompes D, D'Hoore A, Wolthuis A et al (2014) The use of Oxaliplatin or Mitomycin C in HIPEC treatment for peritoneal carcinomatosis from colorectal cancer: A comparative study. J Surg Oncol 109:527-532
62. Kusamura S, Dominique E, Baratti D et al (2008) Drugs, carrier solutions and temperature in hyperthermic intraperitoneal chemotherapy. J Surg Oncol 98:247-252
63. Turaga K, Levine E, Barone R et al (2014) Consensus Guidelines from The American Society of Peritoneal Surface Malignancies on Standardizing the Delivery of Hyperthermic Intraperitoneal Chemotherapy (HIPEC) in Colorectal Cancer Patients in the United States. Ann Surg Oncol 21:1501-1505
64. Zani S, Papalezova K, Stinnett S et al (2013) Modest advances in survival for patients with colorectal-associated peritoneal carcinomatosis in the era of modern chemotherapy. J Surg Oncol 107:307-311
65. Klaver YL, de Hingh IH, Boot H, Verwaal VJ (2011) Results of cytoreductive surgery and hyperthermic intraperitoneal chemotherapy after early failure of adjuvant systemic chemotherapy. J Surg Oncol 103:431-434
66. Passot G, Vaudoyer D, Cotte E et al (2012) Progression following neoadjuvant systemic

chemotherapy may not be a contraindication to a curative approach for colorectal carcinomatosis. Ann Surg 256:125-129
67. Hompes D, Aalbers A, Boot H et al (2014) A prospective pilot study to assess neo-adjuvant chemotherapy for unresectable peritoneal carcinomatosis from colorectal cancer. Colorectal Dis doi:10.1111/codi.12560
68. Eveno C, Passot G, Goere D et al (2014) Bevacizumab Doubles the Early Postoperative Complication Rate after Cytoreductive Surgery with Hyperthermic Intraperitoneal Chemotherapy (HIPEC) for Peritoneal Carcinomatosis of Colorectal Origin. Ann Surg Oncol 21:1791-1800
69. Pelz JO, Doerfer J, Dimmler A et al (2006) Histological response of peritoneal carcinomatosis after hyperthermic intraperitoneal chemoperfusion (HIPEC) in experimental investigations. BMC Cancer 22:6-162
70. Klaver YL, Hendriks T, Lomme RM et al (2010) Intraoperative hyperthermic intraperitoneal chemotherapy after cytoreductive surgery for peritoneal carcinomatosis in an experimental model. Br J Surg 97:1874-1880
71. Elias D, Delperro JR, Sideris L et al (2004) Treatment of peritoneal carcinomatosis from colorectal cancer: impact of complete cytoreductive surgery and difficulties in conducting randomized trials. Ann Surg Oncol 11:518-521
72. Cashin PH, Graf W, Nygren P, Mahteme H (2012) Intraoperative hyperthermic versus postoperative normothermic intraperitoneal chemotherapy for colonic peritoneal carcinomatosis: a case-control study. Ann Oncol 23:647-652
73. Huang CQ, Feng JP, Yang XJ, Li Y (2013) Cytoreductive surgery plus hyperthermic intraperitoneal chemotherapy improves survival of patients with peritoneal carcinomatosis from colorectal cancer: A case-control study from a Chinese center. J Surg Oncol doi:10.1002/jso.23545
74. Chua TC, Yan TD, Saxena A, Morris DL (2009) Should the treatment of peritoneal carcinomatosis by cytoreductive surgery and hyperthermic intraperitoneal chemotherapy still be regarded as a highly morbid procedure?: a systematic review of morbidity and mortality. Ann Surg 249:900-907
75. Kusamura S, Younan R, Baratti D et al (2006) Cytoreductive surgery followed by intraperitoneal hyperthermic perfusion: analysis of morbidity and mortality in 209 peritoneal surface malignancies treated with closed abdomen technique. Cancer 106:1144-1153
76. Maggiori L, Elias D (2010) Curative treatment of colorectal peritoneal carcinomatosis: current status and future trends. Eur J Surg Oncol 36:599-603
77. Scheithauer W, Kornek GV, Marczell A et al (1998) Combined intravenous and intraperitoneal chemotherapy with fluorouracil plus leucovorin vs fluorouracil plus levamisole for adjuvant therapy of resected colon carcinoma. Br J Cancer 77:1349-1354
78. Sugarbaker PH, Gianola FJ, Speyer JC et al (1985) Prospective, randomized trial of intravenous versus intraperitoneal 5-fluorouracil in patients with advanced primary colon or rectal cancer. Surgery 98:414-422
79. Vaillant JC, Nordlinger B, Deuffic S et al (2000) Adjuvant intraperitoneal 5-fluorouracil in high-risk colon cancer: A multicenter phase III trial. Ann Surg 231:449-456
80. Nordlinger B, Rougier P, Arnaud JP et al (2005) Adjuvant regional chemotherapy and systemic chemotherapy versus systemic chemotherapy alone in patients with stage II-III colorectal cancer: a multicentre randomized controlled phase III trial. Lancet Oncol 6:459-468
81. Sammartino P, Sibio S, Biacchi D et al (2012) Prevention of Peritoneal Metastases from Colon Cancer in High-Risk Patients: Preliminary Results of Surgery plus Prophylactic HIPEC. Gastroenterol Res Pract 2012:141585
82. Noura S, Ohue M, Shingai T et al (2011) Effects of intraperitoneal chemotherapy with mitomycin C on the prevention of peritoneal recurrence in colorectal cancer patients with positive peritoneal lavage cytology findings. Ann Surg Oncol 18:396-404
83. Elias D, Honore C, Dumont F et al (2011) Results of systematic second-look surgery plus HIPEC in asymptomatic patients presenting a high risk of developing colorectal peritoneal carcinomatosis. Ann Surg 254:289-293

84. Ripley RT, Davis JL, Kemp CD et al (2010) Prospective randomized trial evaluating mandatory second look surgery with HIPEC and CRS vs. standard of care in patients at high risk of developing colorectal peritoneal metastases. Trials 11:62

Peritoneal Carcinomatosis from Ovarian Cancer

20

Angelo Di Giorgio, Paolo Sammartino, and Pierandrea De Iaco

20.1 Introduction

Peritoneal carcinomatosis (PC) is the most impressive and frequent form of locoregional spread of epithelial ovarian cancer (EOC). For much of its natural history, the disease remains confined to the peritoneal district, thus representing the target for various combinations of surgery and systemic or locoregional chemotherapy (CHT). PC is evident both in the primary setting, i.e., in patients first treated for locally advanced EOC, or as a recurrence in patients previously treated for OC at any Fédération Internationale de Gynécologie et Obstétrique (International Federation of Gynecology and Obstetrics) (FIGO) stage.

20.2 Evolution of Peritoneal Carcinomatosis Treatment

Treating PC from OC is generally based on CRS associated with systemic CHT and, more rarely, on normothermic IP-CHT (Intraperitoneal Chemotherapy). However, it is arduous to identify accurately optimal treatment, or at least the most widely accepted standard treatment, for ovarian carcinomatosis. The therapeutic success of maximal CRS, aimed at complete removal of peritoneal disease, and the high chemosensitivity of EOC for first-line treatment with carboplatin and Taxol, threaten to make these two basic forms of therapy antagonistic (surgery and systemic CHT) and give rise to conflicting therapeutic indications in the same settings. From a surgical point of view, the scenario is complicated further by the inhomogeneity of specialists in charge of surgical proce-

A. Di Giorgio (✉)
Department of Surgery "Pietro Valdoni".
Sapienza University of Rome, Rome, Italy
e-mail: angelo.digiorgio@uniroma1.it

A. Di Giorgio, E. Pinto (Eds), *Treatment of Peritoneal Surface Malignancies*,
Updates in Surgery
DOI: 10.1007/978-88-470-5711-1_20, © Springer-Verlag Italia 2015

dures (gynecologic oncologists vs. surgical oncologists), whereas among medical oncologists, factors that divide opinions are relate to the range of possible strategies for CHT timing compared with surgery, drug choice, and CHT infusion methods, either systemic or locoregional. Moreover identifying at least four different evolutive settings of EOC as targets for therapeutic strategies leaves little room for sharing therapeutic strategies, thus generating a compulsive demand of prospective studies, which for this disease entity are difficult to conduct.

Following a similar pattern for other forms of PSM, from the second half of the 1990s, the choice of peritonectomy (PRT) associated with hyperthermic intraperitoneal chemotherapy (HIPEC) (PRT plus HIPEC) has progressively become more widespread among the wide range of possible therapeutic strategies for ovarian carcinomatosis. This trend derives from a long evolutionary path in the field of surgery and CHT, which is based on a solid rationale and on promising results of phase II studies rather than specific randomized controlled trials.

20.2.1 Evolution of Surgical Treatment: From Debulking to Peritonectomy

Since the 1970s, locally advanced OC was the main field of application of the concept of surgical debulking, understood as a procedure aimed not only at palliate clinical conditions resulting from IP spread of the disease but also at improved survival [1]. The principle of debulking has gradually earned consent by progressively emphasizing the impact of the level of cytoreduction on patient survival–so much so that among gynecologic oncologists, tumor residual dimensions indicative of optimal cytoreduction have progressively decreased from 2 cm to 0.5 cm [2]. Sugarbaker pioneered the concept of PRT, an all-encompassing term for complex surgical exeresis aimed at maximizing cytoreduction of parietal and visceral carcinomatosis with an optimal limit up to a maximum of 2.5 mm. Sugarbaker also standardized PRT procedures, defining protocols for evaluating PC diffusion (the PCI), and level of surgical cytoreduction obtained [Completeness of Cytoreduction (CC) score] [3, 4].

Since the first report by Griffith in 1975 [1], in the setting of primary cytoreduction for locally advanced EOC, the most relevant prospective studies on the role of the extent of cytoreduction have consistently demonstrated that survival progressively decreases as the volume of residual nodules increases (Table 20.1) [5, 6]. The most significant gap is observed between totally cytoreduced cases and those with residue of any size [2]. A meta-analysis of 6,855 cases confirmed these data and showed that each 10 % increase in maximal cytoreduction corresponded to a 5.5 % increase in median survival [7].

More controversial is the role of CRS in the setting of recurrent disease in which the prognosis is related to a large number of factors, such as patient age, interval between initial diagnosis and relapse, presence of ascites, and histologic

Table 20.1 Cytoreduction for locally advanced epithelial ovarian cancer (EOC). Residual tumor size and survival

Setting	Study [Reference]	No.	Residual disease	Survival	
Primary cytoreduction				5-year (%)	Median (months)
	Hoskins (1994) [5]	41	R 0	60	
		62	≤ 1 cm	35	
		77	> 1 cm	20–35	
	Chi (2006) [6]	67	R 0		106
		70	≤ 0,5 cm		66
		328	> 0,5		33–48
	du Bois (2010) [40]	1,046	R 0		99.1
		975	≤ 1 cm		36.2
		1,105	> 1cm		29.6
Secondary cytoreduction					
	Authors[a]	513	R 0		30–63.2
		441	Any residual		7.2–27.6

[a]Eisenkop et al. 1995-2000 [8, 10]; Cormio et al. 1999 [9]; Gadducci et al. 2000 [11]; Tay et al. 2002 [17]; Gronlund et al. 2005 [12]; Onda et al. 2005 [13]; Benedetti et al. 2007 [14]; Oksefjell et al. 2009 [15]; Tian et al. 2010 [16]

subtype. Even in the absence of prospective studies, multiple retrospective studies [8–17] (Table 20.1) and a meta-analysis involving 40 studies and 2,019 patients [18] confirmed the prognostic role of maximal cytoreduction in recurrent cases. Even after tertiary and quaternary cytoreduction, total cancer removal is a reliable prognostic factor, as constantly demonstrated in relevant publications, although this assumption is based on the analysis of retrospective studies only [19–22].

Tumor reduction surgery has evident benefits: it improves the patient's QoL, enhances tumor susceptibility to CHT by stimulating the active division of cells, and decreasing the likelihood of drug-resistant clones by removing gross necrotic tumor masses. Maximum cytoreduction able to permit complete removal of peritoneal disease is therefore the most significant prognostic factor in all settings and currently represents the fundamental aim of surgery when this approach is indicated.

20.2.1.1 Peritonectomy

PC is characterized by neoplastic involvement of both the parietal and visceral peritoneum, and radical surgery involves removing the peritoneal areas affected by carcinomatosis.

In treating ovarian carcinomatosis, debulking, cytoreduction, and PRT—even if considered as synonyms of the same concept, i.e. maximal removal of cancerous tissue—express the progressive evolution toward more extensive surgery and match criteria and techniques described in Chap. 9. All endoperitoneal viscera and parenchyma are susceptible to partial or total excision, according to the degree of invasiveness and the feasibility of in situ cytoreduction of implants, as previously described (Fig. 20.1). However, some aspects need further clarification, as they are related to visceral resection and lymphadenectomy.

Until now, type and extent of visceral resection for locally advanced EOC have reflected the different attitudes of key figures dealing with these procedures; there are clear-cut differences between the approach of oncologic surgeons engaged in PSM treatment and that of gynecologic oncologists. The aim of the surgeon performing PRT is to achieve complete cytoreduction (CC-0) or optimal CRS with residues up to 2.5 mm, whereas gynecologic oncologists—with few exceptions—consider that optimal cytoreduction is achieved even when residual disease includes nodules of 1 or 2 cm. Such limits in many cases can result in residual disease classification of FIGO stage III, the same stage as before cytoreduction. This low aggressive approach toward eradicating the disease is adopted especially when the carcinomatosis involves critical areas difficult to treat, such as the supramesocolic space or when there is an extensive infiltration of the colon and rectum. Such cases of partial cytoreduction are assigned to subsequent chemotherapies that are often carried out by the same gynecologists, with the aim being more toward disease chronicity rather than treatment radicalization. Recently, even oncologic gynecologists have begun recognizing the importance of maximal cytoreduction in the supramesocolic space, but it must be noted that few gynecologic centers have sufficient surgical skills to address this technical challenge [23].

Particularly relevant is the problem of PC treatment when it involves the colon and the rectum, as discussed in specific studies [24, 25] (Fig. 20.2). Widespread pelvic disease, with involvement of the pouch and colorectal wall, entails resection of this viscus with the same criteria of radicality adopted when treating primary CRC (Colorectal Cancer), i.e., including mesorectal excision and sections of mesenteric vessels at their origin. Similar radical colonic resections should be performed when other large-bowel sectors are involved (Fig. 20.3). Using this procedure allows both removal of a large amount of mesocolon—frequently infiltrated by implants—and regional lymphadenectomy that removes lymph node stations, which are metastatic in > 50 % of cases [24, 26]. In primary CRS, pelvic and para-aortic lymphadenectomy must be routinely performed in relation to the high incidence of locoregional metastases. In secondary CRS, locoregional lymph node dissection should be performed if not done during primary cytoreduction or if there is evident of lymph node recurrence (Fig. 20.4).

In patients who undergo NACT and attain a complete or partial response, persistent morphological alterations of the peritoneal membrane identify the sites of previous carcinomatosis, as described in Chap. 4. Accurate evaluation of such morphological alterations is invaluable in planning a correct CRS strategy. If there is no evidence of macroscopic disease, basic hysteroadnexectomy, locoregional lymphadenectomy, complete omentectomy, appendectomy, and resection of the *ligamentum teres* and falciform ligament should be performed

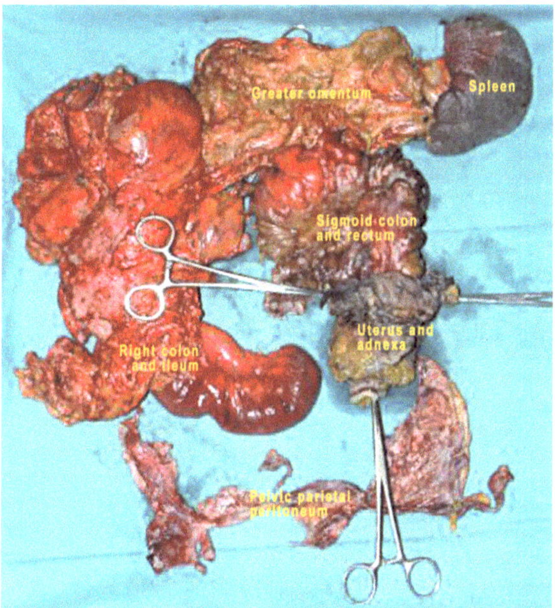

Fig. 20.1 Visceral and parietal peritonectomy for ovarian carcinomatosis

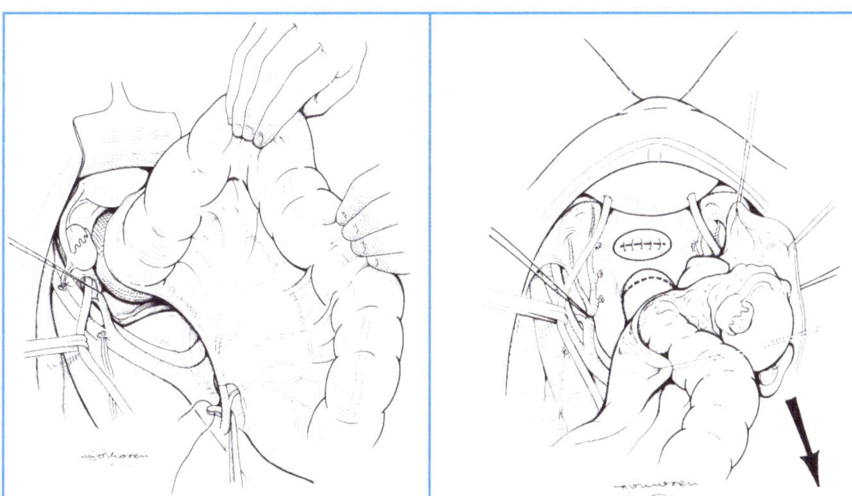

Fig. 20.2 En bloc hysteroadnexectomy, pelvic–parietal peritonectomy, and colorectal resection. Inferior mesenteric artery is ligated at the aortic origin

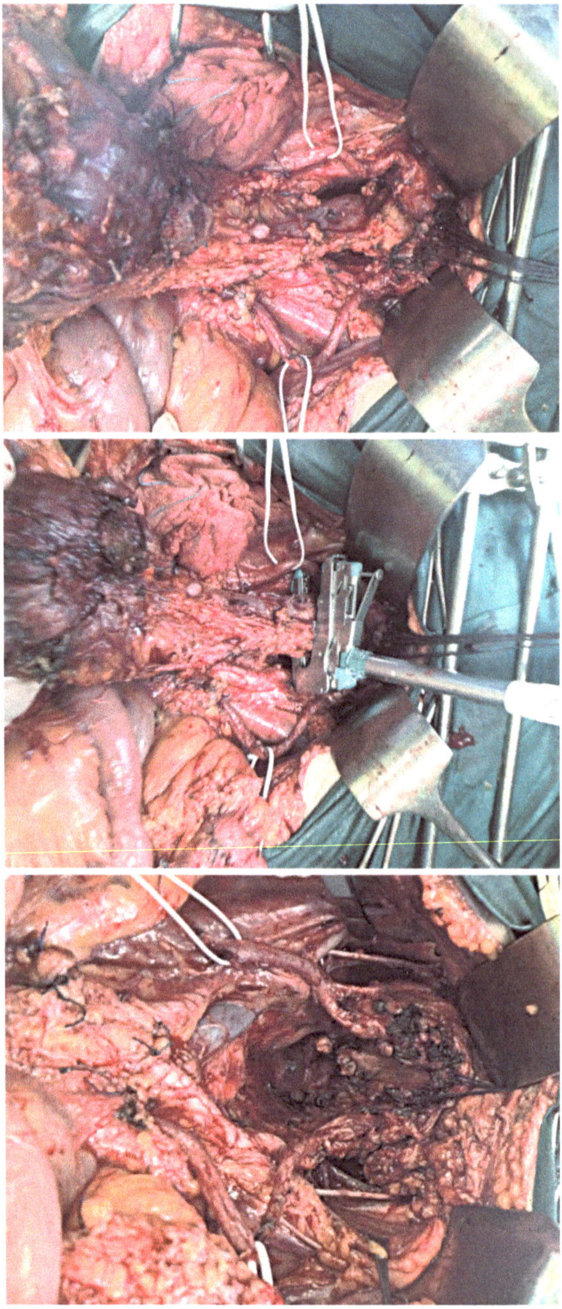

Fig. 20.3 Pelvic peritonectomy: hysteroadnexectomy, colorectal en-bloc resection, and pelvic lymphadenectomy

according to criteria described in Chap. 9. In these cases, it is appropriate in principle to perform a parietal PRT of the lower abdomen and pelvis below the transverse umbilical line to remove the peritoneum, which is often involved in

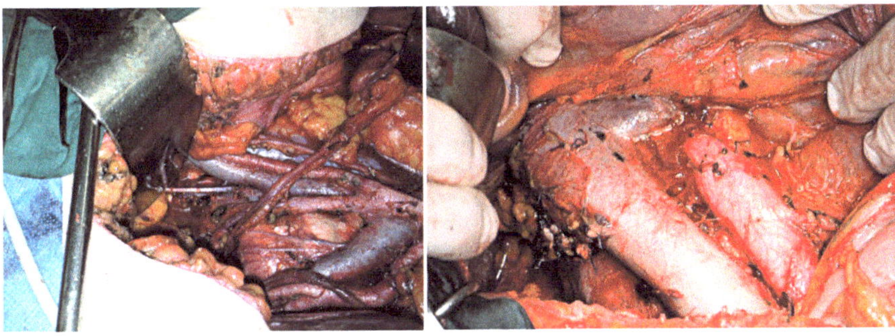

Fig. 20.4 Pelvic, para-aortic, and paracaval lymphadenectomy

carcinomatosis. All other residual peritoneal areas with previously described morphological alterations should be treated superficially and extensively with argon or ball-tip electrosurgery to alter structural continuity of post-CHT fibrosis, thus allowing deeper penetration of drugs into the peritoneal membrane during HIPEC.

20.2.2 Peritonectomy plus Hyperthermic Intraperitoneal Chemotherapy

Removing all macroscopically visible tumor tissue is not an absolute guarantee of neoplastic "sterilization" of the abdominopelvic cavity; persistence of microscopic residual is possible. Therefore, a more suitable means of treatment is required to ensure control over microscopic residual. From this perspective, HIPEC at the end of the surgical phase is a logical method of addressing this problem, as for other forms of PSM. The principles and rationale underlying the association of PRT plus HIPEC, together with results from the largest multi-institutional case studies, are the major factors supporting the adoption of this integrated procedure in treating primary and recurrent ovarian carcinomatosis.

Cisplatin (CDDP), at doses varying from 50 to 100 mg/m^2, is the most widely used drug for HIPEC in ovarian carcinomatosis. The isolated or combined administration of other drugs in association with CDDP is used in some centers. In most centers treating ovarian carcinomatosis with this combined procedure, general criteria for patient inclusion are rather homogeneous and relate to patients without extra-abdominal disease, with optimal American Society of Anesthesiologists (ASA) and performance status (PS) scores and with surgically cytoreducible disease. Patient age is not a matter of absolute exclusion; even patients in their 80s, particularly motivated, with good ASA and PS scores with limited and easily resectable PC can be scheduled for the procedure. The presence of easily resectable and isolated liver metastases is not a contraindication for the procedure if complete cytoreduction is achievable. The role of PCI as a factor conditioning patient inclusion is not uniformly accepted for ovarian carcinomatosis: some authors identify the levels beyond which PRT plus HIPEC is inadvisable [27–29]; for others, limitation is related to the infeasibility of cytoreduction. When the cytoreduction score is suboptimal, HIPEC is theoretically avoidable, as it is not effective in attacking residues > 2.5–3 mm; but if ascites is present, then HIPEC can still be performed, as it is effective in preventing ascites reproduction in a large percentage of cases.

PRT plus HIPEC is applicable in various phases of the disease and in relation to different evolutionary scenarios related to previous treatments. Therefore, four possible treatment settings are predictable:

- Front line
- After NACT (interval debulking) } primary cytoreduction
- Consolidation
- Recurrence/persistence } secondary cytoreduction.

20.3 Role of Peritonectomy plus Hyperthermic Intraperitoneal Chemotherapy in Treating Peritoneal Carcinomatosis from Ovarian Cancer

Since 2000, the use of HIPEC combined with maximum cytoreduction (PRT) for treating PC from OC has gradually become more widespread. Results obtained thus far, although drawn exclusively from phase 1 and 2 studies of small and inhomogeneous case series, encourage the continuation of experience in this field and continue to support the benefits for long-term survival in both primary and recurrent forms, with acceptable morbidity rates when performed in high-volume HIPEC centers. However, inhomogeneity when selecting patients for neoadjuvant and adjuvant treatments and when assessing and classifying PC spread and cytoreduction levels complicates comparative data analysis and opens up the results of multicenter studies to criticism. Moreover PRT requires a high number of surgical resections to eradicate a disease with multiform diffusion, in the face of which surgical attitude is hardly comparable, so that the surgeon is a prognostic factor of considerable significance [30]. Furthermore, the risk of high morbidity and lack of controlled studies further exacerbate this general scepticism, particular regarding the role of HIPEC.

At present—and pending results of future prospective trials—the role and limitations of applying the procedure are drawn from experiences from three basic study types (Table 20.2):

- Collective reviews
- Multicenter studies
- Monocentric case studies produced by high-volume HIPEC centers

Table 20.2 Peritonectomy plus HIPEC for treating ovarian carcitomatosis: literature review and ongoing studies (2,419 cases)

Type of study	Year	Study [Reference]	Study design	No. cases	No. studies/ centers
Collective reviews	2012	de Bree and Helm [33]	Collection of phase II	1,102	22
Multicenter	2010	Helm et al. [34] (HYPER-O)	Retrospective	141	9
	2011	Deraco et al. [35]	Prospective phase II	26	4
	2013	Bakrin et al. [29]	Retrospective	566	13
	2014 (unpublished)	De Iaco, Multi Institutional Italian Study (MIIS)*	Prospective phase II	454	13
Monocentric	2014 (unpublished)	Di Giorgio	Prospective phase II	130	1

*CRO-Aviano; Riuniti Hospitals, Bergamo; Sant'Orsola-Malpighi Hospital, Bologna; Careggi Hospital, Florence; Morgagni-Pierantoni Hospital, Forlì; G. Martino Hospital, Messina; Multimedica, Milan; Infermi Hospital, Rimini; Sapienza University of Rome, Roma; Catholic University, Rome; National Cancer Institute, Rome; Santa Maria Hospital, Terni; Candiolo Institute IRCCS, Turin

20.3.1 Collective Reviews

The most important available collective reviews are the studies by Bijelic et al., Chua et al., and de Bree [31–33]. In their (more recent) review, de Bree and Helm present results of 22 studies, 12 and 9 of which are also considered by Chua et al. and Bijelic et al. in their collections. These collective studies report data from phase I and II studies that are remarkably heterogeneous, particularly in terms of drugs used in HIPEC, post-HIPEC results, and duration of follow-up. The reviews are primarily focused on evaluating survival, morbidity, and postoperative mortality rates but summarize the other results of the individual studies partially and rather inhomogeneously. Concerning survival, base parameters that impact prognosis, such as CC and PCI scores, are either not analyzed or are only marginally considered: concerning morbidity, common risk classifications are not evaluated. Even if with some inaccuracy on data retrieval that have been rectified or not taken into consideration in this analysis, the de Bree/Helm review can be considered the most complete and to best represent current results inferable from collective reviews.

20.3.2 Multicenter Studies

Multicenter studies are the most frequently reported in the literature, but similarly to reviews, they show such a high degree of heterogeneity both in methods and in contents that comparison between them is often difficult. Two studies are retrospective: the first [34] refers to the Hyperthermic Intraperitoneal Chemotherapy In Ovarian Cancer (HYPER-O) US register, which refers to seven centers; the second [29] is currently the major collective clinical report and collects data derived from 13 French centers, including 246 cases already reported in a previous work [28]. Two further studies are considered as prospective by their own authors: the Multi-Institutional Italian Study (MIIS), and Deraco et al.'s Multi-Institutional Study [35]. The Italian study is ongoing, and results reported here are as yet unpublished; to date, that study comprises 454 cases from 13 centers, including 109 cases from clinical records of the senior author of this chapter. The primary aim of all these studies–except Deraco et al.'s, which exclusively analyzes front-line-treated cases–is to evaluate long-term survival and morbidity and consider the various settings in which the PRT plus HIPEC procedure is administered. Survival is analyzed with uniform statistical methodology, and in all studies, several types of prognostic factors are considered in univariate and multivariate analysis–except in Deraco et al.'s study, which exclusively and generically analyzes overall (OS) and progression-free (PFS) survival. Among prognostic factors, PCI and CC scores are the most frequently considered. Heterogeneity is evident when morbidity is analyzed, with the majority of reports referring generically to major complications that are classified with inhomogeneous protocols. Few studies analyze risk factors for complication with univariate or multivariate analyses.

20.3.3 Monocentric Study: Personal Experience

Most relevant single-center studies have been included in the reviews described above and summarized in de Bree and Helm's review [33], but all examine a limited number of cases, with the largest study analyzing 81 patients. The single-center clinical study reported here and until now unpublished represents the largest monocentric study on treating PC from OC with PRT plus HIPEC: 130 cases of PC derived from high-grade and FIGO stages IIIc/IV OC are enrolled in this non-randomized prospective phase II study on treating ovarian carcinomatosis with PRT plus HIPEC. The study analyzes clinical records of treatment performed between November 2000 and December 2013 by a single surgeon as main operator (Di Giorgio) and assisted by the same surgical and anesthesiological staff. The same team of pathologists analyzed surgical samples following a specific protocol implemented at the beginning of the study. The same radiological staff carried out investigations and reviewed morphological CT and MR images both during the preoperative and follow-up phases. The database was organized prospectively. At the beginning of 2013, part of this series was included in the MIIS described above.

20.4 Study Results

Clinical and anatomopathological characteristics and HIPEC techniques inferable from the analysed studies are summarized in Table 20.3.

De Bree and Helm's review [33] does not describe or summarize these types of data, even if they are reported more or less analytically in the original individual studies. Anatomopathological characteristics and FIGO stage seemed rather similar between studies reporting these specific data: the absolute majority of patients had high-grade (G3) and FIGO stage III/IV tumors. Except for Deraco et al.'s study [35], which includes only cases treated as front line, all other studies refer to various settings in which PRT plus HIPEC was performed: distribution of setting results was sufficiently homogeneous.

Chemosensitivity to platinum was analyzed in different ways in four studies: HYPER-O evaluated the response to chemotherapeutic treatments performed as front line in all settings. Bakrin [29] described the pre-HIPEC response exclusively in patients with recurrent or persistent carcinomatosis. In our patients, chemosensitivity was evaluated for adjuvant CHT post-HIPEC performed after both primary and secondary cytoreduction; in addition, NACT sensitivity was considered in the primary setting. This evaluation was also performed in the MIIS.

PCI score differs significantly between studies: in ours and in that of Deraco et al., the median PCI score was the highest; the French study [28] reported the lowest. Optimal cytoreduction scores were homogeneous among these studies. In all studies except ours, combinations of drugs were used for HIPEC, with platinum-based drugs being the most commonly used. Drug doses were very variable: CDDP doses ranged from 50 to 100 mg/m^2. HIPEC duration varied from 30 to 120 min according to the drug used. Both open and closed HIPEC techniques were used, except for in Deraco et al.'s and our studies, in which only the closed technique was applied. In all studies, protocols provided for adjuvant treatments, even if the percentage of their application was significantly different.

20.4.1 Survival and Prognostic Factors

The majority of studies analyzed survival in relation to various settings in which CSR plus HIPEC was performed. Deraco et al.'s study is an exception, as it is totally dedicated to front-line cases. Our monocentric study, the MIIS (unpublished), and de Bree and Helm's [33] review describe similar long-term results after primary and secondary CRS respectively (Tables 20.4 and 20.5). For primary CRS, survival at 5 years was remarkably variable in the de Bree and Helm review, ranging from 33% to 84%; in multicentric analyses and in the monocentric study, survival was more homogeneous, with a median value almost 50 % at 5 years for primary CRS and 40 % for secondary CRS. The HYPER-O registry

Table 20.3 Patient characteristics and hyperthermic intraperitoneal chemotherapy (HIPEC) techniques

Study [Reference]	HYPER-O [34]	Deraco et al. [35]	Bakrin [29]	MIIS (unpublished)	Di Giorgio (unpublished)	de Bree and Helm [33]
No. cases	141	26	566	454	130	1,102
Grade (%)						
1	9.9					NR
2	8.5	15.4			8.7	NR
3	74.5	84.6			85.8	NR
Undetermined or consolidation	7.1				5.5	NR
FIGO (%)						
0 (Consolidation or undetermined)	2.8				5.4	NR
II	7.1				2.3	NR
III	80.1	96.2			85.4	NR
IV	10	3.8			6.9	NR
Liver metastasis (%)			5.5	11.9	3.1	NR
Lymph node metastasis (%)						
Yes				26.2	52.6	
No				73.8	47.4	
Setting (%)						
Frontline	18.5	100	2.1	9.5	17.7	18.4
Interval debulking	13.6		4.2	23.3	29.2	5.6
Consolidation	8.6		9.9	8.8	5.4	8.9

(*cont.*) ↓

Study [Reference]	HYPER-O [34]	Deraco et al. [35]	Bakrin [29]	MIIS (unpublished)	Di Giorgio (unpublished)	de Bree and Helm [33]
Recurrence	59.3		83.8	58.4	47.7	67.1
Platinum response (%)						
Resistant	34		52.1	35	36.8	NR
Sensitive	53.9		47	34.4	53.8	NR
Undetermined	12.1		0.9	30.6	9.4	NR
PCI median		15.5 (5–26)	10.6 (0–31)	10.9 (0–39)	16.3 (0–39)	NR
CC score (%)						
0	58.3	57.7	74.9	71.6	66.7	NR
1	15.1	42.3	17.9	22.3	20	NR
> 1	26.6		7.2	6.1	13.3	NR
HIPEC drugs (%)						
CDDP	37.2*	a	41	17.4	100	NR
Oxaliplatin			21.3	11.5		NR
MMC	38.7*		2.1	0.3		NR
CarboTaxol	14.6*			-		NR
Doxorubicin		b	0.2	-		NR
Adriamycin				4.2		
Combination (≥ 2)	9.5*	100 (a +b)	35.4	66.6		NR

(*cont.*) →

Table 20.3 *(continued)*

Study [Reference]	HYPER-O [34]	Deraco et al. [35]	Bakrin [29]	MIIS (unpublished)	Di Giorgio (unpublished)	de Bree and Helm [33]
HIPEC technique (%)						
Open	12.1		68.4	41.3		NR
Closed	87.9	100	31.6	50.2	100	NR
Semiopen				9.5		
HIPEC duration						
60 min				64.1	100	
60–90 min	45.4	100		35.9		
90–120 min	54.6			-		
Adjuvant CHT (%)						
Yes	93.6?	100	28.3		71.5	NR
No			71.7		28.5	NR

HIPEC, hyperthermic intraperitoneal chemotherapy; *FIGO*, Fédération Internationale de Gynécologie et Obstétrique (International Federation of Gynecology and Obstetrics); *PCI*, Peritoneal Cancer Index; *CC*, Completeness of Cytoreduction score; *CDDP*, cisplatin; *MMC*, mitomycin-C; *CHT*, chemotherapy; *HYPER-O*, Hyperthermic Intraperitoneal Chemotherapy in Ovarian Cancer, US Register; *MIIS*, Multi-Institutional Italian Study; *NR*, not reached
*Some values recalculated to correlate with the total of 141 cases

Fig. 20.4 Part I - PRT plus HIPEC in ovarian carcinomatosis treatment. Survival and prognosis factors

	Multicentre Studies			
Study [Reference]	**HYPER-O [34]**			
	5 yr OS	5 yr PFS	median OS	median PFS
SETTING	%	%	months	months
frontline	33,3	19,7	41,7	24,8
interval debulking	50,2*	9,6*	68,6*	16,8*
consolidation	42,4*	24,2*	53,7*	29,6*
recurrence	18	9,6	23,5	13,7
Primary	25,4	13	30,3	13,7
Recurrence	-	-	-	-
Maximal cytoreduction				
CC 0 (primary)	26,7	-	37	-
CC 0 (recurrence)	-	-	-	-
Prognostic factors	**Univariate or Multivariate Analyses - p value**			
CC score	0.025			
PCI	nr			
PS	nr			
Platinum response	0.048			
setting	ns			
blood loss	0,005			
ca 125	nr			
Lymph-node metastases	nr			
age	nr			
HIPEC drugs number	nr			
HIPEC drug type(carboplatin)	0.011			
duration of perfusion (90 min)	0,047			
Study [Reference]	**DERACO [35]**			
	5 yr OS	5 yr PFS	median OS	median PFS
SETTING	%	%	months	months
frontline	60,7	15,2	not reached	30

* unreliable because of the small number of events

Fig. 20.4 Part II - PRT plus HIPEC in ovarian carcinomatosis treatment. Survival and prognosis factors

	Multicentre Studies			
Study [Reference]	**BAKRIN [29]**		**MIIS (unpublished)**	
	5 yr OS	median OS	5 yr OS	median OS
SETTING	%	months	%	months
frontline	33,7	52,7	43	73
interval debulking	16	36,5	34	53
consolidation	12,5	33,4	-	-
recurrence	37	45,7	32,16,30^	45,29,47^
salvage	-	-	28	30
Primary	17	35,4		
Recurrence	37	45,7		
Maximal cytoreduction				
CC 0 (primary)	23.6	41.5	49,5	54
CC 0 (recurrence)	40.2	51.5	41,8	48,2
Prognostic factors	**Univariate or Multivariate Analyses - p value**			
	Primary	**Recurrence**	**Primary**	**Recurrence**
CC score	0.005	0.0001	ns	0,001
PCI	0.0012*	0.0001**	0,01	0,001
PS	ns	0.0224		
Platinum response	nr	ns	p<0,005	
setting	nr	nr		
blood loss	nr	nr		
ca 125	0.0241	0.2131	ns	ns
lymph-node metastases	nr	nr	ns	ns
age	0.0574	0.0314	ns	ns
HIPEC drugs number	0.9689	0.0176		
HIPEC drug type (carboplatin)	0.2653	0.7098		
duration of perfusion (90 min)	nr	nr		

^ 1ST recurrence Platinum sensitive, insensitive after 2ndchemotherapy;
*multivariate(o,oo5)
**multivariate(0,001)
nr, not referred; ns, not significant

Table 20.5 Peritonectomy and hyperthermic intraperitoneal chemotherapy (HIPEC) in ovarian carcinomatosis treatment. Survival and prognostic factors

	Monocentric study				Collective review			
Study [Reference]	**Di Giorgio (unpublished)**				**de Bree [33]**			
	5 yr OS	5 yr PFS	median OS	median PFS	5 yr OS	5 yr PFS	median OS	median PFS
Setting	%	%	months	months	%	%	months	months
Front-line	57,6	38	63,1	38,5	33-61	15-20	24-42	20-30
Interval debulking	41,2	39,7	37,4	21	50-58	10	69	17
Consolidation	not reached	not reached	not reached	not reached	84	63	64	13-57
Recurrence	45	29,5	40	17,7	15-51	10-13	24-54	10-31
Primary	50,7	43,1	61,1	38,5	33-84	10-63	64-69	13-57
Recurrence	45	29,4	40	17,7	15-51	10-13	28-57	10-31
Maximal cytoreduction								
CC 0 (primary)	59,6	53,7	50,5	56,8	-	-	66*	-
CC 0 (recurrence)	61,3	42,2	66	52				
						*only front-line		
Prognostic factors	**Univariate or multivariate analyses - p value**							
	Primary		Recurrence					
	univariate	multivariate	univariate	multivariate				
CC score	0,000	0,003	0,03	0,009	nr			
PCI	0,008	ns	0,007	0,02	nr			
PS	ns	ns	0,006		nr			
Platinum response	0,0005	ns	ns		nr			

(cont.) →

Table 20.5 *(continued)*

	Monocentric study				Collective review
Study [Reference]	**Di Giorgio (unpublished)**				**de Bree [33]**
Prognostic factors	**Univariate or multivariate analyses - p value**				
	Primary		Recurrence		
	univariate	multivariate	univariate	multivariate	
Setting	ns	ns	ns	ns	nr
Bowel wall infiltration	0,047	0,0002	0,01	0,00	nr
Blood loss	ns	ns	0,0004		nr
Ca 125	ns	ns	ns		nr
Lymph-node metastases	0,0026	0,002	ns	ns	nr
Age	ns	ns	ns	ns	nr
HIPEC drugs number	nr	nr	nr	nr	nr
HIPEC drug type (carboplatin)	nr	nr	nr	nr	nr
Duration of perfusion (90 min)	nr	nr	nr	nr	nr

nr, not referred; ns, not significant

[34] demonstrated significantly lower survival values in secondary CRS (18 % at 5 years and a median of 23.5 months) compared to all other studies. Across studies, PFS values at 5 years range from 13 % to 50 %; in the monocentric study, PFS is higher than other studies and closer to OS (Fig. 20.5).

In conclusion, except for the HYPER-O study, no other substantial difference after primary and secondary CRS in terms of OS and PFS is reported. Also, comparative analysis of survival in relation to single-center settings shows no significant differences in terms of OS or PFS (Fig. 20.6). Nevertheless, in primary cytoreductions, front-line cases tend to have a better prognosis than those treated at interval debulking, except in the HYPER-O study. The scarce number of patients in the setting of consolidation generates less reliable data and makes it difficult to identify a consistent survival trend. In all studies, completely cytoreduced patients demonstrated median survival rates ranging from 37 to 66 months, with small differences between primary and secondary CRS. Two studies [33, 35] did not analyze prognostic factors; in the other four studies (Tables 20.4, 20.5) [48, 53, MIIS (unpublished), Di Giorgio (unpublished)], CC and PCI scores were more constantly analyzed as prognostic factors and significantly influenced survival on univariate and multivariate analysis.

The prognostic significance of platinum chemoresistance was analyzed in four studies (Table 20.3) [29, 33, MIIS (unpublished), Di Giorgio (unpublished)], even though each had different criteria; and in three studies (Tables 20.4, 20.5) [35, MIIS (unpublished), Di Giorgio (unpublished)], chemoresistance was statistically correlated with survival and negatively influenced the prognosis. In our monocentric study, univariate and multivariate analyses showed that the level of carcinomatous infiltration of the intestinal wall from

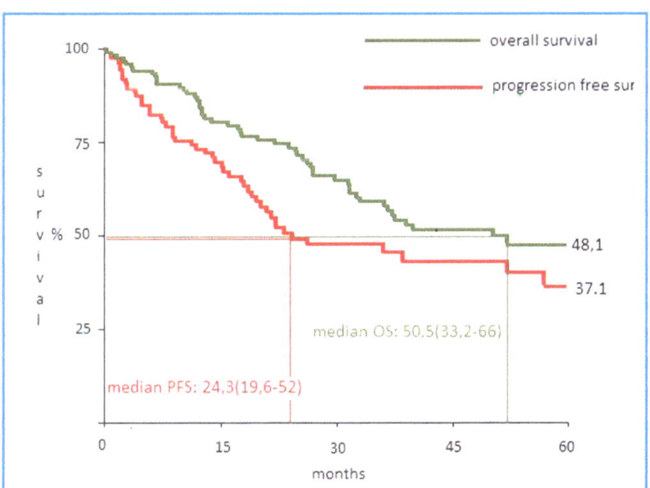

Fig. 20.5 Monocentric study: peritonectomy and hyperthermic intraperitoneal chemotherapy (HIPEC) in ovarian carcinomatosis treatment. Overall and progression-free survival using the Kaplan–Meier method

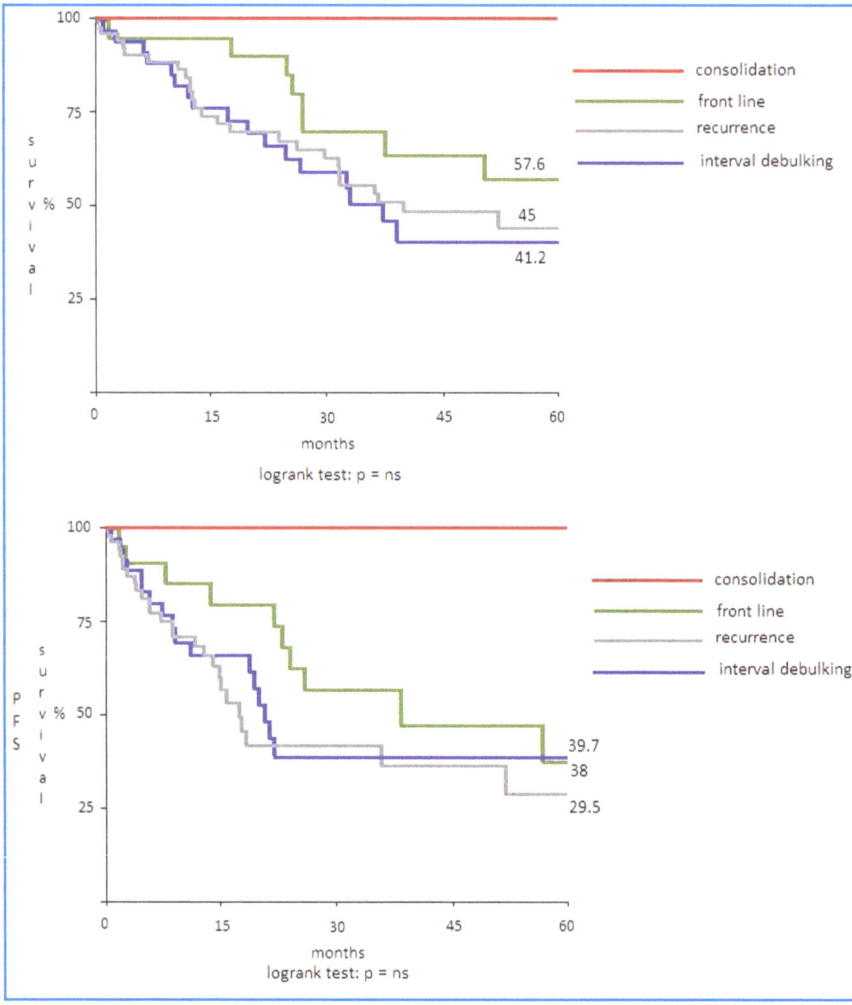

Fig. 20.6 Monocentric study: peritonectomy and hyperthermic intraperitoneal chemotherapy (HIPEC) in ovarian carcinomatosis treatment. Overall and progression-free survival according to all settings; consolidation survival curves are unreliable because of small number of cases

serosa to mucosa negatively influenced the prognosis. HIPEC duration and the use of different drugs had little impact on survival.

Ultimately the analyzed studies permit the evaluation of the overall impact of PRT plus HIPEC on prognosis of patients with ovarian carcinomatosis, even with the methodological limitations previously described. However, two fundamental aspects must be defined:

- The role of HIPEC in comparison with traditional treatments
- The role of HIPEC in various settings

Thus, it is necessary to verify whether the integrated procedure of PRT with HIPEC creates advantages in terms of survival in comparison with CRS associated with systemic or normothermic IP-CHT and whether it is effective in the various settings in which carcinomatosis requires treatment.

20.4.1.1 HIPEC versus No HIPEC

In a general evaluation of treatment for ovarian carcinomatosis, comparison between traditional treatments based on CRS and systemic or, more rarely, IP-CHT and PRT plus HIPEC is difficult and inconclusive due to the lack of specific controlled studies. Therefore, comparison on the basis of results of currently available studies is arduous due to the wide inhomogeneity of patients and methods, and particularly to the different approach between PSM centers that are mainly proponents of HIPEC and gynecologic–oncologic centers that primarily use standard treatments. Indeed, one significant example is sufficient to demonstrate the profound differences between these approaches and refers to the evaluation of optimal debulking. In the gynecological context, a limit of 1 cm is tolerated, whereas in the HIPEC context, this limit is 2.5 mm. This observation alone is sufficient to render insignificant the comparison between such different experiences.

In the first report of the HYPER-O registry [34], Helm compared survival results in 20 front-line cases treated with HIPEC with those obtained from the GOG 172 protocol [36] in patients with similar characteristics and treated with systemic or IP-CHT. This comparison shows consistent results among these studies, even if the comparison was limited to 2-year survival and cases involved in the GOG protocol were far more numerous.

Major clarity is inferred from case–control studies that compare results of CRS plus HIPEC with controls treated with conventional procedures for EOC. In all these studies, HIPEC results were consistently superior, guaranteeing better survival rates than traditional protocols in various settings, both primary and secondary (Table 20.6).

20.4.1.2 HIPEC in Primary CRS-HIPEC in Front-line and Interval-debulking Treatment

In primary CRS plus HIPEC, the most discussed problem is the role of NACT. Theoretically, primary forms with diffuse PC are the ideal target for neoadjuvant treatments based on CarboTaxol due to the high percentage of chemosensitivity in front-line treatment (~ 80 % of cases). However, the expected results do not demonstrate a clear advantage of NACT when compared with front-line treatment with CRS followed by adjuvant CHT, nor with CRS plus HIPEC.

NACT in Traditional Treatment

The EORTC 55971 trial evaluated the role of NACT in patients with stages III and IV ovarian cancer. In that study, patients were randomized in two groups: standard CRS plus adjuvant CHT vs. NACT and interval debulking surgery.

Table 20.6 Treatment of ovarian carcinomatosis with and without hyperthermic intraperitoneal chemotherapy (HIPEC). Overall and progression-free survival

HIPEC vs. NO HIPEC - Comparative non-randomized studies								
Study [Reference]	**Treatment**	**Patients (n)**	**Progression-free survival**			**Overall survival**		
			Median (months)	**5-year (%)**	**P**	**Median (months)**	**5-year (%)**	**P**
			Front-line					
GOG 172 vs. HYPER-O	IV cht	210	18,3	42(2 y)°°	–	49,7	75(2 y)°°	–
(Helm 2010) [34]	IP cht	205	23,8	53°(2 y)°°		65,6	82(2 y)°°	
	HIPEC	20	36,5	47,6(2y)		57,5	66,4(2y)	
			Consolidation					
Gori (2005) [44]	HIPEC	29				64,4	~50°	?
	no HIPEC	19				46,4	0	
Kim (2010) [45]	HIPEC	19	NR	63,1	0,027		84,2	0,0004
	no HIPEC	24	18,5	29,2			41,7	
			Recurrent					
Munoz-Casares	CRS + HIPEC	14	48		nr		58	0.046
(2009) [56]	CRS without HIPEC	12	24				17	
	CRS + HIPEC	optimal CRS (R0)					67	ns
	CRS without HIPEC	optimal CRS (R0)					29	
Fagotti (2012) [57]	CRS + HIPEC	30	26	30*	0,004	NR	68,4	0,017
	no HIPEC	37	15	0*		NR	42,7	

(*cont.*) ↓

			Secondary surgery					
Ryu (2004) [49]	HIPEC (Carbo)	35 (FIGO III)	26,4**	26,9**	0,007	60,9	53,8	0,0015
	no HIPEC	39 (FIGO III)	6,1**	10,3**		22,3	33,3	
	HIPEC (Carbo)	26 (optimal CRS)	40,6**	~35***	0.0027	nr	65,6	0,0046
	no HIPEC	27 (optimal CRS)	13,2**	~15***		nr	40,7	
Bae (2007) [43]	HIPEC	44	56	56,3	0.0028	nr	66	0,0003
	no HIPEC	24	15	16,7		31	33	
	HIPEC	27 (optimal CRS)	74	62.9	0,0079	nr	70,4	0,0007
	no HIPEC	15 (optimal CRS)	17	18,8		31	31,3	

***value estimated from fig 1 in Ryu KS et al. 2004 [47] ° value estimated from Fig.2 in"Gori j et al. 2005 [42] °° value estimeted from Fig. 4 in GOG 172 [5]
**disease free survival
NR: not reached nr: not referred ns: not significant

Results showed an increased rate of optimal cytoreduction (residual ≤ 1 cm; 80.6 % vs. 41.6 %) and a decreased incidence of postoperative complications in patients treated with NACT versus those treated with primary debulking surgery (PDS), without any difference in terms of OS (median 30 vs. 29 months) and PFS (12 months for both arms). The most significant prognostic parameter was optimal cytoreduction [37]. The study is the subject of several criticisms [38] that undermine the overall validity of results. However, conclusions from a practical point of view tend to favor the choice of neoadjuvant treatment in patients with bulky disease and at risk of incomplete cytoreduction or in patients with metastatic disease (stage IV). Alternatively, for patients for whom obtaining optimal cytoreduction is feasible, PDS should be preferred.

NACT in CRS plus HIPEC

Review data in this regard are conflicting, and no evident survival trend with its use emerges (Tables 20.4 and 20.5). However, a better understanding of the role of NACT in this setting can be obtained from analysis of its efficacy on carcinomatosis before cytoreduction. Indeed, patients who undergo NACT present several degrees of response that generate minimal or null variations in staging the initial carcinosis, up to total eradication of ovarian and peritoneal disease. Comparison of prognoses based on different responses to NACT can contribute to specifying its role and identifying patients who may benefit the most from its use.

In our monocentric and the Italian MIIS study, patients who received NACT and nonresponders to a preoperative Taxol plus platinum-based regimen demonstrated a significantly worse prognosis in comparison with patients treated front line or those who responded to NACT both having similar prognoses (Fig. 20.7). In our study and the Italian MIIS study (unpublished), NACT was performed in patients with major peritoneal diffusion or with systemic metastases; thus, the good prognostic result obtained in chemosensitive NACT patients, similar to those obtained with front-line treatment, leads to the positive consideration of NACT in more advanced cases. In NACT nonresponders, prognosis was significantly worse and CRS plus HIPEC did not appear to modify significantly the negative evolution of the disease, even if the rates of optimal cytoreduction were similar to those obtained in front-line cases and in NACT-sensitive cases. In our clinical records, complication rates are similar in the different settings of primary cytoreduction.

The role of NACT appears uncertain also in HIPEC studies, with results similar to those regarding the role of NACT in traditional treatment, thus inducing a personalized choice regarding these treatment options based primarily on PC extent and presence of hematogenous or extra-abdominal metastases susceptible to systemic treatments at first diagnosis. Different therapeutic strategies are worth consideration for NACT unresponsive patients, and results from current clinical trials regarding the role of NACT pre-HIPEC could give more significant indications.

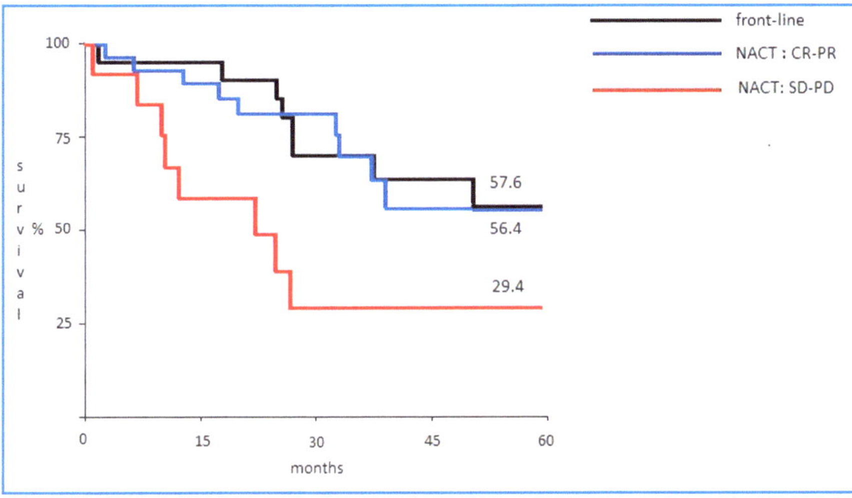

Fig. 20.7 Monocentric study: peritonectomy and hyperthermic intraperitoneal chemotherapy (HIPEC) in ovarian carcinomatosis treatment. Overall survival in primary setting with and without neoadjuvant chemotherapy (NACT)

In our monocentric study, 45.5 % of patients treated with primary cytoreduction had lymph node metastasis, which negatively influenced survival and resulted as a significant prognostic factor in univariate and multivariate analyses. Nevertheless 33.4 % of patients with lymph node metastases showed a 5-year survival, thus confirming the therapeutic role of lymphadenectomy in the presence of locoregional lymphatic diffusion (Table 20.5). The role of lymphadenectomy in advanced ovarian carcinomas is controversial. Some authors support its need on the basis of favorable prognostic results [39–41]; others are sceptical [42] or think that systematic lymphadenectomy should be not performed in principle. The high percentage of locoregional lymph node metastasis and the need to radicalize the intervention in lymph nodes as well as in the peritoneal cavity justify systematic lymphadenectomy in primary settings.

Lymph node diffusion in PC from advanced EOC may also involve other sectors, such as the hepatic pedicle and perigastric and mesenteric stations, rather than locoregional lymph nodes. In these compartments, the extent of lymphadenectomy should be performed as necessary.

20.4.1.3 HIPEC in Consolidation Treatment

Patients treated with PRT plus HIPEC as consolidation therapy are worthy of specific evaluation. First, the concept of consolidation needs to be defined, as this is inhomogeneous in various studies. In general, consolidation therapy is defined as a cancer-specific treatment planned in patients already treated and who show no apparent recurrent disease. Consolidation treatment may be performed after exclusive systemic CHT or after integrated surgical and chemotherapeutic treatment. It can consist of surgery or CHT, either alone or in combination.

In the majority of studies that consider HIPEC as consolidation therapy, the procedure was performed in patients without apparent endoperitoneal recurrence on second-look surgery and after first-line treatment consisting of CRS plus systemic CHT, as in studies by Bae et al., Gori et al., Kim et al., and Pomel et al. [43–46]. In these studies, consolidation is prevalently performed with HIPEC associated with multiple peritoneal biopsies; further secondary cytoreductions are rare and only used in cases with macroscopic recurrence at second look.

Other authors [46–48] identified the use of PRT plus HIPEC as consolidation after NACT. Kim et al. [45], in a series of patients previously treated with PDS and systemic CHT, used PRT plus HIPEC both as consolidation and as secondary cytoreduction, without specific discrimination between the two series. Given that all patients during PRT plus HIPEC presented peritoneal metastases, the study more aptly refers to cases of secondary cytoreduction for recurrence and not for consolidation treatment. The HYPER-O study reports 12 cases treated as consolidation without specifying previous treatment; the relative survival results are reported as being unreliable by the same authors due to the small number of cases examined. These data confirm inappropriateness in identifying the consolidation setting in series treated with HIPEC. More accurate is identifying the use of PRT plus HIPEC as consolidation in patients who undergo NACT for diffuse PC and who obtain complete remission. In our opinion, these patients, even if apparently disease free, require an integrated procedure aimed not only at excising genital organs and other structures described above, but also using HIPEC to treat sites previously affected by peritoneal metastases.

In the analyzed studies, it was not possible to identify significant groups of patients in this specific setting. Cases treated with this procedure in our single-center experience were too few to provide useful indications; however, all seven patients treated with consolidation therapy were alive and disease free at this writing, with a follow up ranging from 2 to 7 years.

It should be also considered that the percentage of cases developing recurrence after negative second-look surgery is significantly high, ranging from 30 % to 56 %, in relation to the risk of undertreatment for the reason previously indicated. Thus, novel treatment strategies should be verified for this peculiar set of patients in future trials [47, 48].

20.4.1.4 HIPEC for Recurrence

In almost all studies dealing with PRT plus HIPEC, patients treated for recurrence are significantly more numerous than those treated for primary forms, except in our monocentric study. These data conflict with traditional treatments, which suggest limited use of CRS for recurrence, using that approach only for patients with intestinal obstruction, with single symptomatic or slow-growing localization, and with platinum-sensitive recurrence. Patients affected by platinum-resistant or platinum-refractory disease with progression during first-line treatment are not considered suitable candidates for CRS.

Concerning traditional treatments, two multicentric randomized studies in progress are aimed at proving the efficacy of surgical treatment in patients with platinum-sensitive recurrence: GOG 213 and AGO-OVAR DESKTOP III studies [38]. In the study by Harter et al. comprising 250 patients who underwent CRS and treated for recurrence from EOC, overall median survival was 29.5 months, which decreased drastically to 19.9 months in patients with diffuse PC [51]. In Bristow et al.'s meta-analysis [18] involving 2,019 patients who underwent secondary CRS for platinum-sensitive recurrence, median OS was 30.3 months. These survival values are significantly lower than those reported in studies summarized in Tables 20.4 and 20.5, in which patients were prevalently treated for diffused carcinomatosis rather than for localized forms, as in Bristow et al.'s study, and without distinguishing first or multiple recurrences. Also, case–control studies in Table 20.6 clearly demonstrate that in secondary forms, CRS plus HIPEC guarantees median survival rates higher than standard treatments without HIPEC.

It is interesting to note that among multicenter studies reported in table 4 and in relation to patients treated for recurrence only, the HYPER-O study showed a negative prognostic influence of platinum resistance; in Bakrin et al.'s study, the most extensive dealing with HIPEC; in this author's monocentric study, and in the MIIS study, platinum resistance showed no significant influence on survival in comparison with chemosensitive cases. In HIPEC studies on recurrence, analogous to primary forms, CC and PCI scores were the most significant prognostic factors. Infiltration grade of the intestinal wall by carcinomatosis resulted in a significant prognostic factor in the monocentric study, confirming results of a previous report and those of other studies [24–26]. In secondary forms, lymphadenectomy is necessary when it has not been performed in previous primary CRS or when metastatic lymph nodes are present; the aim is to radicalize exeresis at the lymphatic level.

In our monocentric study, 62.5 % of recurrent cases presented lymph nodal metastases, but this involvement did not significantly influence prognosis. These data confirm the significance and need for lymphadenectomy, as exeresis of metastatic lymph nodes guarantees similar survival to that observed in patients with negative lymph nodes.

Results of ongoing trials will elucidate the real role of CRS plus HIPEC for treating recurrent ovarian carcinomatosis. On the basis of analyzed experiences, CRS plus HIPEC is a promising choice, which can guarantee long-term survival rates higher than those of standard treatment and similar to those in primary forms. It is also appropriate for both platinum-sensitive and -resistant forms.

20.5 Morbidity and Mortality

Most relevant complications after PRT plus HIPEC primarily involve toxicity derived from CHT during HIPEC and the complexity of adverse events strictly related to the procedure (Table 20.7). Hematological toxicity with grades 3 and

Table 20.7 Peritonectomy and hyperthermic intraperitoneal chemotherapy (HIPEC) in ovarian carcinomatosis treatment. Morbidity and risk factors

Study [Reference]	Hyper-O [34]	Deraco [35]	Bakrin [29]	MIIS (unpublished)	de Bree [33]	Di Giorgio (unpublished)	
Hematologic toxicity	nr	4%	11%		nr		
Renal toxicity	nr	nr	8%		nr	6%	
Major complications (grade III-IV)	nr	15%	31.3%		12%-56%	15%	
Re-operation,interventional radiology or endoscopy		19,2%	13%			13,1%	
Post-operative mortality	0.5%	4%	0.8%		0%-10%	3,8%	
Risk factors	Univariate or multivariate analyses - **p value**						
			Multiple regression			**Univariate analysis**	**Multiple regression**
PCI			0.003			0,0001	0,018
CC score			0.003			0,005	
CDDP (HIPEC)			0.002			ns	
First line tratment			0.008			ns	
No. organ resection						0,008	
Intestinal resections						0,002	
Blood loss						0,0068	
PS						0,0017	
ASA						0,002	
Duration of preocedure > 8 hours						0,001	0,04

4 leukopenia was reported in Deraco et al.'s [35] and Bakrin et al.'s [29] studies, with a maximum incidence of 11 %; renal toxicity ranged from 6 % to 8 %. In Bakrin et al.'s study, 2 % of patients developed a chronic renal failure and 1 % required long-term dialysis. The incidence of major complications (grades 3 and 4) was variable, ranging from 14 % to 56 %, with a mortality rate ranging from 0 % to 10 %. The rate of reintervention with surgical, endoscopic, or radiological procedures varied between 13 % and 19.2 %. Only two studies (Table 20.7) [27, Di Giorgio (unpublished)] used both univariate and multivariate analyses to assess risk factors for complications. High PCI score and incomplete cytoreduction were significantly correlated with increased morbidity in both studies. A study by Cascales Campos et al. involving 91 patients treated with PRT plus HIPEC for ovarian carcinomatosis in various settings [52] used multivariate analysis to determine the role of PCI as a risk factor for major complications associated with performing digestive anastomoses.

It is difficult to compare various experiences mainly because of the different criteria by which complications are defined and the different classifications with which morbidity levels are synthesized. The number of possible complications after PRT plus HIPEC is high, and the possibility of achieving a complete scenario of all adverse events is difficult and depends on the accuracy with which databases are designed and on prospective or retrospective modalities with which data are updated.

Among the criticisms regarding PRT plus HIPEC, the high percentage of major complications and the role of HIPEC as a morbidity risk factor are well known. It is difficult, if not impossible, to establish the precise responsibility of HIPEC, even if its role as cofactor cannot be ignored. Among the analyzed studies, only Bakrin et al.'s multicenter study and the author's monocentric study reported results of multivariate analyses of risk factors, and both studies identified PCI and CC scores as most relevant parameters correlated to the occurrence of major complications.

These results logically correlate with operative mortality and reintervention rates, as reported in Deraco et al.'s [35] and Di Giorgio's monocentric study (unpublished), which include cases with the highest mean PCI value. Such results also correlate with lowest morbidity rates observed in patients treated as consolidation and who were free of disease at second look. An exception is represented by Pomel et al.'s prospective study [46] dedicated to cases treated as consolidation with oxaliplatin-based HIPEC [Hyperthermic Intra-peritoneal Chemotherapy using Oxaliplatin as Consolidation Therapy for Advanced Epithelial Ovarian Carcinoma. Results of a phaseII prospective multicentre trial (CHIPOVAC)]; this study was interrupted for excessive morbidity. Procedure duration was a risk factor in the monocentric study, as in other reports of PRT plus HIPEC treatment in both ovarian and extraovarian carcinosis [53, 54].

In summary, in the presence of notable variability of data from analyzed studies, incidences of complication and mortality appear limited and comparable with those related to major abdominal and pelvic surgery. Controlling morbidity rate is possible in highly active centers with consolidated experience and specialized medical, nursing, and logistic organization, as reported in previous chapters. Results of trials in progress regarding the specific role of HIPEC shall furnish significant data about its related morbidity, whereas the use of specific protocols and prospective databases related to multi-institutional experiences can provide useful data to limit morbidity in the mid-term.

20.6 Conclusions

Using the integrated procedure of PRT plus HIPEC for treating ovarian carcinomatosis is the most discussed issue among PSM. The main criticism regards the use of HIPEC, since the need for maximal cytoreduction is consolidated and does not raise any doubts. Lack of prospective randomized studies on the role of HIPEC and the differing opinions between oncological surgeons, who are more likely to use HIPEC; and oncologic gynecologists and medical oncologists, who are more likely to use standard treatment with cytoreduction associated with systemic CHT or, more rarely, isothermic IP-CHT, plays a relevant role in such a scenario.

Communities of surgeon and oncologic gynecologists who believe in the role of HIPEC have started controlled clinical trials aimed at clarifying the role of PRT plus HIPEC, but conducting these studies with the aim of achieving reliable results is lengthy and difficult. Furthermore, the use of innovative drugs or combinations of drugs to treat OC, which is basically highly sensitive to first-line treatment with CarboTaxol and susceptible to benefits from second- and third-line CHT for attaining disease chronicity, contributes to further questions regarding the role of HIPEC in ovarian carcinomatosis.

To date, the major criticisms of HIPEC involve its potential influence on survival and morbidity. Therefore, it is necessary to verify whether PRT plus HIPEC can guarantee better survival when compared with standard treatments and whether the incidence of related morbidity is acceptable in comparison with other types of treatment. To answer these questions, we must rely on available literature reports and unpublished data of research in progress that maximally corresponds to studies analyzed in this chapter and which comprise almost 2,400 cases, representing a solid base by which to identify a trend in results, regardless of the study limitations discussed above.

On the basis of possible comparison of overall results drawn from the analyzed studies, it is reasonable to state that PRT plus HIPEC guarantees better OS and PFS values than those derived from traditional treatments in all settings. Notwithstanding, some specific aspects, including the role of chemoresistance and neoadjuvant treatment, should be clarified by further experience and results of on-going trials.

Criticism pertaining to morbidity rate is generally poorly posed and tends to attribute to HIPEC responsibilities that it cannot be objectively sustained while decreasing the weighting of morbidity attributable to standard treatments.

Moreover, PRT plus HIPEC and standard treatments are not fully comparable realities: PRT has the fundamental aim of total exeresis of peritoneal disease and tolerates remarkably more severe limits for optimal cytoreduction than standard treatments performed by oncologic gynecologists. For this reason, a greater number of visceral resections, longer procedure duration, and greater blood—loss all related to PRT—may constitute risk factors for postoperative outcomes. Furthermore, as reported in various studies, specialized PSM centers treat patients with more advanced PC than do gynecological centers.

Except for well-tolerated bone marrow and renal toxicity exclusively attributable to HIPEC, it is difficult to discriminate the negative impact on morbidity of the surgical phase from that of chemohyperthermia. The incidence of morbidity from PRT plus HIPEC is no different from that related to major abdominopelvic surgery. Moreover, the impact of traditional systemic and/or IP-CHT on morbidity and the related QoL merits further consideration. In a recent review comparing IP-CHT and IV-CHT treatments, Chan et al. showed that related morbidity and mortality rates were similar to those related to PRT plus HIPEC, which includes the surgical phase. In addition, related complications cause a significant reduction of complete application of both procedures (i.e. IP-CHT and IV-CHT) [55].

On the basis of results analyzed, the following conclusions regarding the current role of PRT plus HIPEC can be drawn:

- PRT plus HIPEC can guarantee significant percentage of long-term PFS and OS survival in primary and recurrent settings.
- In all settings, complete cytoreduction represents the most significant prognostic factor.
- High PCI levels do not constitute a limitation for this procedure if optimal CRS is technically feasible.
- The prognostic role of NACT is uncertain: NACT-chemosensitive cases demonstrate similar prognoses to patients treated with front-line PRT plus HIPEC, whereas chemoresistant patients show a significantly worse prognosis.
- Platinum-based chemoresistance requires a more specific definition and tends to assume a negative prognostic role.
- Major complications and mortality rates are similar to those related to major abdominal pelvic surgery and are not different after primary or secondary cytoreduction. PCI and CC scores represent the most significant risk factors for major complications.

References

1. Griffiths CT (1975) Surgical resection of tumor bulk in the primary treatment of ovarian carcinoma. Natl Cancer Inst Monogr 42:101-104
2. Shih KK, Chi DS (2010) Maximal cytoreductive effort in epithelial ovarian cancer surgery. J Gynecol Oncol 21:75-80

3. Sugarbaker PH (1996) Complete Parietal and Visceral Peritonectomy of the Pelvis for advanced primary and recurrent ovarian cancer. Cancer Treat Res 81-75-87
4. Jacquet P, Sugarbaker PH (1996) Clinical research methodologies in diagnosis and staging of patients with peritoneal carcinomatosisi. Cancer Treat Res 82:359-374
5. Hoskins WJ, McGuire WP, Brady MF et al (1994) The effect of diameter of largest residual disease on survival after primary cytoreductive surgery in patients with suboptimal residual epithelial ovarian carcinoma. Am J Obstet Gynecol 170:974-979
6. Chi DS, Eisenhauer EL, Lang J et al (2006) What is the optimal goal of primary cytoreductive surgery for bulky stage IIIC epithelial ovarian carcinoma (EOC)? Gynecologic Oncology 103:559-564
7. Bristow RE, Tomacruz RS, Armstrong DK et al (2002) Trimble EL, Montz FJ. Survival effect of maximal cytoreductive surgery for advanced ovarian carcinoma during the platinum era: a meta-analysis. J Clin Oncol 20:1248-1259
8. Eisenkop SM, Friedman RL, Wang HJ (1995) Secondary cytoreductive surgery for recurrent ovarian cancer. A prospective study. Cancer 76:1606-1614
9. Cormio G, di Vagno G, Cazzolla A et al (1999) Surgical treatment of recurrent ovarian cancer:report of 21 cases and a review of the literature. Eur J Obstet Gynecol Reprod Biol 86:185-188
10. Eisenkop SM, Friedman RL, Spirtos NM (2000) The role of secondary cytoreductive surgery in the treatment of patients with re- current epithelial ovarian carcinoma. Cancer 88:144-153
11. Gadducci A,Iacconi P, Cosio S, Fanucchi A et al (2000) Complete salvage surgical cytoreduction improves further survival of patients with late recurrent ovar- ian cancer. Gynecol Oncol 79:344-349
12. Gronlund B, Lundvall L, Christensen IJ et al (2005) Surgical cytoreduction in recurrent ovarian carcinoma in pa- tients with complete response to paclitaxel-platinum. Eur J Surg Oncol 31:67-73
13. Onda T, Yoshikawa H, Yasugi T et al (2005) Secondary cytoreductive surgery for recurrent epi- thelial ovarian carcinoma: proposal for patients selection. Br J Cancer 92:1026-1032
14. Benedetti Panici P, De Vivo A, Bellati F et al (2007) Secondary cytoreductive surgery in patients with platinum-sensitive recurrent ovarian cancer. Ann Surg Oncol 14:1136-1142
15. Oksefjell H, Sandstad B, Trope C (2009) The role of secondary cytor- eduction in the management of the first relapse in epithelial ovarian cancer. Ann Oncol 20:286-293
16. Tian WJ, Jiang R, Cheng X et al (2010) Surgery in re- current epithelial ovarian cancer: benefits on Survival for patients with residual disease of 0.1-1 cm after secondary cytoreduction. J Surg Oncol 101:244-250
17. Tay EH, Grant PT, Gebski V, Hacker NF (2002) Secondary cytor- eductive surgery for recurrent epithelial ovarian cancer. Obstet Gynecol 99:1008-1013
18. Bristow RE, Puri I, Chi DS (2009) Cytoreductive surgery for recurrent ovarian cancer: a meta-analysis. Gynecol Oncol 112:265-274
19. Leitao MM Jr, Kardos S, Barakat RR, Chi DS (2004) Tertiary cytoreduction in patients with recurrent ovarian carcinoma. Gynecol Oncol 95:181-188
20. Shih KK, Chi DS, Barakat RR, Leitao MM Jr (2010) Tertiary cytoreduction in patients with recurrent epithelial ovarian, fallopian tube, or primary peritoneal cancer: an updated series. Gynecol Oncol 117:330-335
21. Karam AK, Santillan A, Bristow RE et al (2007) Tertiary cytoreductive surgery in recurrent ovarian cancer: selection criteria and survival outcome. Gynecol Oncol 104:377-380
22. Fotopoulou C, Savvatis K, Kosian P et al (2003) Quaternary cytoreductive surgery in ovarian cancer: does surgical effort still matter? Br J Cancer 108:32-38
23. Chi DS, Eisenhauer EL, Zivanovic O et al (2009) Improved progression-free and overall survival in advanced ovarian cancer as a result of a change in surgical paradigm. Gynecol Oncol 114:26-31
24. Di Giorgio A, Cardi M, Biacchi D et al (2013) Depth of colorectal-wall invasion and lymphnode involvement as major outcome factors influencing surgical strategy in patients with advanced and recurrent ovarian cancer with diffuse peritoneal metastases. World J Surg On-

col 11:64
25. Park JY, Seo SS, Kang S, Lee KB et al (2006) The benefits of low anterior en bloc resection as part of cytoreductive surgery for advanced primary and recurrent epithelial ovarian cancer patients outweigh morbidity concerns. Gynecol Oncol 103:977-984
26. Scarabelli C, Gallo A, Franceschi S (2000) Primary cytoreductive surgery with rectosigmoid colon resection for patients with advanced epithelial ovarian carcinoma. Cancer 88:389-397
27. Fagotti A, Ferrandina G, Fanfani F et al (2006) A laparoscopy-based score to predict surgical outcome in patients with advanced ovarian carcinoma: a pilot study. Ann Surg Oncol 13:1156-1161
28. Bakrin N, Cotte E, Golfier F et al (2012) Cytoreductive surgery and hyperthermic intraperitoneal chemotherapy (HIPEC) for persistent and recurrent advanced ovarian carcinoma: a multicenter, prospective study of 246 patients. Ann Surg Oncol 19:4052-4058
29. Bakrin N, Bereder JM, Decullier E, Classe JM, Msika S, Lorimier G, Abboud K, Meeus P, Ferron G, Quenet F, Marchal F, Gouy S, Morice P, Pomel C, Pocard M, Guyon F, Porcheron J, Glehen O; FROGHI (FRench Oncologic and Gynecologic HIPEC) Group (2013) Peritoneal carcinomatosis treated with cytoreductive surgery and Hyperthermic Intraperitoneal Chemotherapy (HIPEC) for advanced ovarian carcinoma: a French multicenter retrospective cohort study of 566 patients. Eur J Surg Oncol 39:1435-1443
30. Eisenkop SM, Spirtos NM, Lin WC (2006) "Optimal" cytoreduction for advanced epithelial ovarian cancer: a commentary. Gynecol Oncol 103:329-335
31. Bijelic L, Yan TD, Sugarbaker PH (2008) Treatment failure following complete cytoreductive surgery and perioperative intraperitoneal chemotherapy for peritoneal dissemination from colorectal or appendiceal mucinous neoplasms. J Surg Oncol 98:295-299
32. Chua TC, Robertson G, Liauw W et (2009) Intraoperative hyperthermic intraperitoneal chemotherapy after cytoreductive surgery in ovarian cancer peritoneal carcinomatosis: systematic review of current results. J Cancer Res Clin Oncol 135:1637-1645
33. de Bree E, Helm CW (2012) Hyperthermic intraperitoneal chemotherapy in ovarian cancer: rationale and clinical data. Expert Rev Anticancer Ther 12:895-911
34. Helm CW, Richard SD, Pan J, Bartlett D et al (2010) Hyperthermic intraperitoneal chemotherapy in ovarian cancer: first report of the HYPER-O registry. Int J Gynecol Cancer 20:61-69
35. Deraco M, Kusamura S, Virzi S et al (2011) Cytoreductive surgery and hyperthermic intraperitoneal chemotherapy as upfront therapy for advanced epithelial ovarian cancer: multi-institutional phase-II trial. Gynecol Oncol 122:215-220
36. Barlin JN, Dao F, Bou Zgheib N et al (2012) Progression-free and overall survival of a modified outpatient regimen of primary intravenous/intraperitoneal paclitaxel and intraperitoneal cisplatin in ovarian, fallopian tube, and primary peritoneal cancer. Gynecol Oncol 125:621-624
37. Onda, T, Yoshikawa, H (2011) Neoadjuvant chemotherapy for advanced ovarian cancer: overview of outcomes and unanswered questions. Expert Review of Anticancer Therapy 11:1053–1067
38. Goff BA (2013) Advanced ovarian cancer: what should be the standard of care? J Gynecol Oncol 24:83-91
39. Chan JK, Urban R, Hu JM et al (2007) The potential therapeutic role of lymph node resection in epithelial ovarian cancer: a study of 13918 patients. Br J Cancer 96:1817-1822
40. du Bois A, Reuss A, Harter P, Pujade-Lauraine E, Ray-Coquard I, Pfisterer J. Arbeitsgemeinschaft Gynaekologische Onkologie Studiengruppe Ovarialkarzinom; Groupe d'Investigateurs Nationaux pour l'Etude des Cancers Ovariens (2010) Potential role of lymphadenectomy in advanced ovarian cancer: a combined exploratory analysis of three prospectively randomized phase III multicenter trials. J Clin Oncol 28:1733-1739
41. Pereira A, Perez-Medina T, Magrina JF et al (2012) The role of lymphadenectomy in node-positive epithelial ovarian cancer. Int J Gynecol Cancer 22:987-992
42. Sakai K, Kajiyama H, Umezu T (2012) Is there any association between retroperitoneal lymphadenectomy and survival benefit in advanced stage epithelial ovarian carcinoma patients? J Obstet Gynaecol Res 38:1018-1023
43. Bae JH, Lee JM, Ryu KS et al (2007) Treatment of ovarian cancer with paclitaxel- or carbo-

platin-based intraperitoneal hyperthermic chemotherapy during secondary surgery. Gynecol Oncol 106:193-200
44. Gori J, Castano R, Toziano M et al (2005) Intraperitoneal hyperthermic chemotherapy in ovarian cancer. Int J Gynecol Cancer 15:233-239
45. Kim JH, Lee JM, Ryu KS et al (2010) Consolidation hyperthermic intraperitoneal chemotherapy using paclitaxel in patients with epithelial ovarian cancer. J Surg Oncol 101:149-155
46. Pomel C, Ferron G, Lorimier G et al (2010) Hyperthermic intra-peritoneal chemotherapy using oxaliplatin as consolidation therapy for advanced epithelial ovarian carcinoma. Results of a phase II prospective multicentre trial. CHIPOVAC study. Eur J Surg Oncol 36:589-593
47. Frenel JS, Leux C, Pouplin L et al (2011) Oxaliplatin-based hyperthermic intraperitoneal chemotherapy in primary or recurrent epithelial ovarian cancer: A pilot study of 31 patients. J Surg Oncol 103:10-16
48. Di Giorgio A, Naticchioni E, Biacchi D et al (2008) Cytoreductive surgery (peritonectomy procedures) combined with hyperthermic intraperitoneal chemotherapy (HIPEC) in the treatment of diffuse peritoneal carcinomatosis from ovarian cancer. Cancer 113:315-325
49. Ryu KS, Kim JH, Ko HS et (2004) Effects of intraperitoneal hyperthermic chemotherapy in ovarian cancer. Gynecol Oncol 94:325-332
50. Rubin SC, Randall TC, Armstrong KA et al (1999) Ten-year follow-up of ovarian cancer patients after second-look laparotomy with negative findings. Obstet Gynecol 93:21-24
51. Harter P, Hahmann M, Lueck HJ et al (2009) Surgery for recurrent ovarian cancer: role of peritoneal carcinomatosis: exploratory analysis of the DESKTOP I Trial about risk factors, surgical implications, and prognostic value of peritoneal carcinomatosis. Ann Surg Oncol 16:1324-1330
52. Cascales Campos P, Gil J, Parrilla P (2013) Morbidity and mortality outcomes of cytoreductive surgery and hyperthermic intraperitoneal chemotherapy in patients with primary and recurrent advanced ovarian cancer. Eur J Surg Oncol p ii: S0748-7983(13)00752-X
53. Glehen O, Osinsky D, Cotte E et al (2003) Intraperitoneal chemohyperthermia using a closed abdominal procedure and cytoreductive surgery for the treatment of peritoneal carcinomatosis: morbidity and mortality analysis of 216 consecutive procedures. Ann Surg Oncol 10:863-869
54. Hansson J, Graf W, Pahlman L et al (2009) Postoperative adverse events and long-term survival after cytoreductive surgery and intraperitoneal chemotherapy. Eur J Surg Oncol 35:202-208
55. Chan D L, Morris DL, Rao A, Chua TC (2012). Intraperitoneal chemotherapy in ovarian cancer: a review of tolerance and efficacy. Cancer Management and Research 4:413–422
56. Munoz-Casares FC, Rufian S, Rubio MJ et al (2009) The role of hyperthermic intraoperative intraperitoneal chemotherapy (HIPEC) in the treatment of peritoneal carcinomatosis in recurrent ovarian cancer. Clin Transl Oncol 11:753-759
57. Fagotti A, Costantini B, Petrillo M et al (2012) Cytoreductive surgery plus HIPEC in platinum-sensitive recurrent ovarian cancer patients: a case-control study on survival in patients with two year follow-up. Gynecologic Oncology 127:502–505

Other Primary Peritoneal Surface Malignancies

21

Paolo Sammartino, Fabio Accarpio, Tommaso Cornali, Alessio Impagnatiello, Bianca Maria Sollazzo, and Maria Luisa Framarino dei Malatesta

21.1 Introduction

Primary peritoneal surface malignancies (other than mesothelioma) are serous papillary carcinoma (PPSPC) and desmoplastic small round cell tumor (DSRCT). According new histogenetic theories, PPSPC and ovarian cancer (OC) originate from the tubal epithelium. Primary treatment in foreseen as being the application of maximal cytoreduction (peritonectomy procedures) combined with hyperthermic intraperitoneal chemotherapy (HIPEC). Evaluation of results must be done using the staging system comprising Peritoneal Cancer Index (PCI) and Completeness of Cytoreduction (CC) score. DSRCT is a rare and aggressive neoplasm, and patients typically present with an advanced stage with multiple peritoneal-based lesions. Despite multiple therapeutic strategies that include chemotherapy, aggressive debulking surgery, and abdominal-wall radiation, durable remission remains rare. A new staging system is proposed by the MD Anderson Cancer Center in the US, where peritonectomy procedures plus HIPEC are being applied with interesting results.

21.2 Primary Peritoneal Serous Papillary Carcinoma

Primary peritoneal serous papillary carcinoma (PPSPC) has heretofore been considered a rare malignant tumor originating from single or multiple foci starting from the peritoneum and first described by Swerdlow in 1959 [1]. The first

P. Sammartino (✉)
Department of Surgery "Pietro Valdoni", Sapienza University of Rome, Rome, Italy
e-mail: paolo.sammartino@uniroma1.it

A. Di Giorgio, E. Pinto (Eds), *Treatment of Peritoneal Surface Malignancies*, Updates in Surgery
DOI: 10.1007/978-88-470-5711-1_21, © Springer-Verlag Italia 2015

observation identifying PPSPC as a separate clinical entity whose histological and immunohistochemical features overlap those of high-grade ovarian serous tumors came from a paper describing its onset in patients who had undergone prophylactic oophorectomy for a family history of ovarian cancer [2]. The difficulty in distinguishing PPSPC histologically from other high-grade ovarian malignancies made it extremely hard, especially in patients with advanced stage tumors, to assess epidemiologically the true incidence of PPSPC, which is estimated by some as ~ 10 % of all ovarian cancers (OC) [3]. To facilitate the diagnosis and thus avoid possible misclassifications, the Gynecologic Oncology Group (GOG) formulated recommendations intended to make PPSPC easier to identify [4]. These criteria comprised:

- Normal-size or enlarged ovaries due to a benign process;
- Absent ovarian involvement or limited to the surface or superficial cortex or both, with no tumor nodule within the ovarian cortex > 5 × 5 mm;
- Serous histology;
- Extraovarian disease volume significantly exceeding that in ovarian disease.

The histogenetic hypotheses proposed in recent years for ovarian tumors [5–7] now raise doubts as to whether PPSPC exists as a separate clinical entity. Even though the single layer covering the ovarian surface, the ovarian surface epithelium (OSE), accounts for < 1 % of the total glandular mass, > 90 % of ovarian malignant tumors originate from the epithelium. The hypothesis that the OSE might give rise to OC emerged from the paper by Fathalla [8], who identified as the oncogenic stimulus unceasing ovulation, hence trauma and ovarian repair. Arguing against the hypothesis that OSE might act as a source for OC is the observation that these patients constantly lack a precancerous lesion on the ovarian surface. In addition, most OC (serous, mucinous, endometrioid) fit in poorly with the proposed cellular origin (OSE) given the histological features and some biomarkers (*HOXA, PAX8* genes) typically found in Müllerian epithelia but not expressed in the OSE [5, 9]. According to Kurman and Shih [6, 7], who first proposed these new histogenetic criteria, rather than constituting a single disease entity, OC arises through a dualistic ovarian carcinogenesis model comprising two broad categories designated as type I and type II tumors, exhibiting widely differing clinicopathologic features and behaviors, and both types, including PPSPC, originating from the tubal epithelium [10, 11] (Fig. 21.1).

Type I tumors comprise low-grade serous, low-grade endometrioid, mucinous, and clear-cell carcinomas. These tumors typically present as large cystic masses confined to one ovary, have a relatively indolent course, are genetically relatively stable, and typically display various specific mutations, including *KRAS*, *BRAF*, *PTEN*, *PIK3CA*, *CTNNB1*, *ARID1A*, and *PPP2R1A* genes. These molecular alterations result in morphologic changes that progress in a stepwise manner from benign through varying degrees of atypia (borderline tumor) to noninvasive and then invasive carcinoma. Traditional thinking maintains that these low-grade precursor lesions correlate with epithelial inclusion cysts and derive from ovarian surface epithelium invaginations that later, owing to estro-

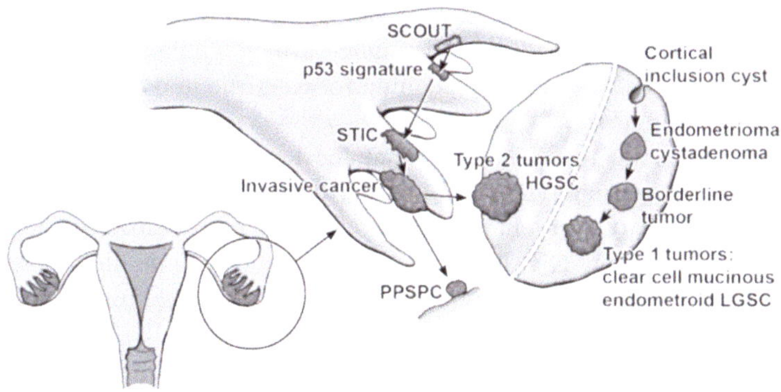

Fig. 21.1 Proposed models for the development of types 1 and 2 tumors of the ovary. *SCOUT*, secretory cell outgrowths; *P53*, tumor protein 53; *STIC*, serous tubal intraepithelial carcinoma; *PPSPC*, primary peritoneal serous papillary carcinoma; *HGSC*, high-grade serous cancer; *LGSC*, low-grade serous cancer. (Modified from [11])

gen hormone stimulation, progress to Müllerian type metaplasia [12]. Observations from a study conducted by Li et al. [13] show that most epithelium lining inclusion cysts are immunohistochemically and phenotypically *PAX8*(+), closely resembling tubal epithelium. Given the close anatomical relationship between the fimbriae and the ovarian surface, when ovulation disrupts the ovarian surface epithelium, tubal mucosa may implant on the ovary and become entrapped within the ovarian cortex [14]. Hence, according to a putative evolutionary model [10], papillary tubal hyperplasia (PTH) of the tubal mucosa through *KRAS*/*BRAF* mutations may be responsible for the development of atypical proliferative serous tumors (APST) and endosalpingiosis. As they progress further, APST subsequently develop into serous borderline tumor and invasive low-grade serous carcinoma.

Type II tumors comprise high-grade serous carcinoma (HGSC), high-grade endometrioid carcinoma, malignant mixed mesodermal tumors (carcinosarcomas), and undifferentiated carcinomas. These tumors are usually in an advanced stage at onset (> 75 %), grow rapidly, and are highly aggressive. Type II tumors are chromosomally highly unstable, in more than 95 % of cases harbor *TP53* mutations, and rarely display mutations found in the type I tumor. *BRCA* is inactivated in up to 40–50 % of HGSC [6]. During the past few years, abundant histological and molecular evidence has emerged that strongly suggests that most high-grade ovarian and peritoneal serous carcinoma originate in the fallopian tube, specifically from a serous tubal intraepithelial carcinoma (STIC), thus implying that ovarian and peritoneal spread is metastatic [15–17]. Despite possible exceptions, including a rare serous borderline tumor evolving into high-grade serous carcinoma [18], histological and molecular evidence shows that nearly all ovarian and peritoneal high-grade serous carcinomas derive from

STIC and arise in the fallopian tube. Tubal carcinogenesis manifests with increased positive immunohistochemical staining for nuclear p53 in the tubal secretory epithelium (so-called p53 signature), which would evolve into STIC characterized by increased positive staining for Ki-67 up to overt HGSC with a *TP53* gene mutation [5].

These histogenetic theories imply that the term pelvic serous carcinoma might be more appropriately applied to describe a single disease characterized by a high-grade serous carcinoma, an entity previously differentiated into PPSPC, tubal cancer, and OC. These findings notwithstanding, the literature on PPSPC in recent years contains numerous case reports, some referring to men [19, 20], and a few case series, most including no more than 10–20 patients [21, 23]. Apart from classification problems, the therapeutic principles overall resemble the treatment schemes applied for OC, the same staging procedures apply [International Federation of Gynecology and Obstetrics (FIGO)], and studies analyzing treatment results or data for follow-up procedures usually combine the two types [24–28]. Equally important, studies conducted in recent years and designed to compare PPSPC (identified according to the GOG criteria) and serous OC, have, as expected, failed to identify substantial differences [22, 29]. Outcome data for patients with PPSPC treated according to GOG criteria and provided by the major international studies [21–23, 29], including experience obtained in our own department (Table 21.1), dictate the following conclusions. First, the advanced intra-abdominal spread already present when PPSPC becomes clinically manifest makes published results extremely difficult to assess without quantifying the amount of disease present at the first therapeutic approach. As Table 21.1 shows, the only groups who assessed this variable with an adequate score [the Peritoneal Cancer Index (PCI)] are research centers used to treating peritoneal surface malignancies. Hence, only they can provide this descriptive variable, without which even the FIGO classification fails to provide all the necessary information. Another essential point to emphasize again, especially given the new histogenetic theories on OC, is that a disease resulting in severe peritoneal spread cannot be staged with the FIGO classification given that FIGO staging considers together in the subgroup IIIc patients with severe peritoneal spread along with those with minimal peritoneal spread and a single lymph-node metastasis [30, 31]. Any disease-staging system that omits the PCI risks losing much information. A second concern is that these patients often undergo preoperative neoadjuvant chemotherapy. Even though the precise role of neoadjuvant chemotherapy in these neoplasias and in the so-called OCs remains undefined [32], peritoneal spread can make complete cytoreduction hard to achieve, so that an optimal surgical outcome means recourse to downstaging chemotherapy. Earlier studies have already used this approach in patients with PPSPC [33]. A final possible concern regards the therapeutic procedures depending on the clinical characteristics of OC. Obviously in these cases, the definition used for surgical cytoreduction, albeit integrated with the adjective "optimal" (a term that apart from anything else

Table 21.1 Literature review

Study [Reference]	No. cases	Age (years)	Stage of disease	Surgical procedures	Cytoreduction obtained	Pre-operative chemo therapy	Survival
Liu et al. 2011 [21]	22	56.2	FIGO IIIC (54.5 %)	Pelvic peritonectomy + lymphadenectomy	-	22.7 %	21 months
Kawaguchi et al. 2012 [29]	22	67	-	Pelvic peritonectomy + lymphadenectomy	Optimal cytoreduction < 1 cm, 54.5 %	90.9 %	26.5 months
Chao et al. 2013 [22]	38	63	FIGO IIIC (81.6%)	Cytoreduction NOS	Optimal cytoreduction < 1 cm, 71.9 %	- -	62 months
Bakrin et al. 2013 [23]	36	60.5	Median PCI 10	PRT + HIPEC	Complete cytoreduction 75 %	97.2 %	5-year OS 57.4 %
Di Giorgio (unpublished data)	12	59.7	Median PCI 14.8	PRT + HIPEC	Complete cytoreduction 75 %	50 %	61 months

FIGO, International Federation of Gynecology and Obstetrics; *PCI*, Peritoneal Cancer Index, *PRT*, peritonectomy; *HIPEC*, hyperthermic intraperitoneal chemotherapy; *OS*, overall survival

foresees substantial residual disease), provides few elements for judgment. In a disease such as PPSPC, inherently involving extensive peritoneal involvement, the only approach that seems to answer the need for a rational therapeutic program is to use peritonectomy procedures, hence defining the extent of surgical cytoreduction obtained according to standardized criteria [Completeness of Cytoreduction (CC) score]. Among the studies we review in Table 21.1, the only series to report obtaining in most patients a percentage of complete cytoreduction without macroscopically evident residual disease, thus yielding an acceptable outcome, is the case series collected by Bakrin et al. [23] and data collected in our department. A final consideration merits integrating the peritonectomy procedure with hyperthermic intraperitoneal chemotherapy (HIPEC), as generally done when surgery ends in centers specialized in treating peritoneal surface malignancy [34]. Although this combined approach is now considered standard care for treating pseudomyxoma peritonei (PMP) [35], malignant peritoneal mesothelioma (MPM) [36], and selected patients with colorectal carcinomatosis [37], HIPEC combined with cytoreduction surgery (CRS) remains highly controversial in patients with peritoneal spread

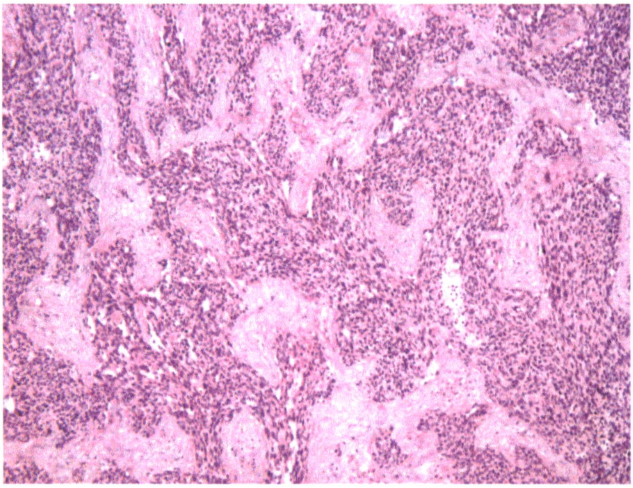

Fig. 21.2 Desmoplastic small round cell tumor (DSRCT)

from gynecological malignancies, and the controversy concerns HIPEC itself [38]. The chief objection regards a possible increase in morbidity and the lack of randomized controlled studies to assess the eventual benefits accruing from HIPEC plus CRS. While awaiting the results of numerous ongoing trials, to which this book devotes a specific chapter, the increasingly encouraging results obtained with normothermic adjuvant intraperitoneally applied chemotherapy (IP-CHT) seem to envisage an ever growing space for using HIPEC when surgical cytoreduction ends, especially insofar as the two techniques, rather than being alternatives, could be complementary [39, 40].

21.3 Desmoplastic Small Round Cell Tumor

Desmoplastic small round cell tumor (DSRCT) is a rare and highly aggressive neoplasm involving children, adolescents, and young adults that begins and spreads on the peritoneal surface. Approximately 300 DSRCT cases have been reported in the literature since the tumor was initially described by Gerald and Rosai in 1989 [41]. Histologically, DSRCT consists of desmoplastic stroma containing small round blue cells in nests (Fig. 21.2) and is associated with a characteristic chromosomal translocation, t(11;22)(p13;q12), which fuses the N-terminus of the Ewing sarcoma (*EWS*) gene to the C-terminus on the Wilms tumor (*WT-1*) gene [42, 43]. The reference standards for diagnosis include cytogenetic evaluation to confirm the characteristic translocation and *EWS–WT-1* fusion. DSRCT usually arises from abdominal or pelvic peritoneum as a diffuse multifocal disease similar to carcinomatosis, even though it sometimes arises also in solid organs, such as ovaries, liver, kidneys, pancreas, and brain [44]. Patients typically present in an advanced stage with multiple peritoneal-based lesions and, despite multiple strategies that include several chemotherapy regimens, aggressive debulking surgery, and whole abdominal radiation, durable remission remains rare, with a 15 % 5-year overall survival [45]. Current guidelines include neoadjuvant chemotherapy, debulking surgery, adjuvant chemotherapy, and radiation therapy. The MD Anderson Cancer Center group was the first to apply the HIPEC procedure when satisfactory (CC-0/1) cytoreduction ended [46]. The standard regimen is dose-intense neoadjuvant chemotherapy (recently combined with irinotecan and bevacizumab) with cyclophosphamide, doxorubicin, vincristine alternating with ifosfamide, and etoposide [47, 48]. According to the MD Anderson Cancer Center, case series patients were evaluated after receiving chemotherapy for 4–6 months; those having a partial response and found to be candidates for complete cytoreduction underwent surgery including HIPEC using cisplatin at 100 mg/m^2 with a maximum dose of 130 mg for 90 min [45]. One of the main prognostic factors is the completeness of surgical resection. In their Cox regression analysis, Zhang et al. identified this variable as the only independent outcome indicator (Table 21.2) [49]. After chemotherapy and maximal surgical debulking, multimodal protocols included whole-abdomino-

Table 21.2 Cox regression analysis for overall survival in desmoplastic small round cell tumor (DSRCT) patients. (Reproduced from [49], with permission)

Parameter	SE	OR	95 % CI	*P* value
Age	.442	.587	0.247—1.397	.228
Gender	.496	.986	0.373–2.606	.977
Site	.528	.769	0.273–2.163	.618
Size	.335	.698	0.348–1.401	.312
Complete surgery	.470	.266	0.106–0.670	.005
Chemotherapy	.380	.529	0.251–1.114	.094

SE, standard error; *OR*, odds ratio; *CI*, confidence interval

Table 21.3 Proposed desmoplastic small round cell tumor (DSRCT) staging criteria. (Reproduced from [51], with permission)

Stage	PCI	Liver metastasis	Extra-abdominal metastasis
I	< 12	No	No
II	> 12	No	No
III	Any PCI	Yes	No
IV	Any PCI	Yes or no	Yes

PCI, Peritoneal Cancer Index

pelvic radiation therapy (WAP-RT) (30 Gy) with or without focal boost according to the minimal residual disease eventually present [46]. A recent report from the Memorial Sloan-Kettering Cancer Center shows that intensity-modulated radiation therapy (IMRT) for consolidative WAP-RT after surgical debulking reduces toxicity and improves the therapeutic index [50].

Despite several efforts, therapy for DSRCT achieves disappointing results, and new approaches are therefore urgently needed to treat this devastating and refractory disease. An appropriate strategy for managing DSRCT might be one that includes HIPEC in the therapeutic schedule and applies the treatment criteria generally used in peritoneal surface malignancy. Seeking a new staging system for patients with DSRCT, Hayes-Jordan et al. used the PCI, even though it does not in itself predict outcome, together with the extent of liver and extra-abdominal disease (Table 21.3) [51]. They showed, despite a small study sample, that this new classification stratified recurrence-free survival and identified a trend toward stage-specific survival. According to this staging system, a patient with a large tumor burden but no liver metastases or extra-abdominal disease when neoadjuvant chemotherapy ends can still have a prolonged disease-free interval after CRS plus HIPEC. Investigating HIPEC in a small cohort of patients, Hayes-Jordan et al. showed an increased 3-year survival in patients in whom they combined this procedure with cytoreduction than in those who underwent debulking surgery alone [46, 51].

References

1. Swerdlow M (1959) Mesothelioma of the pelvic peritoneum resembling papillary cystadenocarcinoma of the ovary; case report. Am J Obstet Gynecol 77:197-200
2. Tobacman JK, Greene MH, Tucker MA et al (1982) Intra-abdominal carcinomatosis after prophylactic oophorectomy in ovarian-cancer-prone families. Lancet 2:795-797
3. Fromm GL, Gershenson DM, Silva EG (1990) Papillary serous carcinoma of the peritoneum. Obstet Gynecol 75:89-95
4. Bloss JD, Liao SY, Buller RE et al (1993) Extraovarian Peritoneal Serous Papillary Carcinoma: A Case-Control Retrospective Comparison To Papillary Adenocarcinoma Of The Ovary. Gynecol Oncol 50:347-351
5. Levanon K, Crum C, Drapkin R (2008) New insights into the pathogenesis of serous ovarian cancer and its clinical impact. J Clin Oncol 26:5284-5293
6. Kurman RJ, Shih IeM (2011) Molecular pathogenesis and extraovarian origin of epithelial ovarian cancer—shifting the paradigm. Hum Pathol 42:918-931
7. Nik NN, Vang R, Shih IeM et al (2014) Origin and pathogenesis of pelvic (ovarian, tubal, and primary peritoneal) serous carcinoma. Annu Rev Pathol 9:27-45
8. Fathalla MF (1971) Incessant ovulation—a factor in ovarian neoplasia? Lancet 2:163
9. Li J, Fadare O, Xiang L, Kong B, Zheng W (2012) Ovarian serous carcinoma: recent concepts on its origin and carcinogenesis. J Hematol Oncol 5:8
10. Vang R, Shih IeM, Kurman RJ (2013) Fallopian tube precursors of ovarian low- and high-grade serous neoplasms. Histopathology 62:44-58
11. Sama AR, Schilder RJ (2014) Refractory fallopian tube carcinoma – current perspectives in pathogenesis and management. Int J Women Health 6:149-157
12. Hennessy BT, Coleman RL, Markman M (2009) Ovarian cancer. Lancet 374:1371-1382

13. Li J, Abushahin N, Pang S et al (2011) Tubal origin of 'ovarian' low-grade serous carcinoma. Mod Pathol 24:1488-1499
14. Kurman RJ, Shih IeM (2010)The origin and pathogenesis of epithelial ovarian cancer: a proposed unifying theory. Am J Surg Pathol 34:433-443
15. Carlson JW, Miron A, Jarboe EA et al (2008) Serous tubal intraepithelial carcinoma: its potential role in primary peritoneal serous carcinoma and serous cancer prevention. J Clin Oncol 26:4160-4165
16. Kindelberger DW1, Lee Y, Miron A, et al (2007) Intraepithelial carcinoma of the fimbria and pelvic serous carcinoma: Evidence for a causal relationship. Am J Surg Pathol 31:161-169
17. Przybycin CG, Kurman RJ, Ronnett BM et al (2010) Are all pelvic (nonuterine) serous carcinomas of tubal origin? Am J Surg Pathol 34:1407-1416
18. Garg K, Park KJ, Soslow RA (2012) Low-grade serous neoplasms of the ovary with transformation to high-grade carcinomas: a report of 3 cases. Int J Gynecol Pathol 31:423-428
19. Shmueli E, Leider-Trejo L, Schwartz I et al (2001)Primary papillary serous carcinoma of the peritoneum in a man. Ann Oncol 12:563-567
20. Canbay E, Ishibashi H, Sako S et al (2014) Photodynamic detection and management of intraperitoneal spreading of primary peritoneal papillary serous carcinoma in a man: report of a case. Surg Today 44:373-377
21. Liu Q, Lin JX, Shi QL et al (2011) Primary peritoneal serous papillary carcinoma: a clinical and pathological study. Pathol Oncol Res 17:713-719
22. Chao KC, Chen YJ, Juang CM et al (2013) Prognosis for advanced-stage primary peritoneal serous papillary carcinoma and serous ovarian cancer in Taiwan. Taiwan J Obstet Gynecol 52:81-84
23. Bakrin N, Gilly FN, Baratti D et al (2013) Primary peritoneal serous carcinoma treated by cytoreductive surgery combined with hyperthermic intraperitoneal chemotherapy. A multi-institutional study of 36 patients. Eur J Surg Oncol 39:742-747
24. Look M, Chang D, Sugarbaker PH (2004) Long-term results of cytoreductive surgery for advanced and recurrent epithelial ovarian cancers and papillary serous carcinoma of the peritoneum. Int J Gynecol Cancer 14:35-41
25. Ramirez PT, Schmeler KM, Milam MR et al (2008) Efficacy of letrozole in the treatment of recurrent platinum- and taxane-resistant high-grade cancer of the ovary or peritoneum. Gynecol Oncol 110:56-59
26. Levy T, Weiser R, Boaz M et al (2012) Prognostic significance of rising serum CA-125 levels within the normal range in patients with epithelial ovarian, primary peritoneal, and tubal cancers, who, after initial treatment, had a complete clinical response. Int J Gynecol Cancer 22:1344-1348
27. Luyckx M, Leblanc E, Filleron T et al Maximal cytoreduction in patients with FIGO stage IIIC to stage IV ovarian, fallopian, and peritoneal cancer in day-to-day practice: a Retrospective French Multicentric Study. Int J Gynecol Cancer 22:1337-1343
28. Rettenmaier NB, Rettenmaier CR, Wojciechowski T et al (2010) The utility and cost of routine follow-up procedures in the surveillance of ovarian and primary peritoneal carcinoma: a 16-year institutional review. Br J Cancer 103:1657-1662
29. Kawaguchi R, Tanase Y, Haruta S et al (2012) Paclitaxel plus Carboplatin Chemotherapy for Primary Peritoneal Carcinoma: A Study of 22 Cases and Comparison with Stage III-IV Ovarian Serous Carcinoma. Case Rep Oncol 5:173-180
30. Cliby WA, Aletti GD, Wilson TO et al (2006) Is it justified to classify patients to Stage IIIC epithelial ovarian cancer based on nodal involvement only? Gynecol Oncol 103:797-801
31. Berek JS (2009) Lymph node-positive stage IIIC ovarian cancer: a separate entity? Int J Gynecol Cancer 19:S18-20
32. da Costa Miranda V, de Souza Fêde ÂB, Dos Anjos CH et al (2014) Neoadjuvant chemotherapy with six cycles of carboplatin and paclitaxel in advanced ovarian cancer patients unsuitable for primary surgery: Safety and effectiveness. Gynecol Oncol 132:287-291
33. Dubernard G, Morice P, Rey A et al (2004) Prognosis of stage III or IV primary peritoneal serous papillary carcinoma. Eur J Surg Oncol 30:976-981

34. Glehen O, Gilly FN, Boutitie F et al (2010) Toward curative treatment of peritoneal carcinomatosis from nonovarian origin by cytoreductive surgery combined with perioperative intraperitoneal chemotherapy: a multi-institutional study of 1,290 patients. Cancer 116:5608-5618
35. Chua TC, Moran BJ, Sugarbaker PH et al (2012) Early- and long-term outcome data of patients with pseudomyxoma peritonei from appendiceal origin treated by a strategy of cytoreductive surgery and hyperthermic intraperitoneal chemotherapy. J Clin Oncol 30:2449-2456
36. Yan TD, Deraco M, Baratti D et al (2009) Cytoreductive surgery and hyperthermic intraperitoneal chemotherapy for malignant peritoneal mesothelioma: multi-institutional experience. J Clin Oncol 27:6237-6242
37. Elias D, Gilly F, Boutitie F et al (2010) Peritoneal colorectal carcinomatosis treated with surgery and perioperative intraperitoneal chemotherapy: retrospective analysis of 523 patients from a multicentric French study. J Clin Oncol 28:63-68
38. Herzog TJ (2012) The role of heated intraperitoneal chemotherapy (HIPEC) in ovarian cancer: hope or hoax? Ann Surg Oncol 19:3998-4000
39. Landrum LM, Java J, Mathews CA et al (2013) Prognostic factors for stage III epithelial ovarian cancer treated with intraperitoneal chemotherapy: a Gynecologic Oncology Group study. Gynecol Oncol 130:12-18
40. Eskander RN, Cripe J, Bristow RE (2014) Intraperitoneal chemotherapy from Armstrong to HIPEC: challenges and promise. Curr Treat Options Oncol 15:27-40
41. Gerald WL1, Rosai J (1989) Case 2. Desmoplastic small cell tumor with divergent differentiation. Pediatr Pathol 9:177-1783
42. Gerald WL, Ladanyi M, de Alava E et al (1998) Clinical, pathologic, and molecular spectrum of tumors associated with t(11;22)(p13;q12): desmoplastic small round-cell tumor and its variants. J Clin Oncol 16:3028-3036
43. Ladanyi M, Gerald W (1994) Fusion of the EWS and WT1 genes in the desmoplastic small round cell tumor. Cancer Res 54:2837-2840
44. Rekhi B, Ahmed S, Basak R et al (2012) Desmoplastic small round cell tumor-clinicopathological spectrum, including unusual features and immunohistochemical analysis of 45 tumors diagnosed at a tertiary cancer referral centre, with molecular results t(11; 22) (p13; q12) (EWS-WT1) in select cases. Pathol Oncol Res 18:917-927
45. Lal DR, Su WT, Wolden SL et al (2005) Results of multimodal treatment for desmoplastic small round cell tumors. J Pediatr Surg 40:251-255
46. Hayes-Jordan A, Green HL, Lin H et al (2014) Complete cytoreduction and HIPEC improves survival in desmoplastic small round cell tumor. Ann Surg Oncol 21:220-224
47. Kushner BH, LaQuaglia MP, Wollner N et al (1996) Desmoplastic small round-cell tumor: prolonged progression-free survival with aggressive multimodality therapy. J Clin Oncol 14:1526-1531
48. La Quaglia MP (2014) State of the art in oncology: high risk neuroblastoma, alveolar rhabdomyosarcoma, desmoplastic small round cell tumor, and POST-TEXT 3 and 4 hepatoblastoma. J Pediatr Surg 49:233-240
49. Zhang J, Xu H, Ren F et al (2014) Analysis of clinicopathological features and prognostic factors of desmoplastic small round cell tumor. Pathol Oncol Res 20:161-168
50. Desai NB, Stein NF, LaQuaglia MP et al (2013) Reduced toxicity with intensity modulated radiation therapy (IMRT) for desmoplastic small round cell tumor (DSRCT): an update on the whole abdominopelvic radiation therapy (WAP-RT) experience. Int J Radiat Oncol Biol Phys 85:e67-72
51. Hayes-Jordan A, Green H, Fitzgerald N et al (2010) Novel treatment for desmoplastic small round cell tumor: hyperthermic intraperitoneal perfusion. J Pediatr Surg 45:1000-1006

Other Secondary Peritoneal Surface Malignancies

22

Maurizio Cardi, Joseph Maher Fouad Atta, Valentina Mingarelli, Enzo Naticchioni, Daniele Biacchi, and Angelo Di Giorgio

22.1 Introduction

Patients with peritoneal metastasis (PM) are typically considered as having a terminal and incurable disease [1–3]. Since the late 1990s, a novel therapeutic approach, has emerged combining cytoreductive surgery (CRS) performed to treat all visible disease, plus hyperthermic intraperitoneal chemotherapy (HIPEC) used to treat microscopic residual disease [4, 5]. This treatment radically changed the therapeutic approach to patients with peritoneal surface malignancies and is regarded as the standard of care for pseudomyxoma peritonei from appendiceal cancer and peritoneal mesotheliomas [6, 7]. It also provides improved survival rates for treating PM from ovarian [8–10], gastric [11, 12], and colorectal cancers [13–15].

PM often complicates the clinical course of many patients with other primary digestive and non-digestive-system cancers [16, 17], for which CRS plus HIPEC has not yet shown a survival advantage over standard treatments [18–21]. The main reasons may be that CRS plus HIPEC is still regarded by many oncologists with scepticism, mostly due to treatment complexity, the reported high complication rate, and because reports of CRS plus HIPEC for PM from unusual primary tumors is sporadic and the numbers are too small to draw conclusions on survival benefit.

This chapter reports our single-institution experience with CRS plus HIPEC for patients with PM from rare or unusual primary tumors and discusses possible indications, results, and peculiar issues related to each tumor type, with the

M. Cardi (✉)
Department of Surgery "Pietro Valdoni", Sapienza University of Rome, Rome, Italy
e-mail: maurizio.cardi@uniroma1.it

A. Di Giorgio, E. Pinto (Eds), *Treatment of Peritoneal Surface Malignancies*, Updates in Surgery
DOI: 10.1007/978-88-470-5711-1_22, © Springer-Verlag Italia 2015

aim of contributing to the body of knowledge about treating PM using this combined approach.

22.2 Managing Peritoneal Metastases from Breast Cancer

Breast cancer (BC) is among the most frequent malignancies in Western countries [22, 23]. As local and systemic treatments improve, BC metastasis patterns change so that metastatic disease now manifests in unusual ways. Among them, peritoneal carcinomatosis (PC) is a rare event but one that carries high morbidity and mortality rates [24–26]. No clear guidelines are available regarding the role of CRS with or without HIPEC in PC from BC [22, 27]. Literature reports are sporadic, and only Gusani et al. (one patient in 2008) and Glehen et al. (two patients in 2010) [1, 12] report PM from BC treated by CRS plus HIPEC. In our institution, we treated five patients with PM from BC with CRS plus HIPEC [28]; no patient carried the *BRCA*. The Peritoneal Cancer Index (PCI) score ranged from 15 to 24. Optimal cytoreduction [Completeness of Cytoreduction score (CC0, CC1)] was achieved in fur patients. Patients with residual disease (two with CC1 and one with CC2) were advised to undergo adjuvant systemic treatment according to tumor biological features [estrogen receptor (ER), progesterone receptor (PR), human epidermal growth factor receptor (HER)-2 expression] and patients' overall clinical condition. Aromatase inhibitors were used for postmenopausal ER- or PR-positive peritoneal disease or both, and patients with HER-2-positive tumor expression at histology underwent combination therapy with trastuzumab. Patients with no residual disease (CC0) were advised to undergo adjuvant systemic treatment as a precautional option. The clinical characteristics and related treatments are reported in Table 22.1. Of the five patients, four were alive and disease free at 13, 45, 74, and 128 months, respectively.

Our study provides previously unavailable information on treating women with PM from BC. In our patients, a median of 18 years (range 10–30) elapsed after BC was diagnosed and PC developed, which accords with previous reports describing breast carcinoma as one of the most slowly growing solid tumors given that metastases may appear many years, even decades, after the initial diagnosis [22, 29]. Of the five patients treated, four achieved long-term survival, with one of them surviving for 10 years.

In patients with PC and an ovarian mass and history reporting previous BC, reaching a correct diagnosis can be difficult but is essential. As reported by other authors [30], immunohistochemical staining showing combined negative wild-type 1 (WT1) and cancer antigen (CA-125) tumor expression associated with positive GCDFP-15 expression in peritoneal disease invariably strengthened the diagnosis.

Our study extends current knowledge, showing that once the correct diagnosis is established, these patients can benefit from treatment. The study also possibly argues against previous reports describing poor prognosis. After max-

Table 22.1 Peritonectomy plus HIPEC for PC from various primary tumors (Di Giorgio, unpublished)

Patient	Age	Sex	Primary	HIPEC	PCI	CC	FU	Surv
1	72	M	Sarcoma	Oxal	20	1	DOD	12
2	77	F	Sarcoma	Oxal	16	0	AWD	11
3	61	M	Sarcoma	Oxal	14	1	AWD	9
4	68	F	Small bowel	CDDP	26	0	QDF	23
5	51	M	Small bowel	CDDP	15	0	AWD	23
6	59	M	Small bowel	Oxal	20	1	AWD	8
7	46	F	Small bowel	Oxal	7	0	AWD	3
8	67	M	Pancreas	Oxal	23	1	ADF	5
9	67	M	Pancreas	Oxal	22	2	AWD	4
10	74	F	Pancreas	Oxal	3	0	ADF	8
11	70	F	GIST	CDDP	6	0	ADF	34
12	53	F	GIST	CDDP	12	0	ADF	108
13	73	M	GIST	CDDP	20	0	DOD	38
14	58	F	Breast IDC	CDDP 75 m	15	0	ADF	128
15	54	F	Breast ILC	CDDP	22	1	ADF	74
16	55	F	Breast ILC	CDDP	22	2	DOD	56
17	77	F	Breast IDC	CDDP	24	1	ADF	45
18	53	F	Breast IDC	CDDP	18	0	ADF	13
19	6	M	Bladder	CDDP	19	2	DOD	9
20	68	F	Uterus ADC	CDDP	5	0	DOD	46
21	56	F	Uterus ADC	CDDP	6	0	DOD	24
22	64	F	Uterus ADC	CDDP	23	0	AWD	12
23	58	F	Uterus ADC	CDDP	17	0	AWD	52
24	61	F	Uterus ADC	CDDP	9	0	ADF	95
25	67	F	Uterus ADC	CDDP	30	1	DOD	15
26	59	F	Uterus ADC	CDDP	29	1	DOD	15
27	65	F	Uterus ADC	CDDP	19	0	DOD	12
28	51	M	Lung	CDDP	19	0	DOD	7

GIST, gastrointestinal stromal tumor; *IDC*, invasive ductal carcinoma; *ILC*, invasive lobular carcinoma; *ADC*, adenocarcinoma; *HIPEC*, hyperthermic peritoneal cytoreduction; *Oxal*, oxaliplatin; *CDDP*, cisplatin; *PCI*, Peritoneal Cancer Index; *CC*, Completeness of Cytoreduction score; *Surv* survival; *DOD*, dead of disease; *AWD*, alive with disease; *ADF*, Alive Disease Free; *FU*, follow-up

imal cytoreduction plus HIPEC, morbidity and mortality rates in our patients were in line with those reported for similar procedures. This combined treatment allowed good survival and quality of life (QOL). Although maximal cytoreduction plus HIPEC cannot be proposed as standard care for patients with PM from primary BC, survival rates observed in our small series suggest that in highly selected patients with no extraperitoneal disease and in whom surgery can achieve adequate cytoreduction, this combined procedure can offer patients with PC from BC a promising approach for long-term survival. This finding merits further investigation in larger studies.

22.3 Managing Peritoneal Carcinomatosis from Small-bowel Adenocarcinoma

Management strategy for patients with PM from small-bowel adenocarcinoma is unclear, and literature reports are episodic, even though PM is a frequent manifestation of small-bowel carcinoma [31]. Typically, these tumors present after a significant delay in diagnosis due to symptom vagueness and imaging difficulty, leading to poor prognosis and survival rates varying from 10 to 40 months. Marchettini and Sugarbaker [32] reported a median survival of 12 months in two of their patients treated with CRS plus HIPEC, with prolonged survival of 57 and 59 months, respectively. Chua et al. [33] published a review of seven patients treated with CRS plus HIPEC [mitomycin C and early postoperative intraperitoneal chemotherapy (EPIC) with 5-fluorouracil (FU)], reporting a median disease-free survival (DFS) of 12 months. They also reported a Kaplan–Meier analysis for a combined group of 19 patients treated with CRS plus HIPEC with a median overall survival (OS) of 29 months. Shen et al. [34] reported a median OS of 45 months after treatment with CRS plus HIPEC. A large, multi-institutional experience is reported by the French Association of Surgery [35], with a median OS for patients treated by CRS plus HIPEC of 32 months. In the four patients treated in our institution, one, who presented with intestinal obstruction, had a mean PCI of 17 (range 7–26). Mean OS was 31.2 months, with two patients alive and disease free at 43 and 22 months, respectively, and two alive with disease at 33 (pulmonary metastases) and at 27 (abdominal recurrence) months, respectively. The rarity of small-bowel carcinoma makes impossible the design of prospective trials. However, all series reported show better results compared with conventional treatments. Moreover, it must be considered that CRS plus HIPEC could represent the only valid surgical option for palliation in obstructed patients in whom a simple surgical procedure aimed at bowel decompression is often impossible due to small-bowel mesentery retraction or in those with associated ascites. Although it is impossible to conclude that CRS plus HIPEC is a treatment option for patients with PM from small-bowel adenocarcinoma, this combined treatment modality should be considered as a valid alternative in selected patients.

22.4 Managing Peritoneal Carcinomatosis from Endometrial Cancer

Endometrial cancer remains the most common cancer of the female reproductive tract. Treatment is surgery alone or in combination with brachytherapy and/or radiotherapy. Survival rates are approximately 90% at 5 years [36]. However, in cases of PM, patient management becomes more complex and prognosis is poor, with a median survival < 1 year. Bakrin et al. [37] reported on five patients with endometrial cancer treated by this combined modality, with a median survival of 19.4 months. Two patients experienced recurrent disease and died; three patients were alive and disease free at 7, 23, and 39 months, respectively after treatment. Glehen et al. [38], in a multi-institutional review of the French Surgical Association of 1,290 patients with PM from various primary tumors, reported in 2010 the treatment of 17 patients with uterine adenocarcinoma (13) and epidermoid carcinoma (four); however, their report did not provide specific survival data for this specific group of patients. Delotte et al. [36], in 2014, reported CRS plus HIPEC treatment in 13 patients with endometrial cancer. Five patients died of disease, three were alive with disease at 14, 26, and 28 months, and four were alive and disease free at 1, 60, 60, and 124 months, respectively. In our institution, from 2002, we treated eight patients with a diagnosis of uterine adenocarcinoma using CRS plus HIPEC. Mean PCI was 16, and complete cytoreduction was achieved in five patients; three patients had residual CC1 disease. In four patients, we observed recurrent disease: two died of disease at 9 and 13 months; two were alive with disease at 19 and 26 months; four were alive and disease free at 9, 14, 26, and 33 months. Treatment strategies for stage IV endometrial cancer remain controversial. Some reports highlight the histologic characteristics and extent of the disease as the main prognostic determinants; others favor the effects of a more aggressive surgical cytoreduction. Long-term survival reported in these observational studies were higher compared with those reported in the literature using conventional treatments, which seems to justify a more aggressive surgical approach with the aim of leaving patients without residual visible disease. CRS plus HIPEC could therefore represent a valid alternative to more conservative treatments, and survival results seem to justify future randomized trials.

22.5 Managing Peritoneal Carcinomatosis from other Unconventional Miscellaneous Tumors

The increased interest in and reports of increased survival in treating PM with CRS plus HIPEC led many specialized centers to treat rarer and unusual primary tumors metastatic to the abdominal cavity and for which there no clear and accepted indications. The optimal management of these patients is a matter of intense debate. Systemic chemotherapy for PM has improved but remains

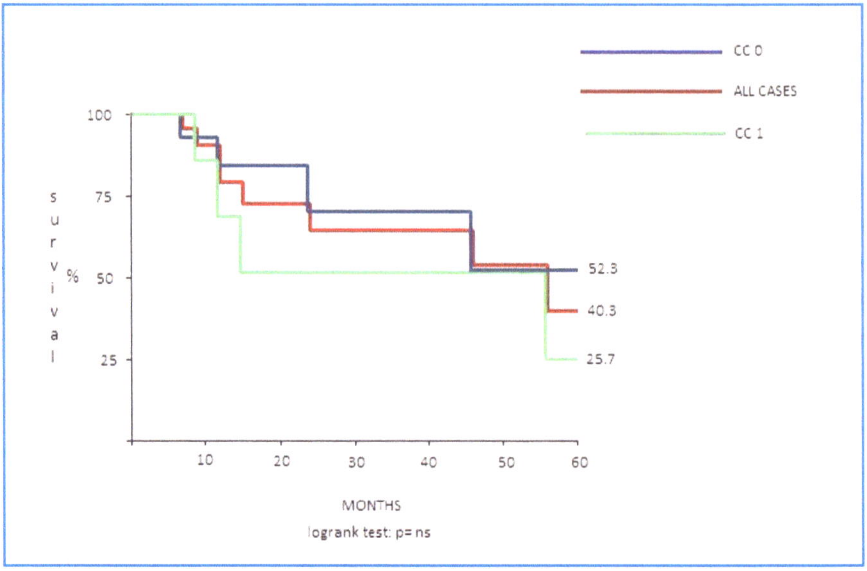

Fig. 22.1 Peritonectomy plus hyperthermic intraperitoneal chemotherapy (HIPEC) for various primary tumors: 5-year survival (Di Giorgio, unpublished). *CC*, Completeness of Cytoreduction score

limited because of poor drug diffusion into the peritoneum; however, the frequent tumor localization within the peritoneal cavity makes an appealing therapeutic option for selected cases. This is why many authors [1, 28, 34, 39–46] report small observational series of patients with PM from various unconventional tumors treated by CRS plus HIPEC (Table 22.1). This combined treatment modality has been used in PM from pancreatic, gastrointestinal stromal tumor (GIST), abdominal sarcomas, and gallbladder, liver, cholangiocarcinoma, adrenal, urachal, esophageal, and kidney tumors. In a multi-institutional review of the French Surgical Association on 1,290 cases of PM from various primary tumors treated with CRS plus HIPEC [38], there were 29 unconventional indications. Mortality was 4.1%, with a rate of major (grades 3 and 4) complications of 33%, similar to those reported after other major surgical procedures. Obviously, the numbers are too small to draw conclusion on survival figures for each specific primary tumor, but an overall median survival of 34 months, with a 5-year DFS of 22% compares favorably with survival figures reported in the literature regarding palliative treatment for the same tumor types.

Results of peritonectomy plus HIPEC at our institution for treating PC from various primary tumors are summarized in Fig. 22.1 and Table 22.2. Differently from other authors, we treated a significant number of PC from BC (five patients) and uterus cancer (eight patients). Median survival was 56 months, and 5-year OS rates were 40.3 %. Ten patients were alive and disease-free at the time of this writing, and eight were alive with disease.

Table 22.2 Peritonectomy plus HIPEC for PC from various primary tumors (literature review)

Study [Reference]	Primary	No.	Survival			
			Median (months)	1 year (%)	3 years (%)	5 years (%)
Jacks et al. 2005 [45]	Small bowel	6	30	-	-	-
Gusani 2008 [1]	Unknown	2				-
	Breast	1				
	GIST	6				
	Gallbladder	1	26.2	-	49	-
	Liver	1				
	Adrenal	1				
	Esophagus	1				
Shen et al. 2009 [34]	Unknown	2				
	Pancreas	5				
	GIST	11				
	Sarcoma	10				
	Gallbladder	3	22.2	66	40	27
	Adrenal	1				
	Small bowel	6				
	Urachus	5				
Chua et al. 2009 [33]	Small bowel	7	25	57	20	-
Kerscher et al. 2010 [39]	Small bowel	3	-	-	-	-
Glehen et al. 2010 [38]	Unknown	8				
	Breast	2				
	GIST	3				
	Sarcoma	28				
	Liver	2				
	Adrenal	3	34	77	49	37
	Urachus	4				
	Small bowel	45				
	Esophagus	1				
	Kidney	2				
Randle et al. 2010 [46]	Sarcoma	10	21	-	-	43
Turrini et al. 2012 [41]	Pancreas	1	-	-	-	-

HIPEC, hyperthermic intraperitoneal chemotherapy

22.6 Conclusions

Disseminated malignant PM has traditionally been considered a terminal disease and justifiably approached only with palliative therapeutic options. An increasing interest since the late 1990s led many centers to develop a combined treatment modality in which CRS is used to remove all visible abdominal disease, followed by HIPEC to treat microscopic residual disease. This treatment option shows promising results in treating PM from many primary tumors and is regarded as the standard attempt to cure PM from pseudomyxoma peritonei, malignant peritoneal mesothelioma, and–for some authors–from colorectal cancer. It is also under evaluation for treating PM from ovarian, gastric, and neuroendocrine cancers. A number of studies suggest a survival benefit, but oncologists remains sceptical mostly because of treatment complexity, the perceived high complication rate, and the need to treat patients in highly specialized centers only.

Despite such scepticism, as described in this chapter, there are many reports of using CRS plus HIPEC in treating PM from unconventional primary tumors for which no clinical controlled study showed a survival benefit. Fist, the small number of these observational series makes it unlikely that prospective trials will be designed. Second, diagnosis of the primary tumor is often very difficult, becoming clear only after CRS. Third, death in these patients typically occurs after intractable bowel obstruction, as the disease is frequently confined to the peritoneal cavity. A regional approach therefore appears reasonable. Moreover, the presence of intractable malignant ascites and bowel involvement with mesentery retraction make it impossible to perform even limited palliative surgery, such as a simple ostomy. Fourth, most observational studies report a clear survival benefit over patients treated by conventional palliative treatments.

We conclude that CRS plus HIPEC should not be excluded a priori for treating PM from unconventional primary tumors. This combined multimodal therapeutic approach, when performed in a highly experienced peritoneal surface malignancy center, is safe, and it provides survival benefit over conventional palliative treatments.

References

1. Gusani NG, Sung WC, Colovos C et al (2008) Aggressive surgical management of peritoneal carcinomatosis with low mortality in a high volume tertiary center. Ann surg oncol 15:654-663
2. Chu DZ , Lang NP, Thomson C et al (1989) Peritoneal carcinomatosis in non gynecologic malignancies. A prospective study of prognostic factors. Cancer 63:364-367
3. Jayne DG, Fook S, Loi C et al (2002) Peritoneal carcinomatosis from colorectal cancer. Br J Surg 89:1545-1550
4. Sugarbaker PH, Cunliffe WJ, Beliveau JF et al (1988) Rationale for perioperative intraperitoneal chemotherapy as a surgical adjuvant for gastro-intestinal malignancies. Reg Cancer Treat 1:66-79
5. Sugarbaker PH (1988) Intraperitoneal chemotherapy and cytoreductive surgery for the prevention and treatment of peritoneal carcinomatosis and sarcomatosis. Semin Surg Oncol 14:254-261
6. Chua T, Moran B, Sugarbaker PH (2012) Early and long-term outcome on 2298 patients with psudomyxoma peritonei of appendiceal origin treated by a strategy of cytoreductive surgery and hyperthermic intraperitoneal chemotherapy. J Clin Oncol 30:2449-2456
7. Yan TD, Deraco M, Baratti D (2009) Cytoreductive surgery and hyperthermic intraperitoneal chemotherapy for malignant peritoneal mesothelioma: multi institutional experience. J Clin Oncol 27:6237-6242
8. Di Giorgio A, Naticchioni E, Biacchi D et al (2008) Cytoreductive surgery (peritonectomy procedures) combined with hyperthermic intraperitoneal chemotherapy (HIPEC) in the treat-

ment of diffuse peritoneal carcinomatosis from ovarian cancer. Cancer 113:315-325
9. Chang SJ, Bristow R, Tyu HS (2012) Impact of complete cytoreduction leaving no gross residual disease associated with radical cytoreductive surgical procedures on survival in advanced ovarian cancer. Ann Surg Oncol 19:4059-4067
10. Helm WC (2012) Current status and future directions of cytoreductive surgery and HIPEC in the treatment of ovarian cancer. Surg Oncol Clin N Am 21:645-663
11. Yonemura Y, Kawamura T, Bardon E et al (2005) Treatment of peritoneal dissemination from gastric cancer by peritonectomy and chemo-hyperthermic peritoneal perfusion. Br J Surg 92:370-375
12. Glehen O, Gilly F, Arvieux C (2010) Peritoneal carcinomatosis from gastric cancer: a multi institutional study of 159 patients treated by cytoreductive surgery combined with perioperative intraperitoneal chemotherapy. Ann Surg Oncol 17:2370-2377
13. Verwaal VJ, Van Ruth S, de Bree E et al (2003) Randomized trial of cytoreduction and hyperthermic intraperitoneal chemotherapy versus systemic chemotherapy and palliative surgery in patients with peritoneal carcinomatosis of colorectal cancer. J Clin Oncol 21:3737-3743
14. Sammartino P, Sibio S, Biacchi D et al (2012) Prevention of peritoneal metastases from colon cancer in high risk patients: Preliminary results of surgery plus prophylactic HIPEC. Gastroenterol Res Pract 2012:141585
15. Elias D, Lefevre JH, Chevalier J et al (2009) Complete cytoreductive surgery plus intraperitoneal chemo-hyperthermia with oxaliplatin for peritoneal carcinomatosis of colorectal origin. J Clin Oncol 27:681-685
16. Glehen O, Osinski D, Baujard AL et al (2003) Natural history of peritoneal carcinomatosis from non gynecological malignancies. Surg Oncol Clin N Am 12:729-739
17. Carmignani CP, Sugarbaker TH, Bromley CN (2003) Intraperitoneal cancer dissemination: mechanism of patterns of spread. Cancer Metastasis Rev 22:4105-4172
18. Elias D, David A, Sourrouille I et al (2013) Neuroendocrine carcinomas: optimal surgery of peritoneal metastasis (and associated intra-abdominal metastasis). Surgery (in press) http://dx.doi.org/10.106/jsurg 2013.05.030
19. Munene G, Lloyd A, Temple WJ (2011) Systematic review of the efficacy of multimodal treatment of sarcomatosis with cytoreduction and intraperitoneal chemotherapy. Ann Surg Oncol 18:207-213
20. Baratti D, Pennacchioli E, Kusamura S et al (2012) Peritoneal sarcomatosis: is there subset of patients who may benefit from cytoreductive surgery and hyperthermic intraperitoneal chemotherapy Ann Surg Oncol 17:3220-3228
21. Kalliampust AA, Shukla NK, Deo SV et al (2012) Updates on the multimodality management of desmoplastic small round cell tumors. J Surg Oncol 105:617-621
22. Abu-Rustum NR, Aghajanian CA, Venkatraman ES et al (1997) Metastatic breast carcinoma to the abdomen and pelvis. Gynecol Oncol 66:41-44
23. Parker SL, Tong T, Bolden S et al (1996) Cancer statistics 1996, CA. Cancer J Clin 46:5-27
24. Tuthill M, Pell R, Giuliani R et al (2009) Peritoneal disease in breast cancer: A specific entity with an extremely poor prognosis. Eur J Cancer 45:2146-2149
25. Saunders Y, Stebbing J, Broadley K et al (2001) Recurrent locally advanced breast cancer. The treatment of chest wall disease with further chemotherapy. Clin Oncol (R Coll Radiol) 13:195-199
26. Stebbing J, Crane J, Gaya A (2006) Breast cancer (metastatic). Clin Evid 15:2331-2359
27. Eitan R, Gemignani ML, Verkatraman ES et al (2003) Breast cancer metastatic to abdomen and pelvis. Role of surgical resection. Gynecol Oncol 90:397-401
28. Cardi M, Sammartino P, Framarino ML et al (2013) Treatment of peritoneal carcinomatosis from breast cancer by maximal cytoreduction and HIPEC : a preliminary report on 5 cases. Breast 22:845-849
29. Sheen-Chen SM, Liu YW, Sun CK et al (2008) Abdominal carcinomatosis attributed to metastatic breast carcinoma. Dig Dis Sci 53:3043-3045
30. Tornos C, Soslow R, Chen S et al (2005) Expression of WT1, Ca125 and GCDFP-15 as useful markers in the differential diagnosis of primary ovarian carcinomatosis versus metastat-

ic breast cancer to the ovary. Am J Surg Pathol 20:1482-1489

31. Disario JA, Burt BW, Vargas H et al (1994) Small bowel cancer: epidemiological and clinical characteristics from population-based registry. Am J Gastroenterol 89:699-701
32. Marchettini P, Sugarbaker PH (2002) Mucinous adenocarcinoma of the small bowel with peritoneal seeding. Case report and review of the literature. Eur J Surg Oncol 28:19-23
33. Chua TC, Kohl JL, Yan TD et al (2009) Cytoreductive surgery and perioperative intraperitoneal chemotherapy for peritoneal carcinomatosis from small bowel adenocarcinoma. J Surg Oncol 100:139-143
34. Shen P, Stewart JH 4th, Levine EA (2009) Cytoreductive surgery and intraperitoneal hyperthermic chemotherapy for peritoneal surface malignancy: non colorectal indications. Curr Probl Cancer 33:168-193
35. Glehen O, Elias D, Gilly FN (2008) Presentation du rapport de l'Association Francaise de Chirurgie. In: Elias D, Gilly EN, Glehen O Eds. Carcinoses peritoneales d'origine digestive et primitives. France. Arnette Walkers Kluwer, pp.101-152
36. Delotte J, Desantis M, Frigenza M et al (2014) Cytoreductive surgery with hyperthermic intraperitoneal chemotherapy for the treatment of endometrial cancer with peritoneal carcinomatosis. Eur J Obstet Gynocol Reprod Biol 172:111-114
37. Bakrin N, Cotte E, Sayag-Beaugard A et al (2010) Cytoreductive surgery with hyperthermic intraperitoneal chemotherapy for the treatment of recurrent endometrial carcinoma confined to the peritoneal cavity. Int J Gynecol Cancer 20:809-814
38. Glehen O, Gilly F, Bouttle F et al (2010) Toward curative treatment of peritoneal carcinomatosis from non-ovarian origin by cytoreductive surgery combined with perioperative intraperitoneal chemotherapy. Cancer 16:5608-5618
39. Kerscher AG, Mallalieu J, Pitroff A et al (2010) morbidity and mortality of 109 consecutive cytoreductive procedures with hyperthermic intraperitoneal chemotherapy (HIPEC) performed at a community hospital. World J Surg 34:62-69
40. Levine EA, Stewart JH, Shin P et al (2014) Intraperitoneal chemotherapy from peritoneal surface malignancy : experience with 1000 patient. J Am Coll Surg 218:573-587
41. Turrini O, Lambaudie E, Faucher M et al (2012) Initial experience with hyperthermic intraperitoneal chemotherapy. Arch Surg 147:919-923
42. Yoon W, Alame A, Beni R (2014) Peritoneal surface disease severity score as a predictor of resectability in the treatment of peritoneal surface malignancies. Am J Surg 207:403-407
43. Votanopoulos KI, Newman NA, Russel G et al (2013) Outcomes of cytoreductive surgery (CRS) with hyperthermic intraperitoneal chemotherapy (HIPEC) in patients older than 70 years: survival benefits at considerable morbidity and mortality. Ann Surg Oncol 20:3497-3503
44. Sun Y, Chen P, Stewart JH et al (2013) Cytoreductive surgery and hyperthermic intraperitoneal chemotherapy for peritoneal carcinomatosis from small bowel adenocarcinoma. Am Surg 79:644-648
45. Jacks SP, Hundley JC, Shen P et al (2005) Cytoreductive surgery and hyperthermic intraperitoneal chemotherapy for peritoneal carcinomatosis from small bowel adenocarcinoma. J Surg Oncol 9:112-17
46. Randle RW, Swett KR, Shen P et al (2013) Cytoreductive surgery with hyperthermic intraperitoneal chemotherapy in peritoneal sarcomatosis. Am Surg 6:620-4

Palliative Treatments

23

Simone Sibio, Joseph Maher Fouad Atta, Daniele Biacchi,
Enzo Naticchioni, and Maurizio Cardi

23.1 Introduction

During the last two decades, cytoreductive surgery associated with hyperthermic intraperitoneal chemotherapy (CRS plus HIPEC) has received increasing attention as a promising treatment for peritoneal carcinomatosis (PC) from several primary tumor types. However, many patients with advanced disease have no indications to be treated either by this procedure or by any other systemic therapy. Chronic pain, development of malignant ascites (MA), and bowel obstruction are often reported by the majority of those patients, with detrimental physiological and psychological status affecting quality of life (QoL) and leading to very poor prognosis [1–6]. Even if still controversial, CRS plus HIPEC may play an important role in palliative treatment, especially when associated with a less invasive approach to obtain the best results with limited morbidity and mortality.

23.2 Malignant Ascites and Palliative HIPEC

MA is a condition in which fluids originating from and containing cancer cells accumulate in the peritoneal cavity. Pathogenesis is multifactorial, and several factors such as tumor burden, portal pressure, oncotic pressure, lymphatic resorption, and increased microvascular permeability play a role in its onset [7, 8]. In general, ascites complicating an intra-abdominal malignancy accounts for 10 % of all ascites [9]. The presence of MA is estimated to occur in ~ 90 % of

S. Sibio (✉)
Department of Surgery "Pietro Valdoni", Sapienza University of Rome,
Rome, Italy
e-mail: simone.sibio@uniroma1.it

A. Di Giorgio, E. Pinto (Eds), *Treatment of Peritoneal Surface Malignancies*,
Updates in Surgery
DOI: 10.1007/978-88-470-5711-1_23, © Springer-Verlag Italia 2015

patients with PC, with a reported median survival of 5.7 months, being better for ovarian carcinoma (OC) (median 30 weeks) and worse for gastrointestinal (GI) adenocarcinomas (10 weeks) [10]. Furthermore, in 52–54 % of patients, MA represents the first sign of an intra-abdominal malignancy [11, 12]. Cytologic examination results of peritoneal fluid are still a controversial issue: some authors report it to be highly sensitive (up to 97 %) [13], whereas a more recent study reports it should not be considered as conclusive for a definitive diagnosis [14]. Onset of MA affects QoL and carries poor prognosis. Most symptoms reported are due to progressive abdominal distension that causes abdominal pain, dyspnea, anorexia, hemorrhagic complications, bowel obstruction, and systemic disorders such as protein depletion and hydroelectrolyte disorders [15, 16].

Standard treatments include salt-restricted diets, diuretics, repeated paracentesis, permanent drains, and peritoneal venous shunts in resistant cases [17]. Their real efficacy in treating ascites and improving QoL is difficult to assess due to scarce reports and knowledge about the natural history of MA formation [18]. Due to the lack of randomized controlled trials, no treatment can be considered the standard of care. Nevertheless, traditionally, paracentesis is the most frequently used (98 %) and the most effective (89 %) procedure [19]. It is considered simple and safe, providing at least temporary symptom relief in 93 % of patients [20, 21] However, benefits are time limited (often within 72 h) [18], and potential complications such as bowel perforation, hypotension, and peritonitis can occur in a small but significant number of patients. Peritoneal–venous shunt is used to reduce the need for repeated paracentesis in patients with rapid ascites formation and poor response to diuretics and diet. It provides ascites control in 75–78 % of patients, but the operative mortality rate is high (10–20 %) [22] and complications are frequent [10]. Diuretics when administered in high doses [20, 21] appear to be effective in 43–44 % of patients but with relevant systemic side effects. New treatments are emerging, mainly directed to intraperitoneal (IP) delivery of chemotherapeutic drugs or biological agents, but no definitive selection criteria, guidelines, or results (ascites reduction, QoL evaluation) are yet available [23].

In the last two decades, CRS plus HIPEC has gained increasing attention as a promising treatment in patients with PC from various primary tumor types. Administering chemotherapy directly to the tumor site can achieve higher tissue concentration than can systemic treatments, and association of hyperthermia enhances tissue penetration of cytotoxic agents, with lower systemic absorption and therefore less toxicity [24–32]. Hyperthermia increases drug tissue penetration up to 5 mm and directly inhibits cellular mechanisms of replication and repair [18]. HIPEC can be administered by an open or closed technique: the open technique is believed to achieve homogeneous distribution of thermal energy; the closed technique accounts for increased intra-abdominal pressure, which is believed to drive deeper drug penetration. In patients with PC with symptomatic MA who are not candidates for CRS, HIPEC can be administered by laparoscopy to provide ascites control. The advantages are less pain, lower morbidity and mortality rates, shorter hospitalization, and maintaining the possibility of performing a minimal adhesiolysis to achieve homogeneous drug spatial distribution. In the literature, laparoscopic HIPEC for MA palliation is reported in small retrospective studies as having a high rate of success, low morbidity, and no mortality (Table 23.1) [33–39]. Drugs and procedural duration vary depending upon primary tumor type and other parameters, such as tumor burden, ascites volume, patient's general condition, previous chemotherapies, drug resistance, and personal experience of care providers. No clear data are available on the effects on QoL after laparoscopic HIPEC, although some studies reported a generic improvement in performance status [34, 35]. Literature data report control of MA in almost 100 % of patients, with no improvement in survival rates. A large study by Randle et al. on the efficacy of CRS plus HIPEC in MA management demonstrated that HIPEC alone is highly effective in long-term MA control in patients with macroscopic residual disease after surgery, although, again, the treatment does not provide any survival advantages [40]. This is also reported by other studies, regardless of primary tumor and drugs used, and the reason for these results is not clear. Drugs such as doxorubicin seem to produce sclerosis of the peritoneal surface, preventing capillary extravasation and inducing peritoneal adhesions [41]. Cisplatin and mitomycin-C do not seem to cause this same activity [42, 43] and have a direct cytotoxic effect on cancer cells, occluding lymphatic vessels and producing capillary permeability mediators; however, evidence of these results is merely experimental [44].

New drugs and new IP administration modalities are being studied: Kobold et al. reviewed current evidence suggesting that IP administration of the anti-vascular endothelial growth factor (VEGF) antibody, bevacizumab, might prevent local fluid accumulation [45–48]. Other studies considered the possibility drug delivery using a nebulized aerosol driven throughout the abdominal cavity by the pneumoperitoneal pressure [pressurized IP aerosol chemotherapy (PIPAC)]. Tempfer et al. applied compassionate treatment to 18 patients affected by unresectable PC from platinum-resistant OC, primary malignant peritoneal (PMP), and fallopian-tube cancers: Ten underwent PIPAC only; in eight, CRS was associated. Cisplatin at 7.5 mg/m^2 and doxorubicin at 1.5 mg/m^2 were perfused for 30 min at 37°C. In eight patients, PIPAC was repeated up to six times. Treatment was well tolerated and achieved an objective tumor response in six of eight patients who underwent more than one PIPAC treatment, although the rate of ascites control was not reported [49]. These results match with other, similar studies, on CRC, GC, and appendiceal cancers, suggesting PIPAC is a feasible and promising new modality of IP drug delivery [50, 51].

In conclusion, in patients with PC and MA who are not candidates for CRS, laparoscopic HIPEC can be safely and effectively administered, achieving satisfactory results, good MA control, and improved QoL. Other benefits are short hospitalization and very low morbidity and mortality rates, but there is no survival benefit. New drugs and new perfusion modalities are being studied to improve these promising results.

Table 23.1 Laparoscopic HIPEC for malignant ascites

Study [Reference]	No. (PSM origin)	Drugs	Operative time (min)	HIPEC duration (min)	Hospital stay (days)	Mortality	Morbidity	Ascites resolution	Median survival (months)
Chang et al. 2001[33]	2 (1 MPM, 1 BL)	CDDP	282	90	3–8	0	No	50 %	-
Facchiano et al. 2008 [34]	5 (GI)	MMC + CDDP	-	60–90	23	0	1 (delayed GI emptying)	100 %	3
Patriti et al. 2008 [35]	1 (PM)	CDDP + DOXO	-	60	7	0	No	100 %	6
Valle et al. 2009 [36]	52 (15 GI, 11 colon, 13 ovarian, 8 breast lobular)	CDDP + DOXO	147	90	2.3	0	3 (2 wound infection, 1 deep vein thrombosis)	94 %	3
Ba et al. 2010 [37]	16 (GI)	5-FU + OXA	80	90	NR	0	1 (grade 2 bone marrow suppression)	100 %	5
Graziosi et al. 2009 [38]	1 (PM)	CDDP + DOXO	-	60	7	0	1 (hyponatremia)	100 %	11
De Mestier et al. 2012 [39]	2 (1 GI, 1 OC)	MMC + CDDP	120	25	-	0	-	100 %	7 GI, 3 OC
Di Giorgio 2013 (unpublished)	13 (4 GI, 1 PMP, 8 OC)	MMC, 5-FU + OXA CDDP	157	60	5	0	No	92.3 %	8 OC, 4 GI, 2 PMP

HIPEC, hyperthermic intraperitoneal chemotherapy; *PSM*, peritoneal surface malignancy; *GI*, gastrointestinal; *BL*, breast lobular; *PM*, pulmonary mesothelioma; *OC*, ovarian cancer; *MPM*, malignant peritoneal mesothelioma; *PMP*, pseudomyxoma peritonei; *CDDP*, cisplatin; *MMC*, mitomycin-C; *DOXO*, doxorubicin; *OXA*, oxaliplatin; *5-FU*, 5-fluoroucil

23.3 Palliative Surgery and Managing Bowel Obstruction in Peritoneal Carcinomatosis

Malignant bowel obstruction is a common event in patients with locally advanced cancers, reaching an incidence of 28 % in GI cancer and 51 % in OC [1, 2]. Symptoms are related to the level of obstruction and usually include severe abdominal pain and distension, nausea, vomiting, and inability to pass gas and stool [52]. In patients with advanced or end-stage digestive or gynecological cancers, the onset of bowel obstruction may be insidious, evolving over several weeks and presenting spontaneous remissions between acute relapses [53]. Malignant bowel obstruction may have both mechanical and functional origin: the former is related to direct compression or infiltration by tumor masses of bowel loops, and the latter is related to impaired intestinal motility, resulting from tumor infiltration of mesenteries, nerves involved in intestinal motility, massive ascites, or chronic opioid therapies. Computed tomography is the gold standard for diagnosing malignant bowel obstruction, as it has a specificity and sensitivity > 90 % [54]. CT can exclude nonneoplastic causes of obstruction, which can occur in 15–30 % of patients with carcinomatosis and are mostly related to adhesions, hernias, and eventration [55, 56]. It can also identify the presence of a surgical emergency, such as perforation, volvulus, or strangulation, all of which are surgical indications even for palliative care. Decision making is very difficult in these patients. Medical conservative treatment is often not effective to relieve symptoms, and major surgical procedures should be avoided in patients who have limited life expectancy and who are poor surgical candidates because of malnutrition and underlying disease [57]. A large review by Laval et al. proposed recommendations and practical clinical guidelines to guide decision making, reserving surgery for patients with nonneoplastic mechanical obstruction, emergency situations, and limited obstruction with no indications to endoscopic prosthesis. Conservative medical management is preferred for patients with single stenosis suitable for endoscopic treatment, in poor general condition, or with extensive carcinomatosis, multiple areas of stenosis, or mesentery-root invasion. Age, comorbidities, nutritional status, previous radiotherapy, and level of obstruction are also identified as poor prognostic factors for surgical treatment [52] (Table 23.2).

Conservative management of patients with malignant bowel obstruction includes fasting, intravenously delivered rehydration, total parenteral nutrition, nasogastric tube (NGT) placement, and antiemetic, antisecretory, analgesic, and corticosteroid drug administration. Antisecretory drugs, which reduce digestive secretions such as octreotide, are particularly important in relieving patient distress; if vomiting does not stop, a venting gastrostomy rather than long-term NGT may be considered [52]. Endoscopic prosthesis must be preferred to surgery when technically possible due to its lower morbidity and mortality rates; PC must not be considered a contraindication to stent placement in patients with a single-site bowel obstruction [58]. Complications are rare and include perforation (0.5–4 %) and stent migration (8–12 %) and obstruction (0.5–10 %).

Table 23.2 Prognostic factors influencing surgical treatment of malignant bowel obstruction in unresectable peritoneal carcinomatosis

- Advanced age
- Presence of comorbidities
- Poor performance status
- Extent of peritoneal carcinomatosis; particularly, presence of multiple levels of obstruction
- Small-bowel rather than large-bowel obstruction
- Previous abdominal or pelvic radiotherapy

Technical failure is more frequent in long-standing stenosis [59].

A surgical approach should be carefully considered when conservative treatment fails or is not possible. Surgical procedures include ostomies (colostomy, ileostomy, jejunostomy), small- or large-bowel resections and/or bypass, and lysis of either malignant or inflammatory adhesions. Surgical strategy is determined upon intraoperative findings, and no standard guidelines are available. Several studies demonstrated benefits in symptoms relief with resumption of oral intake after palliative surgery for malignant bowel obstruction in 32–100 % of patients [60–66]. QoL measures are not reported by any available study. The literature reports that perioperative morbidity and mortality and rates are high, ranging from 7 % to 44 % and from 6 % to 32 %, respectively [60–62, 65, 67–69]. A frequent complication, occurring in from 6 % to 47 % of patients, is reobstruction [61–63, 66, 69]. Furthermore, duration of symptom relief may be short [66, 69] and hospital stay considerable in relation to patients life expectancy, which ranges from 1 to 94 days [70]. When obstructive symptom resolution is achieved and is long lasting, survival advantage may be significant, rising from 26 to 36 days to 154 to 192 days in some series [62, 71]. Table 23.3 summarizes the most relevant experiences and results in surgical treatment of malignant bowel obstruction in patients with PC. Authors experience is detailed in Table 23.4: overall median survival was 96.1 days (OC 100.3 days, GI cancer 83.5 days, CRC 104.5 days), and mean hospital stay was 9.6 days (range 6–14). Operative mortality occurred in two patients (17 %): one died after reoperation for bleeding, and reobstruction occurred in one, who died after 28 days.

23.4 Conclusions

In conclusion, palliative surgery may resolve obstructive symptoms and allow oral intake resumption and the patient to return home, even if for a short time; however, it has high mortality and morbidity rates. Moreover hospital stay may be long, affecting the quality of the remainder of the patient's life. Therefore, surgical palliation can be a valid option but should be carefully considered, taking into consideration patient preferences and compliance ability and providing complete information about risks and benefits.

Table 23.3 Malignant bowel obstruction in peritoneal carcinomatosis: outcomes (%) of palliative surgery

Study [Reference]	No.	Primary	Symptom relief	30-day mortality	Morbidity	60–90 days reobstruction
McCarthy [60]	12	OC 7, GI 5	75	25	25	NR
Turnbull et al. [61]	89	GI 84, HPB 5	74	13	43	38
Lau and Laurentz [62]	30	GI 30	57–63	17	27	47
Van Ooijen et al. [71]	59	GYN 46, GI 8, HPB 1, other 4	34–76	NR	NR	15
Blair et al. [67]	63	GI 44, HPB 5, other 14	45	21	44	NR
Legendre et al. [72]	109	GYN 37, GI 46, other 26	61	NR	NR	NR
Abbas and Merrie [68]	79	GI 34, GYN 19, other 25	NR	10	35	NR
Piver et al. [73]	60	OC 60	NR	17	31	NR
Lund et al. [63]	25	OC 25	32	32	32	38
Rubin et al. [74]	52	OC 52	65–87	17	15	NR
Bais et al. [75]	19	OC 19	68	11	32	21
Jong et al. [64]	53	OC 53	68	32	NR	40
Pothuri et al. [76]	64	OC 64	58	6	22	6
Mangili et al. [65]	47	OC 47	59	22	33	NR
Chi et al. [66]	14	OC 14	100	NR	7	29–36
Kim et al. [77]	23	OC 23	48	NR	13	NR
Kolomainen et al. [69]	90	OC 90	66	18	27	17
Di Giorgio (unpublished)	12	OC 6, GI 6	100	17	25	8

OC, ovarian carcinoma; *GI*, gastrointestinal; *GYN*, gynecological; *HPB*, hepatobiliary; *Other*, kidney, bladder, breast, gastrointestinal stromal tumor, melanoma, prostate, lung, sarcoma, unknown; *NR*, not reported

Table 23.4 Palliative surgery for malignant bowel obstruction in peritoneal carcinomatosis: personal experience

Patient no.	Primary tumor	PCI (mean = 26)	Surgical procedure	Morbidity	Hospital stay (days) mean = 9.6	Survival (days) Mean = 96.1
1	GI	24	Mesenteric implants resections	None	14	94
2	OC	27	Left colostomy	None	6	112
3	OC	28	Adhesiolysis	Reobstruction	13	28
4	OC	26	Right ileostomy	None	13	163
5	OC	30	Adhesiolysis	Bleeding	12	12
6	Colic	28	Left colostomy	None	7	127
7	GI	26	Gastroenteric anastomosis	Wound infection	11	73
8	Colic	29	Mesenteric implants resection	None	6	82
9	Colic	25	Gastroenteric anastomosis	Pleural effusion	12	159
10	Colic	24	Colic resection	None	10	50
11	OC	29	Right ileostomy	None	5	173
12	OC	27	Right ileostomy	None	6	114

OC, ovarian carcinoma; *GI*, gastrointestinal

References

1. Feuer DJ, Broadley KE, Shepherd JH et al (2000) Surgery for the resolution of symptoms in malignant bowel obstruction in advanced gynaecological and gastrointestinal cancer. Cochrane Database Syst Rev CD002764
2. Chakraborty A, Selby D, Gardiner K et al (2011) Malignant bowel obstruction: natural history of a heterogeneous patient population followed prospectively over two years. J Pain Symptom Manage. 41:412-420
3. Ripamonti C, Mercadante S (2005) Pathophysiology and management of malignant bowel obstruction. In: Doyle D, Hanks GW, McDonald N, Cherny N, eds. Oxford textbook of palliative medicine, 3rd edn., Oxford University Press, New York, pp 496-506
4. Feuer DJ, Broadley KE (1999) Systematic review and meta-analysis of corticosteroids for the resolution of malignant bowel obstruction in advanced gynaecological and gastrointestinal cancers. Systematic Review Steering Committee. Ann Oncol 10:1035-1041
5. Feuer DJ, Broadley KE, Shepherd JH et al (1999) Systematic review of surgery in malignant bowel obstruction in advanced gynecological and gastrointestinal cancer. The Systematic Review Steering Committee. Gynecol Oncol 75:313-322
6. McQuellon RP, Loggie BW, Fleming RA et al (2001)Quality of life after intraperitoneal hyperthermic chemotherapy (IPHC) for peritoneal carcinomatosis. Eur J Surg Oncol 27:65–73
7. Chung M, Kozuch P (2008)Treatment of malignant ascites. Curr Treat Options Oncol 9:215-233
8. Tamsma JT, Keizer HJ, Meinders AE (2001) Pathogenesis of malignant ascites: Starling's law of capillary hemodinamics revisited. Ann Oncol 12:1353-1357
9. Runyon BA (1994) Care of patients with ascites. N Engl J Med 330:337-342
10. Mackey JR, Venner PM (1996) Malignant ascites: demographics, therapeutic efficacy and predictors of survival Can J Oncol 6:474-480
11. Ayantunde AA, Parsons SL (2007) Pattern and prognostic factors in patietns with malignant ascites: a retrospective study. Ann Oncol 18:945-949
12. Garrison RN, Kaelin LD, Galloway RH et al (1986) Malignant ascites. Clinical and experimental observations. Ann Surg 203:644–651
13. Parsons SL, Watson SA, Steele RJ (1996) Malignant ascites. Br J Surg 83:6–14
14. Sugarbaker PH, Welch LS, Mohamed F et al (2003) A review of peritoneal mesothelioma at the Washington Cancer Institute. Surg Oncol Clin N Am 12:605-621
15. Knutsen A, Sielaff TD, Greeno E et al (2006) Staged laparoscopic infusion of hyperthermic intraperitoneal chemotherapy after cytoreductive surgery. J Gastrointestinal Surg 10:1038-1043
16. Garofalo A, Valle M, Garcia J et al (2006) Laparoscopic intraperitoneal hyperthermic chemotherapy for palliation of debilitating malignant ascites. Eur J Surg Oncol 32:682-685
17. Sommariva A, Zagonel V, Rossi CR (2012) The role of laproscopy in peritoneal surface malignancies selected for hyperthermic intraperitnoeal chemotherapy (HIPEC). Ann Surg Oncol 19:3737-3744
18. Sangisetty SL, Miner TJ (2012) Malignant ascites: a review of prognostic factors, pathophysiology and therapeutic measures. World J Gastrointest Surg 4:87-95
19. Lee CW, Bociek G, Faught W (1998) Asurvey of practice in management of malignant ascites. J Pain Symptom Manage 16:96-101
20. Becker G, Galandi D, Blum HE (2006) Malignant ascites: systematic review and guideline for treatment. Eur J Cancer 42:589-597
21. Smith EM, Jayson GC (2003) The current and future management of malignant ascites. Clin Oncol 15:59-72
22. Adam RA, Adam YG (2004) Malignant ascites: past, present and future. J Am Coll Surg 198:999-1011
23. Heiss MM, Murawa P, Koralewski P et al (2010) The trifunctional antibody catumaxomab for the treatment of malignant ascites due to epithelial cancer: results of a prospective randomized phase II/III trial Int J Cancer 127:2209-2221

24. Sommariva A, Pilati P, Rossi CR (2012) Cytoreductive surgery combined with hyperthermic intraperitoneal chemotherapy for peritoneal surface malignancies: current treatment and results. Cancer Treat Rev 38:258-268
25. Sugarbaker PH (1995) Peritonectomy procedures. Ann Surg 221:29-42
26. Esquivel J (2009) Technology of hyperthermic intraperitoneal chemotherapy in the United States, Europe, China, Japan, and Korea. Cancer J 15:249-254
27. Yan TD, Deraco M, Baratti D et al (2009) Cytoreductive surgery and hyperthermic intraperitoneal chemotherapy for malignant peritoneal mesothelioma: multi-institutional experience. J Clin Oncol 27:6237-6242
28. Cao C, Yan TD, Black D (2009) A systematic review and meta-analysis of cytoreductive surgery with perioperative intraperitoneal chemotherapy for peritoneal carcinomatosis of colorectal origin. Ann Surg Oncol 16:2152-2165
29. Chua TC, Robertson G, Liauw W et al (2009) Intraoperative hyperthermic intraperitoneal chemotherapy after cytoreductive surgery in ovarian cancer peritoneal carcinomatosis: systematic review of current results. J Cancer Res Clin Oncol 135:1637-1645
30. Yan TD, Balck D, Sugarbaker PH et al (2007) A systematic review and meta-analysis of the randomized controlled trials on adjuvant intraperitoneal chemotherapy for resectable gastric cancer. Ann Surg Oncol 14:2702-2713
31. Verwaal VJ, Van Ruth S, De Bree E et al (2003) Randomized trial of cytoreduction and hyperthermic intraperitoneal chemotherapy versus systemic chemotherapy and palliative surgery in patients with peritoneal carcinomatosis of colorectal cancer. J Clin Oncol 21:3737-3743
32. Sugarbaker PH, Cunliffe WJ, Belliveau J et al (1989) Rationale for integrating early postoperative intraperitoneal chemotherapy into the surgical treatment of gastrointestinal cancer. Semin Oncol 16:83-97
33. Chang E, Alexandr HL, Libutti SK et al (2001) Laparoscopic continuous hypertermic peritoneal perfusion. J Am Coll Surg 193:225-229
34. Facchiano, Scaringi S, Kianmanesh R et al (2008) Laparoscopic hypertermic intraperitoneal chemotherapy (HIPEC) for the treatment of malignant ascites secondary to unresectable peritoneal carcinomatosis from advanced gastric cancer. Eur J Surg Oncol 34:154-158
35. Patriti A, Cavazzoni E, Graziosi L et al (2008) Successful palliation of malignant ascites from peritonela mesothelioma by laparoscopi intraperitoneal hypertemric chemotherapy. Surg Laparosc Endosc Percutaneous Tech 18:426-428
36. Valle M, Van der Speeten K, Garofalo A (2009) laparoscopic hypertermic intraperitoneal peorperative chemotherapy (HIPEC) in the management of refractory malignant ascites: a multi-institutional retrospective analysis in 52 patients. J Surg Oncol 100:331-334
37. Ba MC, Cui SZ, Lin SQ et al (2010) Chemotherapy with laparoscope-assisted continuous circulatory Hyperthermic intraperitoneal perfusion for malignant ascites. World J Gastroenterol 16:1901-1907
38. Graziosi L, Bugiantella W, Cavazzoni E et al(2009) Laparoscopic intraperitoneal hyperthermic perfusion in palliation of malignant ascites; a case report. G Chir 30:237-9
39. De Mestier L, Volet J, Scaglia E et al (2012) Palliative Laparoscopic Hyperthermic Intraperitoneal Chemotherapy Effective in Patients with Malignant Hemorrhagic Ascites? Case Rep Gastroenterol 6:166–170
40. Randle RW, Swett KR, Swords DS et al (2013) Efficacy of Cytoreductive Surgery with Hyperthermic Intraperitoneal Chemotherapy in the Management of Malignant Ascites. Ann Surg Oncol 21: 1474-1479
41. Valle M, Federici O, Garofalo A (2012) Patient selection for cytoreductive surgery and hyperthermic intraperitoneal chemotherapy and role of laparoscopy in diagnosis, staging and treatment. Surg Oncol Clin N Am 21:515-531
42. Ozols RF, Young RC, Speyer JL et al (1982) Phase I and pharmacological studies of Adriamycin administered intraperitoneally to patients with ovarian cancer. Cancer Res 42:4265-4269
43. Sugarbaker PH (1996) Early post-operative intraperitoneal Adriamycin as an adjuvant treatment for visceral and retroperitoneal sarcoma. Cancer Treat Res 81:7-14

44. Hagiwara A, Takahashi T, Sawai K et al (1993) Milky spots as the implantation site for malignant cells in peritoneal dissemination in mice. Cancer Res 53:687-692
45. Kobold S, Hegewish-Becker S, Oechsle K et al (2009) Intraperitoneal VEGF inhibition using bevacizumab: a potential approach for the symptomatic treatment of malignant ascites? The Oncologist 14:1242-1251
46. Hamilton CA, Maxwell GL, Chernofsky MR et al (2008) Intraperitoneal bevacizumab for the palliation of malignant ascites in refractory ovarian cancer. Gynecol Oncol 111:530-532
47. Ströhlein MA, Siegel R, Jäger M et al (2009) Induction of anti-tumor immunity by trifunctional antibodies in patients with peritoneal carcinomatosis. J Exp Clin Cancer Res 28:18
48. Numnum TM, Rocconi RP, Whitworth J et al (2006)The use of bevacizumab to palliate symptomatic ascites in patients with refractory ovarian carcinoma. Gynecol Oncol 102:425–428
49. Tempfer CB, Celik I, Solass W et al (2014) Activity of pressurized intraperitoneal aerosol chemotherapy (PIPAC) with cisplatin and doxorubicin in women with recurrent, platinum resistant ovarian cancer: preliminary clinical experience. Gynecol Oncol 132:307-311
50. Solass W, Kerb R, Muerdter T et al (2014) Intraperitoneal chemotherapy of peritoneal carcinomatosis using pressurized aerosol as an alternative to liquid solution: first evidence for efficacy. Ann Surg Oncol 21:553-559
51. Blanco A, Giger-Pabst U, Solass W et al (2013) Renal and hepatic toxicity after pressurized intraperitoneal aerosol chemotherapy (PIPAC). Ann Surg Oncol 20:2311-6
52. Laval G, Marcelin-Benazech B, Guirimand F et al (2014) Recommendations for bowel obstruciotn with peritnoneal carcinomatosis. J pain symptom manage May 4. pii: S0885-3924(14)00232-2
53. Baines MJ (2000) Symptom control in advanced gastrointestinal cancer. Eur J Gastroenterol Hepatol 12:375-379
54. Silva AC, Pimenta M, Guimares LS (2009) Small bowel obstruction: what to look for? Radiographics 29:423-439
55. Osteen RT, Guyton S, Steele G et al (1980) Malignant intestinal obstruction. Surgery 87:611-615
56. Woolfson RG, Jennings K, Whalen GF (1997) Management of bowel obstruction in patients with abdominal cancer. Arch Surg 132:1093-1097
57. Helyer L, Easson AM (2008) Surgical approaches to malignant bowel obstruction. J Support Oncol 6:105-113
58. Mendelsohn RB, Gerdes H, Markowitz AJ et al (2011) Carcinomatosis is not a contraindication to enteral stenting in selected patients with malignant gastric outlet obstruction. Gastrointest Endosc 3:1135 1140
59. Manes G, De Bellis M, Fuccio L et al (2011) Endoscopic palliation in patients with incurable malignant colorectal by means of self-expanding metal stents. Arch Surg 146:1157-1162
60. McCarthy JD (1986) A strategy for intestinal obstruction of peritoneal carcinomatosis. Arch Surg 121:1081-1082
61. Turnbull AD, Guerra J, Starnes HF (1989) Results of surgery for obstructing carcinomatosis of gastrointestinal pancreatic or biliary origin. J Clin Oncol 7:381-386
62. Lau PW, Lorentz TG (1993) Results of surgery for malignant bowel obstruction in advanced unresectable recurrent colorectal cancer. Dis Colon Rectum 36:61-64
63. Lund B, Hansen M, Lundvall F et al (1989) Intestinal obstruction in patients with advanced carcinoma of the ovaries treated with combination chemotherapy. Gynecol Obstet 169:213-218
64. Jong P, Sturgeon J, Jamieson CG (1995) Benefit of palliative surgery for bowel obstruction in advanced ovarian cancer. Can J Surg 38:454-457
65. Mangili G, Aletti G, Firgerio L et al (2005) Palliative care for intestinal obstruction in recurrent ovarian cancer: a multivariate analysis. Int J Gynecol Cancer 15:830-835
66. Chi DS, Phaeton R, Miner TJ et al (2009) A prospective outcomes analysis of palliative procedures performed for malignant intestinal obstruction due to recurrent ovarian cancer. Oncologist 14:835-839

67. Blair SL, Chu DZJ, Schwartz RE (2001) Outcome of palliative operations for malignant bowel obstruction in patients with peritoneal carcinomatosis from nongynaecological cancer. Ann Surg Oncol 8:632-637
68. Abbas SM, Merrie AE (2006) Palliative small bowel surgery in patients with history of malignancy. Int J Cancer Res 2:42-46
69. Kolomainen DF, Daponte A, Barton DPJ et al (2012) Outcomes of surgical management of bowel obstruction in relapsed epithelial ovarian cancer (EOC). Gynecol Oncol 125:31-36
70. OlsonTJP, Pinkerton C, Brasel K et al (2014) Palliative surgery for malignant bowel obstruction from carcinomatosis. A systematic review. JAMA surg 149:383-392
71. Van Ooijen B, Van Der Burg MEL et al (1993) Planting AS et al Surgical treatment or gastric drainage only for intestinal obstruction in patients with carcinoma of the ovary or peritoneal carcinomatosis of other origin. Surg Gynecol Obstet 176:469-474
72. Legendre H, Vanhuyse F, Caroli-Bosc FX, Pector JC (2001) Survival and quality of life after palliative surgery for neoplastic gastrointestinal obstruction. Eur J Surg Oncol 27:364-367
73. Piver MS, Barlow JJ, Lele SB et al (1982) Survival after ovarian cancer induced intestinal obstruction. Gynecol Oncol 13:44-49
74. Rubin SC, Hoskins WJ, Benjamin I et al (1989) Palliative surgery for intestinal obstruction in advanced ovarian cancer. Gynecol Oncol 34:16-19
75. Bais JMJ, Schiltuis MS, Slors JFM et al (1995) Intestinal obstruction in patients with advanced ovarian cancer. Int J Gynecol Cancer 5:346-350
76. Pothuri B, Vaidya A, Aghajanian C et al (2003) Palliative surgery for bowel obstruction n recurrent ovarian cancer: an updated series. Gynecol Oncol 89:306-313
77. Kim K, Kang SB, Kim MJ et al (2009) Factors associated with successful palliation and improved survival in patients with malignant bowel obstruction caused by ovarian cancer. J Women Med 2:54-58

Part IV

Perspectives

Main Topics of Discussion and New Trends 24

Angelo Di Giorgio

24.1 Introduction

In the previous chapters, we analyzed the most relevant aspects related to peritoneal surface malignancy (PSM) classification and treatment by integrated cytoreductive surgery plus hyperthermic intraperitoneal chemotherapy (CRS plus HIPEC). Many of the issues dealt with in previous chapters are common to various forms of PSM; others are more specific to single pathological forms. Recent experience has provided greater clarity for the role of CRS plus HIPEC, albeit partial and nondefinitive, but has also emphasized problems requiring solutions for greater reliability and effectiveness of the combined procedure and to dispel doubts and criticisms regarding its application. The main focus of ongoing studies and of this chapter is on both general and specific issues of HIPEC and its application in specific forms of PSM.

24.2 General Issues

24.2.1 Peritoneal Surface Malignancy Staging Classification

In most cases and for different forms of PSM, the extent of peritoneal diffusion associated with the Completeness of Cytoreduction (CC) score is a significant prognostic indicator and is useful for assessing complication risk. Chapter 5 discusses advantages and limitations of the various classifications applied in PSM staging in the pre-CRS plus HIPEC phase and the evaluation of residual

A. Di Giorgio (✉)
Department of Surgery "Pietro Valdoni", Sapienza University of Rome,
Rome, Italy
e-mail: angelo.digiorgio@uniroma1.it

A. Di Giorgio, E. Pinto (Eds), *Treatment of Peritoneal Surface Malignancies*,
Updates in Surgery
DOI: 10.1007/978-88-470-5711-1_24, © Springer-Verlag Italia 2015

endoperitoneal disease in the post-CRS plus HIPEC phase. These advantages and limitations have been exhaustively discussed and give valuable indications to surgeons operating in this sector regarding choice of therapeutic strategy.

Obviously, commonly accepted classifications need to be applied to standardize the interpretation and comparison of results obtained from different studies. Despite specific limits shown by various studies, the Peritoneal Cancer Index (PCI) and CC score classifications proposed by Jacquet and Sugarbaker [1] are the most validated for all PSM forms. The main aim of the Fagotti score [2], specifically devised and widely applied for ovarian carcinomatosis (OC), is to predict the feasibility of optimal cytoreduction; thus, this criteria is used by some surgeons who consider widespread peritoneal diffusion as a contraindication for CRS, independent of any other parameters.

An interesting fact is the inclusion of the PCI in the new classification system for staging malignant peritoneal mesothelioma (MPM), proposed by the Peritoneal Surface Oncology Group International (PSOGI) [3]. In the near future, therefore, the Sugarbaker classifications are expected to be the most frequently used, and its application will be more reliable when comparative studies are conducted comparing it with magnetic resonance imaging/computed tomography (MRI/CT) and anatomopathological staging. For the future, however, greater consensus is needed regarding the application by surgeons of the PCI classification, which—being a complex procedure—runs the risk of nonhomogeneous scoring.

The PCI score is reported and calculated on a 2D model classically represented by drawings of the abdominal cavity divided into regions; in the near future, 3D imaging technologies will permit 3D lesion mapping and provide useful morphological data invaluable for remote diagnosis and comparison with radiological imaging (Fig. 24.1).

Finally, the methods of assessing scores also requires reconsideration; PCI classification refers to the maximum size of tumor implants in a given region but not to the number of implants or total quantity of tumoral mass resulting from the sum of all nodules present in the same region. The same applies when assessing the CC score, which should refer to either the volume of a single residue or the sum of all residues after CRS rather than to the greatest volume of one of several residual neoplastic nodules.

24.2.2 Diagnosis and Staging

Over the past 20 years, as peritonectomy (PRT) plus HIPEC has progressively become widely used, diagnostic imaging has also shown great technological advancement. Dramatic improvement in the quality of imaging and the possibility of analyzing complex anatomical areas in detail—often significantly altered by size, shape, and conformation of the peritoneal carcinomatosis (PC)—have substantially contributed to diagnosis and staging. Tangible proof of this is the

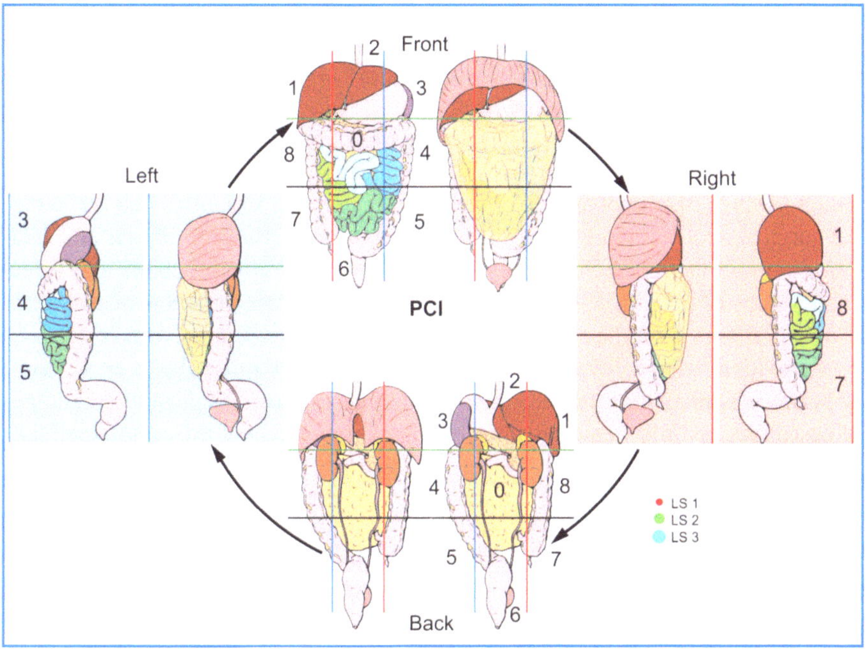

Fig. 24.1 Peritoneal Cancer Index (PCI) classification: Three-dimensional imaging simulation for PCI mapping and scoring. An imaging database can furnish all useful images to place the lesions; dedicated software calculates overall PCI. Images can be used to compare intraoperative and radiological score

high rate of optimal CRS achieved in all forms of PC treated with peritonectomy procedures. Although the merit of these results should be ascribed to surgeon ability, it is indisputable that an 80–90 % success rate for optimal cytoreduction is also partially attributable to the degree of fidelity and specificity of the technology imaging used in diagnosis.

CT, MRI, and positron emission tomography-CT (PET-CT) are now basic diagnostic procedures, but the contribution of endorectal and vaginal ultrasonography (US), particularly in cases of pelvic organ infiltration, together with clinical evaluation via direct vaginal and rectal examination, should not be disregarded.

Laparoscopy (LPS) occupies a relevant role in the diagnostic phase by allowing direct visualization and biopsy of tumor lesions, which is essential when histological or cytological assessment is not otherwise feasible. The utility of LPS in staging intraperitoneal carcinomatosis, however, is more controversial. This procedure is invasive and can potentially be associated with specific risks; therefore, its use must be correlated against the cost–benefit of the possible result.

PSM staging together with histological analysis is essential in planning a general treatment strategy, as regardless of the classification applied, a high PCI score is an indicator of increased risk of complications and lower survival rates. The most accurate staging is fundamental to surgeons or centers that consider high PCI or Fagotti scores as negative indicators for PRT, whereas it is less important for certain PSM, such as low-grade pseudomyxoma peritonei (PMP) or mesotheliomas, for which the assessment of surgical resectability rather than peritoneal disease extent is more useful.

Those surgeons or centers for which a high level of PCI is not an absolute contraindication for peritonectomy must complete a thorough diagnostic investigation to verify the involvement of sensitive anatomical structures that could render surgical excision inadvisable. The complexity of peritoneal disease and limitations of radiological technologies discussed in the previous chapters may affect the accuracy of diagnosis; however, the indiscriminate use of LPS is questionable and is a reflection on the attitude of surgeons or centers dealing with PSM.

As evident from relevant publications, the mean PCI may differ significantly between studies, but the majority of studies includes significant percentages of cases successfully treated for carcinomatosis staged over the established limits for certain specific PSMs. When staging the extent of PSM, the utility of laparoscopy must be assessed against more traditional morphological investigation procedures and its possible role in identifying the involvement of adjacent anatomical structures constituting negative indicators for excision of the disease, regardless of staging limits. Aside from its valuable diagnostic role under certain circumstances, overall assessment of LPS must also consider the complication and procedure impracticality risks, including risks associated with neoplastic contamination by trocar access sites. The use of LPS, considered by some practitioners as a routine and essential procedure, deserves further evaluation, and prospective studies should be planned to define further its role and potential risks.

24.2.3 Eligibility Criteria

Eligibility criteria regarding the patient's clinical status before admission to the procedure are rather homogeneous and are extensively discussed in Chap. 13. Over the years, patient age threshold for treating PSM has continuously varied, and at present there is no specific limit; even patients in their 80s and in optimal physical and psychological condition, with easily resectable disease and a good prognosis, are routinely scheduled for the procedure.

The most avidly discussed eligibility criterion is preoperative PC staging, which is particularly relevant in centers in which high peritoneal spread associated with elevated levels of PCI are considered contraindications for CRS. These centers adopt strict selection criteria and more complex diagnostic procedures, which may also involve routine LPS. In centers in which a high extent of PC is not an absolute negative indicator for procedure execution, rather than the presence of unequivocal signs of infiltration of unresectable anatomical structures, staging has a significantly more important role in determining whether neoadjuvant chemotherapy (NACT) should be part of the general treatment strategy.

Progress in molecular biology, genetics, and pathology, as previously described for mesothelioma and OC, as well as chemosensitivity testing applied in the pre-HIPEC phase, will permit more articulated classification of some PSM forms and identification of subtypes, with differing prognoses and variable responses to specific forms of treatment. All these factors will condition eligibility criteria and will guide drug choice for HIPEC and appropriate adoption of NACT. Results from a number of prospective trials in progress at the time of this writing, and improved adherence to multicenter protocols planned on the basis of past experience, will help refine and standardize eligibility criteria, as well as data comparison from case studies.

24.2.4 Peritonectomy

Peritonectomy is a fundamental and irreplaceable procedure in the treatment of PSM. In all forms of PSM and in all settings in which PRT plus HIPEC can be adopted, complete cytoreduction (CC) is the most significant prognostic factor. Maximum cytoreduction improves HIPEC and early postoperative intraperitoneal chemotherapy (EPIC) efficacy and is the main factor responsible for the results widely reported in the previous chapters for survival rates.

No change in treatment orientation is predictable in the near future; maximal cytoreduction is the main treatment goal in all PSM forms and settings. Maximal cytoreduction will always be the preserve of dedicated PSM surgeons and experts in this field with specific training in surgical oncological procedures and knowledge of the rules of peritoneal cytoreduction. More thought, however, should be given to treatment of patients in which PC can be completely or partially reduced by NACT. This treatment option is most applicable to PSM from gastric cancer (GC) and OC, which are PSM forms with the highest application rates of NACT.

The effects of chemical cytoreduction are evident at post-NACT peritonectomy or at second-look surgery, and their evaluation in combination with pre-NACT PC imaging forms the basis for optimizing the choice of CRS. In ovarian carcinomatosis, primary tumor exeresis conducted according to basic radical criteria with total omentectomy, appendectomy, and lymphadenectomy should also include adequate parietal peritonectomy within the lower half of the abdominal cavity. In these cases, peritonectomy must envisage removing the parietal peritoneum from the transverse umbilical line to the pelvis and include pouch stripping. Any other suspicious peritoneal area bearing signs of chemoreduction, such as fibrosis, thickening, and red spots, should be treated with ball-tip electrosurgery or argon in order to alter peritoneal membrane integrity and improve HIPEC efficacy, as previously described.

In gastric carcinomatosis responsive to intraperitoneally and/or systemically delivered NACT, basic radical primary treatment should be associated with appendectomy, bilateral oophorectomy, and extensive supramesocolic parietal peritonectomy, including stripping the peritoneum of the omental bursa, hepatic pedicle, and diaphragms.

Advances in instrumentation technology used in peritonectomy procedures will increase the efficacy and safety in performing carcinomatosis cleanup of complex anatomical areas, expanding limits of resectability and chances of optimal cytoreduction. Training surgeons in these techniques can only be done in highly specialized centers with high-volumes of activity, which permit the acquisition of specific experience over a reasonably short time period.

A laparoscopic approach to this procedure is and will remain a topic of discussion: its role can be considered only for very limited PC.

However, a general lack of information derived from manual assessment in limited carcinomatosis and the difficulty of full abdominal access for comprehensive assessment of diffuse carcinomatosis render the effectiveness of the laparoscopic approach questionable.

A further criticism concerning the laparoscopic approach is neoplastic involvement of trocar access sites, for which conflicting data exist. In this scenario, some conclusions on the subject appear inconsistent and censurable, such as conclusions that metastases of trocar access sites can be easily excised allowing prognosis, similarly to patients subjected to open peritonectomy [4]. Experienced PSM surgeons know very well the severity of tumor diffusion within the abdominal wall, especially when more than one trocar access site is involved, causing complications in treatment and significantly reduced prognosis. Regardless, the laparoscopic approach will be the subject of future controlled studies, which likely will not be conclusive in resolving disagreements among experts in the field.

24.2.5 Hyperthermic Intraperitoneal Chemotherapy

Most criticisms about PSM treatment focus on HIPEC. Except for disseminated MPM (DMPM), PMP, and localized colorectal cancer (CRC) carcinomatosis, the use of PRT plus HIPEC for other types of PSM is questioned mainly in relation to potential morbidity and therapeutic efficacy.

Scepticism regarding HIPEC is supported mainly by the lack of RCTs, which are complicated to conduct; thus, HIPEC is supported mainly on a strong rationale for its use and on available results derived almost exclusively from phase I and II studies. Although PRT plus HIPEC is considered the treatment of choice for few PSM, its application is progressively increasing for a wider variety of PSM forms.

HIPEC techniques are described in Chap. 9 and in subsequent chapters, as is its role in combination with CRS for treating major forms of PSM. Overall results drawn from past experience in all forms of PSM, including the meagre data from prospective studies, appear to validate the benefits in terms of survival compared with traditional treatments but do nothing to counteract the vehement criticism and scepticism regarding HIPEC. Indeed, the perception among sceptics is that only peritonectomy, undertaken as maximum cytoreduction, is the commonly accepted procedure by which to improve survival rather than traditional treatment based on salvage surgery and systemic chemotherapy or, more rarely, intraperitoneal normothermic chemotherapy. Pending results of randomized prospective studies on the role of HIPEC in treating various types of PSM, HIPEC continues to be widely used, and the various related studies concerning the development of new technologies and new drugs are clear proof of the scientific community's interest in this method.

HIPEC techniques, described in detail in Chap. 10, analyze the difference between open, closed, or semiclosed methods. To date, all studies agree that the choice of technique does not influence procedure efficacy or indicate any need for controlled studies in this regard. The choice is therefore left to the operators, who must also take into account environmental assessments and logistic factors.

Over the years, HIPEC-supporting technologies have been constantly modified to improve performance in terms of maintenance of carrier-solution temperatures, temperature monitoring in the various abdominal regions subjected to treatment, and creation of new systems for abdominal-cavity expansion to contain a higher volume of chemotherapy solutions. New insights into intra-abdominal pressure and the effect of temperature on pharmacokinetics and pharmacodynamics in HIPEC applications have pioneered new techniques of conducting intraperitoneally delivered chemotherapy (IP-CHT) and the use of new cytotoxic agents.

In experimental animal models, increased intra-abdominal pressure enhances the cytotoxic effects of platinum-based drugs and doxorubicin (DOXO) [5, 6]. New technologies to increase intra-abdominal pressure have been introduced to optimize drug spread within the peritoneal cavity and pharmacological penetration of tumor nodules. Using pressurized intraperitoneal aerosol chemotherapy (PIPAC) via laparoscopy involves the application of IP-CHT as a pressurized aerosol to take advantage of the physical properties of gas and pressure. This appears to be an innovative technique of major interest [7].

New drugs applied intraperitoneally benefit from association with hyperthermia: interaction between intraperitoneal use of monoclonal antibodies (MAbs) and hyperthermia suggests a high increase in drug–target interactions and uniform intratumoral drug distribution; new-generation thermosensitive liposomes has been developed that reliably enable drug liberation into heated tissue at a predefined temperature [8–13].

In previous chapters, we analyzed the pharmacokinetic and pharmacodynamic principles that underlie the rationale for HIPEC, possible interactions between drugs and hyperthermia, and characteristics and dosage of drugs used for HIPEC in various forms of PSM. Current research is focused on identifying a greater number of chemotherapeutic or other agents to be applied in bidirectional chemotherapy (intraperitoneal plus intravenous application).

HIPEC, EPIC, and bidirectional chemotherapy are increasingly being used and are now considered consolidated treatment options for carcinomatosis from

GC and CRC.

Published data indicate that the optimal intraperitoneal temperature for drug delivery is 41–42°C. The main purpose for future studies should be to standardize HIPEC techniques and answer questions that remain open regarding optimal duration, drug choice, carrier-solution volume, and drug type. As discussed in Chap. 23, HIPEC via laparoscopic or open approach is significantly effective in palliative treatment of malignant ascites (MA) in all forms of PSM: laparoscopic PIPAC seems to be an interesting alternative technique.

In the near future, a strong commitment will be made to identify shapes and setting of malignancies at high risk of causing PC and susceptible to prophylactic HIPEC treatment. Regarding the use of prophylactic HIPEC, studies to date have focused particularly on CRC, as analyzed in Chap. 19. Further studies should be conducted to assess the effectiveness of prophylactic HIPEC in patients treated with resection for primary T3–4 gastric mucinous cancer, which is a risk for the development of late carcinomatosis.

24.3 Specific Issues

24.3.1 Malignant Peritoneal Mesothelioma

CRS plus HIPEC is the gold standard for treating diffuse DMPM on the basis of results of major centers that deal with PSM. Since it is a rare form of tumor, no prospective studies are likely, as there is little chance they could be concluded. In 2011, a new MPM stage classification that incorporates the PCI was proposed by the PSOGI group [3]. At present, the use of cisplatin (CDDP) in combination with other drugs—mainly with DOXO—represents the most widely used drug regimen for HIPEC.

Although it is not possible to discern the role of HIPEC from that of CRS, success in ascites control in 90 % of cases amply justifies its use in the treatment of DMPM. CRS plus HIPEC has allowed an increase in median survival rate from 12 months in the pre-HIPEC era to 53 months. Taking into account limitations regarding planning and conducting prospective randomized controlled studies, in the near future, more accurate characterization of the different primary tumor subtypes using molecular biology, genetic, and chemosensitivity studies may contribute to optimizing patient management and to personalize treatment.

24.3.2 Pseudomyxoma Peritonei

CRS plus HIPEC should be considered the standard care for diffuse PMP (DPMP), but data from prospective studies analyzing the role of HIPEC are lacking. Even for PMP, maximum cytoreduction is recognized as the primary means of care, whereas the role of HIPEC is uncertain. Analysis of the literature seems show that HIPEC positively influences progression-free survival (PFS) rather than overall survival (OS) [14], and at present, major revisions in PMP treatment indicates HIPEC has a positive predictive value for PFS [15].

PMP treatment is conducted inhomogeneously: HIPEC techniques, drug type, and temperatures vary between specialized HIPEC centers. Future prospective studies on the basic forms of PMP, i.e., disseminated peritoneal adenomucinosis (DPAM), peritoneal mucinous carcinomatosis (PMCA), and intermediate forms, however, are unrealistic because of the low incidence of these pathologies. Therefore only improvement in the identification of different subtypes through genetic typing (genetic signature) may help improve selection and identification of patients susceptible to CRS plus HIPEC, even in the presence of high peritoneal spread with high PCI levels. An improvement in overall results may also results from referring PMP cases to highly specialized centers.

24.3.3 Carcinomatosis from Colorectal Cancer

Similarly to other forms of PSM, such as carcinomatosis from OC and GIC, the specific role of HIPEC in treating CRC carcinomatosis is still a major point of discussion, although a randomized study and many nonrandomized trials demonstrate the multiple advantages of associating CRS with HIPEC over traditional treatments. Results of ongoing trials will validate the effectiveness of CRS plus HIPEC. Despite criticism, the use of HIPEC is earning greater consent, and its acceptance is progressively increasing. CRS plus HIPEC is widely recommended as the treatment of choice for carcinomatosis with PCI < 20. Strong interest in the use of HIPEC is emerging in specialized PSM centers for preventing PC in patients treated for cancer types that pose a high risk of peritoneal metastasis. To date, HIPEC use in this context is applied to inhomogeneous therapeutic programs and in different settings:

- During a second look scheduled for patients treated with exeresis for CRC at risk of metachronous PC [16]
- During primary resection in patients with CRC at high risk of metachronous peritoneal metastasis (T3, T4, mucinous) [17]
- In the presence of positive peritoneal lavage cytology and without evidence of macroscopic PC [18]

Many prospective phase II and III trials are in progress on these specific topics worldwide and are analytically described in Chaps. 19 and 25. Results from these studies will test the role of HIPEC in various settings. The use of oxaliplatin (OXA) combined with IV 5-fluorourocil (5-FU) and leucovorin (LV) in bidirectional chemotherapy is emerging as the treatment of choice during HIPEC.

In the near future, as is currently occurring in part, a significant positive impact on survival will be provided by the introduction of new chemotherapy protocols and the integration of systemic chemotherapy with biologic drugs (targeted therapy), which give competitive results compared with the best HIPEC performance. New drugs or new combinations in systemic chemotherapy that can improve survival rates will create the necessity of comparison between these new schemes and HIPEC in various settings, whereas the role of CRS will remain unchanged.

24.3.4 Carcinomatosis from Gastric Cancer

Prospective randomized trials and retrospective studies of patients with carcinomatosis from gastric cancer (GC) treated with PRT plus HIPEC or POC (perioperative chemotherapy) demonstrate advantages in terms of survival compared with conventional treatments. In particular is the significant increase in long-term survival with acceptable morbidity rates. Despite these findings, the role of PRT plus HIPEC remains controversial, and the procedure is recommended for selected cases with PCI ≤ 12.

For this reason, laparoscopy plays a key role in evaluating disease spread in order to exclude cases with a high PCI or which are unresectable and to identify cases susceptible to NACT. The use of PRT plus HIPEC in GC carcinomatosis is effective only in cases with limited peritoneal diffusion; therefore, NACT plays a strategic and essential role in increasing the possibility of treating a greater number of cases. A new neoadjuvant aggressive treatment with intraperitoneal chemotherapy combined with systemic chemotherapy (NIPS) seems promising in ensuring long-term survival in patients undergoing complete cytoreduction and in containing malignant ascites in cases that are not cytoreducible, with success rates close to 100 %. The promising prophylactic use of HIPEC in patients with GC at risk for postoperative carcinomatosis is expected to lead to further HIPEC diffusion in Western countries.

Intraperitoneal administration of the monoclonal antibody catumaxomab seems to ensure significant success in treating malignant ascites from GC and provides additional benefits as adjuvant treatment after resection for locally advanced GC [19].

24.3.5 Carcinomatosis from Ovarian Cancer

The role of PRT plus HIPEC for treating PC from OC is questioned more frequently than for other forms of PSM. The main criticisms concern the use of HIPEC, whereas maximal cytoreduction is widely accepted as the fundamental goal of therapy when surgical exeresis is indicated. Criticism about HIPEC, analogously to gastric and colorectal carcinomatosis, relates to the potential risk of morbidity and unproven benefit in terms of survival. The lack of controlled studies contributes to foment scepticism toward the procedure. Prospective controlled trials aimed at verifying the role of HIPEC in primary and secondary cytoreduction are in progress at the time of this writing.

The adoption of systemic or intraperitoneal treatments based on biological drugs leads us to expect increasingly complex comparisons between such regimens and HIPEC in the near future.

High chemosensitivity to first-line chemotherapy and good response rates to subsequent lines of treatment were the rational for treating carcinomatosis from OC with less aggressive therapeutic strategies than PRT plus HIPEC, with the aim being to make the disease become chronic rather than radicalize the treatment. However, compared with the results from CRS plus HIPEC, complications resulting from traditional treatments based on CRS and systemic and/or normothermic IP-CHT are often underestimated and may decrease the overall rate of application of such treatments.

Results of ongoing trials will undoubtedly help confirm the role of HIPEC but will probably be insufficient to resolve any controversy regarding the issue of efficacy; adoption of new drugs and new combinations outside the HIPEC setting will contribute to controlling disease progression and prolonging survival, even in the presence of residual disease. Therefore, new, comparative studies and controlled trials for HIPEC will be required, even if difficult to conduct.

The role of NACT and platinum sensitivity are under study, and ongoing trials evaluating HIPEC will provide significant insights even for these factors. The role of PRT plus HIPEC in all the most recent studies is related to various disease settings for treatment; future prospective studies should take account of this issue.

In the near future, the classification of ovarian tumors will take into account the progress achieved using molecular biology and genetic techniques that allowed identifying the extraovarian origin of so-called papillary serous ovarian tumors and classifying together under a unique condition all forms of ovarian, tubal, and peritoneal cancer, as described above. Application of these new classifications and wider diffusion of studies on molecular and genetic profiles of these tumors will enable identification of tumor subtypes as targets for more specific and personalized treatment regimens.

References

1. Jacquet P, Sugarbaker PH (1996) Clinical research methodologies in diagnosis and staging of patients with peritoneal carcinomatosis. Cancer Treat Res 82:359-374
2. Fagotti A, Ferexidina D, Fanfani F et al (2006) A laparoscopy-based score to predict surgical outcome in patients with advanced ovarian carcinoma: a pilot study. Ann Surg Oncol 13:1156-1161
3. Yan TD, Deraco M, Elias D et al (2011) Peritoneal Surface Oncology Group. A novel tumour-node-metastasis (TNM) staging system of diffuse malignant peritoneal mesothelioma using outcome analysis of a multi-institutional database. Cancer 117:1855-1863
4. Vergote I, Marquette S, Amant F et al (2005) Port-site metastases after open laparoscopy: a study in 173 patients with advanced ovarian carcinoma. Int J Gynecol Cancer 15:776-779

5. Thomas F, Ferron G, Gesson-Paute A et al (2008) Increased tissue diffusion of oxaliplatin during laparoscopically assisted versus open heated intraoperative intraperitoneal chemotherapy (HIPEC). Ann Surg Oncol 15:3623-3624
6. Jacquet P, Stuart OA, Chang D, Sugarbaker PH (1996) Effects of intra-abdominal pressure on pharmacokinetics and tissue distribution of doxorubicin after intraperitoneal administration. Anticancer Drugs 7:596-603
7. Tempfer CB, Celik I, Solass W et al (2014) Activity of Pressurized Intraperitoneal Aerosol Chemotherapy (PIPAC) with cisplatin and doxorubicin in women with recurrent, platinum-resistant ovarian cancer: preliminary clinical experience. Gynecol Oncol 132:307-311
8. Hauck ML, Zalutsky MR (2005) Enhanced tumour uptake of radiolabelled antibodies by hyperthermia: Part I: Timing of injection relative to hyperthermia. Int J Hyperthermia 21:1-11
9. Hauck ML, Zalutsky MR (2005) Enhanced tumour uptake of radiolabelled antibodies by hyperthermia. Part II: Application of the thermal equivalency equation. Int J Hyperthermia 21:13-27
10. Kinuya S, Yokoyama K, Hiramatsu T et al (2000) Optimal timing of administration of hyperthermia in combined radioimmunotherapy. Cancer Biother Radiopharm 15:373-379
11. Kinuya S, Yokoyama K, Michigishi T, Tonami N (2004) Optimization of radioimmunotherapy interactions with hyperthermia. Int J Hyperthermia 20:190-200
12. Kong G, Dewhirst MW (1999) Hyperthermia and liposomes. Int J Hyperthermia 15:345-370
13. Lindner LH, Eichhorn ME, Eibl H et al (2004) Novel temperature-sensitive liposomes with prolonged circulation time. Clin Cancer Res 10:2168-2178
14. Votanopoulos KI, Shen P, Stewart JH 4th, Levine EA 2012) Current status and future directions in appendiceal cancer with peritoneal dissemination. Surg Oncol Clin N Am 21:599-609
15. Chua TC, Moran BJ, Sugarbaker PH (2012) Early and long-term outcome data of patients with pseudomyxoma peritonei from appendiceal origin treated by a strategy of cytoreductive surgery and hyperthermic intraperitoneal chemotherapy. J Clin Oncol 30:2449-2456
16. Elias D, Honoré C, Dumont F et al (2011) Results of systematic second-look surgery plus HIPEC in asymptomatic patients presenting a high risk of developing colorectal peritoneal carcinomatosis. Ann Surg 254:289-293
17. Sammartino P, Sibio S, Biacchi D et al (2012) Prevention of Peritoneal Metastases from Colon Cancer in High-Risk Patients: Preliminary Results of Surgery plus Prophylactic HIPEC. Gastroenterol Res Pract 2012:141585
18. Noura S, Ohue M, Shingai T (2011) Effects of intraperitoneal chemotherapy with mitomycin C on the prevention of peritoneal recurrence in colorectal cancer patients with positive peritoneal lavage cytology findings. Ann Surg Oncol 18:396-404
19. Goéré D, Gras-Chaput N, Aupérin A et al (2014) Treatment of gastric peritoneal carcinomatosis by combining complete surgical resection of lesions and intraperitoneal immunotherapy using catumaxomab. BMC Cancer 14:148

New Trials

25

Barbara Costantini, Anna Fagotti, Giulia Montori,
Federico Coccolini, Luca Ansaloni, and Giovanni Scambia

25.1 Background

Primary or secondary peritoneal surface involvement represents an important occurrence in the history of patients with gastrointestinal and gynecological tumors, representing a clinical entity grouped under the name of peritoneal surface malignancies (PSM). Patient life expectancy and quality of life (QoL) are very poor when the disease had reached this phase. In the past, oncologists considered peritoneal carcinosis (PC) as a distant metastasis and therefore as an incurable intra-abdominal disease. Definitely, notwithstanding the advances in systemic chemotherapy regimens, the effects on PC are still limited, probably because of the peritoneal–plasma barrier, which prevents effective drug delivery from the systemic circulation into the peritoneal cavity [1–3]. However, novel therapeutic approaches have been attempted for patients with isolated peritoneal metastases of PSM. Indeed, disease is often restricted to the peritoneal cavity without extra-abdominal involvement, and therefore, it is possible to consider PC as a locoregional disease, and a locoregional approach is thus reasonable for treating these malignancies in humans [4].

In recent years, aggressive cytoreductive surgery (CRS) consisting of peritonectomy with multivisceral resection of all involved viscera eventually combined with hyperthermic intraperitoneal chemotherapy (HIPEC) has been developed as locoregional treatment with curative intent. Since its first appearance in 1980 [5], HIPEC associated with surgery has had an increasingly important role in the treatment of several types of cancer with peritoneal dissemination [6–8].

B. Costantini (✉)
Department of Gynecology and Obstetrics, Division of Gynecologic Oncology,
Catholic University of Sacred Heart,
Rome, Italy
e-mail: Barbara.costantini@rm.unicatt.it

A. Di Giorgio, E. Pinto (Eds), *Treatment of Peritoneal Surface Malignancies*,
Updates in Surgery
DOI: 10.1007/978-88-470-5711-1_25, © Springer-Verlag Italia 2015

The use of such a therapeutic approach find its rationale in the typical spread of this clinical entity that remains confined in the peritoneal cavity for most of its natural history and in achieving higher drug concentrations that come in contact with the peritoneal surface, with lower systemic concentrations resulting in a decrease in systemic toxicity. Hyperthermia is proved to exert a cytotoxic effect directly and indirectly on tumor cells and displays a synergistic effect with several cytotoxic agents, increasing drug penetration up to 3–6 mm into malignant nodules, with an antimitotic effect [9–11].

25.2 Role of Surgery in Primary and Recurrent Ovarian Cancer

Epithelial ovarian carcinoma (EOC) is the ninth most common malignancy and one of the most challenging health issues in women. This tumor type represents the fifth leading cause of cancer-related deaths among female patients. Most EOC cases are diagnosed at an advanced disease stage, when large intraperitoneal diffusion has already occurred [12]. Standard treatment for EOC in the initial stage is bilateral salpingo-oophorectomy, hysterectomy, multiple peritoneal biopsies of all abdominal fields, at least infracolic omentectomy, appendectomy (in case of mucinous histology), and pelvic and para-aortic lymph node dissection up to the renal veins [13]. In advanced EOC, the aim is cytoreductive surgery (CRS) (involving, if is necessary, intestinal resection, peritoneal stripping, diaphragmatic resection, removal of bulky para-aortic lymph nodes, and splenectomy) to improve overall (OS) and progression-free (PFS) survival [13]. However, the role of systematic pelvic and para-aortic lymph node dissection in advanced disease remains controversial.

Completeness of cytoreduction (CC) after primary surgery is one of the most important prognostic factors and in advanced EOC can improve OS between 24 and 106 months, as shown in different series, vs. 11–31 months in patients with a residual disease > 1 cm. It also seems to achieve survival results comparable with the standard treatment [14].

Drug regimens combining platinum–taxane chemotherapy are considered the standard approach to patients with primary EOC. However, only a slight improvement has been achieved in survival rates in patients with advanced ovarian cancer (AOC). Even after optimal cytoreduction followed by platinum–Taxol-based chemotherapy, ~ 60–70 % of stage III patients develop a recurrence and ultimately die of chemoresistant disease [15, 16].

Contrary to what occurs in the primary disease, it is not yet clear what the standard treatment for recurrent EOC should be. Patients who experience recurrence within 6 months from the end of first-line chemotherapy are considered platinum resistant and appropriate for salvage treatment with second-line drugs; however, response rates are low and survival poor. Patients who recur after 6 months are considered suitable for further treatment with platinum-based chemotherapy possibly in combination with paclitaxel (platinum-sensitive patients). Recently, surgery attained a major role in recurrent chemosensitive OC: A meta-analysis of 2,019 patients shows that obtaining optimal secondary cytoreduction independently correlates with survival after recurrence [17]. Despite the lack of randomized studies, a recent Cochrane review [18] suggests that optimal secondary cytoreduction may be associated with improved outcomes in terms of prolonging life in patients with platinum-sensitive recurrent OC.

25.3 Role of Surgery in Gastric Cancer

Gastric cancer (GC) is the fourth most common cancer and the second leading cause of cancer death in the world. Global incidence of primary tumor location and histological types are constantly changing between the lowest rates in Unites States and Western Europe and the highest rates in East Asia, South America, and Eastern Europe. GC remains a tumor with a poor prognosis, with a 5-year OS near 25 % [3, 11].

Standard surgical treatment of GC is total gastrectomy (in case of tumor localization in middle third and superior third) and partial gastrectomy (in case of distal localization, with proximal margin 5–8 cm between tumor and cardias), with a D2 lymphadenectomy (> 16 lymph nodes). Standard chemotherapy regimen used in GC comprises epirubicin, 5-fluorouracil (5-FU), and cisplatin (ECF) as neoadjuvant chemotherapy (NACT) (in case of T3, N+); in advanced tumor, capecitabine (ECX) replaces 5-FU. In the postoperative setting, chemoradiation could compensate for suboptimal surgery, pT4–pT3, N+, and pT2 with high risk. However, due to worse performance status in patients after surgery and NACT, only 40 % of patients receive adjuvant therapy [3, 11, 19].

Penetration of gastric serosa and lymphatic spread are the two most important factors affecting prognosis in GC. Indeed, PC from GC can occur in up to 20% of patients explored for potentially curative resection and peritoneum is the recurrent site in up to 40% [14].

25.4 Role of HIPEC in Primary and Recurrent Ovarian Cancer

In EOC, many patients who undergo optimal cytoreduction may benefit from adjuvant chemotherapy administered intraperitoneally (IP). Several randomized trials have demonstrated improved survival associated with IP platinum-based chemotherapy as first-line adjuvant therapy after optimal cytoreduction, although it is still unclear which patients might benefit most or what would be the most effective drug, dose, and appropriate number of cycles. Adjuvant IP therapy, however, seems to have more side effects than intravenous therapy and consequently worsening of patients' quality of life (QoL) [9, 20, 21]. This treatment has been applied at a different time point in the history of the disease: as upfront therapy, as interval debulking surgery, at first recurrence, and at second or subsequent recurrence.

The broad variety of dosages and drug combinations used at different time points in the history of the disease accounts for the difficulty in drawing conclusions about the best time point for CRS plus HIPEC. Although evidence regarding CRS plus HIPEC efficacy has been established for gastrointestinal cancer [14], controversy remains concerning whether IP chemotherapy, including HIPEC, is a standard treatment option or an experimental approach in other PSM, due to the difficulty in performing randomized controlled trials (RCT).

25.5 Role of HIPEC in Gastric Cancer

In patients with GC, peritoneal washing could be positive for malignant cells of up to 24 % in stage Ib and up to 40 % in stage II or III [3]. Prognosis in patients with GC is therefore poor, with 5-year OS between 6.5 and 12 months in patients with advanced GC and with a similar survival in patients with free peritoneal tumor cells and in patients with macroscopical peritoneal disease. For this reason, chemotherapy regimens given IV seem to result in worse results than IP treatment (12 months at 5 years versus 15–48 months) [22]. Particularly in Asian studies, where the incidence of GC is greater, results are encouraging, but compared with other tumors, GC remains a disease with shorter survival times and higher mortality and morbidity rates.

A number of studies have been conducted to evaluate the role of CRS plus HIPEC in patients with advancer GC, and a significant reduction in PC recurrence have been demonstrated [14]. A recent meta-analysis [23] of 20 RCTs between 1987 and 2009 reported a significant increase in OS at 1, 2, and 3 years in patients who underwent HIPEC, lower peritoneal recurrence, and reduced risk of hematogenous metastasis. HIPEC does not modify the rates of lymph node recurrence, but in patients with lymph node metastasis, it reduces mortality rates at 2 and 3 years. Patients with serosal infiltration are still considered as an intermediate and undefined group due to the impossibility of including them in the group that may benefit from HIPEC prophylaxis or treatment. For this reason, further studies are needed. Yonemura et al. [24] proposed a multimodal approach based on an association with neoadjuvant intraperitoneal and systemic chemotherapy (NIPS), CRS plus HIPEC, and early postoperative intraperitoneal chemotherapy (EPIC). The rational is to attack both sides of the peritoneum with bidirectional chemotherapy: the peritoneal cavity and subperitoneal blood vessels.

25.6 Role of HIPEC in Colorectal Cancer

PC of colorectal origin is frequent (10–35 % of patients), and in 25 % of cases, it is the initial location. PC is the second most common cause of death in patients with colorectal cancer (CRC) after liver metastasis. However, due to the difficulty of performing RCTs and to standardize the HIPEC technique, there is no level I or II evidence that HIPEC increases survival rates in patients with PC from CRC; also, the role of CC in these cases is not supported by RCTs [14]. The multidisciplinary treatment of CRC is standardized up to stage IIIC, whereas the role of this approach is less clear in stages IVa and IVb [14]. This lack of evidence is due to different approaches: in United States, HIPEC is not considered an option for PC from CRC, whereas French guidelines recommend it.

The only RCT in existence regarding HIPEC in treating CRC was published in 2003 from The Netherlands [25]. This study of 105 patients analyzed survival: standard treatment with systemic chemotherapy (5-FU–leucovorin) with or without palliative surgery versus experimental therapy with CRS plus HIPEC, followed by the same systemic treatment. Results reported an increased survival twofold higher in the experimental arm (12.6 versus 22.3 months), with a treatment-related mortality rate of 8 %. Moreover, the authors found that survival was related to macroscopically complete cytoreduction and with the number of abdominal regions involved by the disease (0–5 vs. 6–7 regions). Nevertheless, the value of this RCT is limited by several factors: the chemotherapy scheme was not the actual gold standard (consider irinotecan and oxaliplatin), appendiceal and rectal tumors were not balanced in the two arms, mitomycin-C only was used for perfusate during HIPEC, and the role of surgery in the control arm was not clear. However, other case–control and retrospective studies, particularly in France, were performed in recent years, reporting low mortality rates following CRS plus HIPEC, particularly in patients with a PCI < 10 (patients with a median expected survival of 31–48 months) [26].

25.7 New Trials in Primary and Recurrent Ovarian Cancer

A recent multicenter phase II trial by Deraco et al. [27] reported results of CRS plus HIPEC in first-line treatment of EOC. From 2004 to 2010, 26 patients enrolled in four different Italian centers attained complete cytoreduction (15 with CC-0 and 11 CC-1) and underwent closed-abdomen HIPEC with cisplatin and doxorubicin. Although major complications occurred in four patients, 25 of the 26 started systemic chemotherapy within a median of 46 days after surgery. Moreover, considerable positive results were achieved in terms of 5-year OS (60.7 %) and PFS (15.2 %). Based on this encouraging report and other literature data [28, 29], CRS plus HIPEC could be considered a strategy for upfront treatment of advanced EOC. Several RCTs are ongoing to confirm the role of this approach; among them, patients who underwent interval debulking surgery after NACT may represent an interesting subset. Patients excluded for this treatment modality are those with extra-abdominal disease, high American Society of Anesthesiologists (ASA) score, an unfavorable PFS, and demonstrated chemoresistance.

Another study analyzed CRS plus HIPEC in first-line treatment [30]. This was a phase II Korean trial evaluating the efficacy of HIPEC in treating either primary or recurrent OC. Patients first underwent CRS, and if CC-0 was achieved, they received HIPEC (platinum 75 mg/m^2 at 41.5°C for 90 min) only. Those with primary disease were randomized to or not to receive HIPEC. The primary endpoint was PFS, the secondary end point OS, and adjuvant chemotherapy was added after HIPEC according to the patients' clinical outcomes.

An ongoing Belgian trial [31] is evaluating the possibility of adding HIPEC to the standard first-line treatment for advanced OC (inclusion criteria: stage III or only pleural stage IV; exclusion criteria: incomplete CRS or poor performance status). The study is testing three courses of preoperative chemotherapy with carboplatin plus paclitaxel 175mg/m^2 every 3 weeks, followed by debulking surgery plus HIPEC with cisplatin 50 mg/m^2 and after three courses of postoperative chemotherapy with the same protocol of preoperative chemotherapy.

An Italian trial [32], is a multicenter phase III prospective RCT (Phase 3) Trial Evaluating Hyperthermic Intraperitoneal Chemotherapy in Upfront Treatment of Stage IIIC Epithelial Ovarian Cancer (CHORINE) comparing CRS plus HIPEC (cisplatin plus paclitaxel) versus CRS alone in patients with stage IIIc (FIGO) disease attaining partial or complete response after three cycles of first-line chemotherapy (carboplatin plus paclitaxel). Both groups underwent adjuvant chemotherapy (carboplatin plus paclitaxel). The objective of this study is to evaluate the role of HIPEC after NACT. Only patients with CC with a residual disease < 2.5 mm (CC-0, CC-1) are enrolled. If they receive HIPEC, the drugs used are cisplatin 100 mg/m^2 and paclitaxel 175 mg/m^2 over 90 min. Primary outcome is disease-free survival (DFS); secondary outcomes are morality, morbidity, time chemotherapy began after surgery, OS, 1, 3, and 5-year DFS, and 1, 3, and 5-year OS. The advantages of the CHORINE study are the selection of patients in whom there is a clinical response (test of in vivo chemosensitivity) and then an anticipated response to HIPEC. Moreover, the response to NACT should increase the likelihood of optimal cytoreduction with complete tumor eradication and presumably lower morbidity rates [33]. To evaluate the efficacy of CRS plus HIPEC in different types of tumors it is also very important assess the impact of this combined procedure on patient QoL; European and US studies have evaluated that [34, 35].

Despite optimal upfront surgery and first-line chemotherapy, ~ 70 % of patients will relapse in the first 3 years. Data from published trials [36, 38] regarding the use of HIPEC in platinum-sensitive recurrent EOC patients showed a median DFS and OS of 24 and 38 months, respectively, with an estimated PFS and OS at 3 years of 44 % and 92 %, respectively. These data not only confirmed previously reported data but are more significant, probably because of the highly selected population—a characteristic that contrasts with the wide heterogeneity of patients enrolled in most other trials until now. Therefore, treatment with CRS plus HIPEC in platinum-sensitive recurrent EOC patients would seem to offer similar opportunities in terms of prognosis as those attained by primary treatment, with acceptable complication rates (morbidity and mortality ~ 35 % and 0 %, respectively) if complete tumor resection is obtained [36, 38].

Despite the presence of strong biological and pharmacological rationale and > 10 years of its application in patients with EOC, the use of HIPEC in clinical practice continues to receive mixed reviews. To obtain consistent confirmation of CRS plus HIPEC in treating PC in patients with recurrent OC, several RCTs are ongoing in this subset of patients. In fact, at the time of this writing, six ongoing studies are evaluating the role of HIPEC in patients with recurrent EOC.

The primary objective of the Hyperthermic Intra-peritoneal Chemotherapy (HIPEC) in Ovarian Cancer Recurrence (HORSE) protocol [39] is to assess whether the use of CRS in combination with HIPEC is able to offer an effective advantage in terms of survival compared with exclusive optimal CRS in patients with platinum-sensitive recurrent EOC who potentially could undergo CC on the basis of preoperative and intraoperative evaluation. This prospective phase III randomized multicenter trial is evaluating progression-free interval (PFI) and OS after treatment with CRS (arm 1) versus CRS plus HIPEC (arm 2). Patients attaining optimal cytoreduction (CC-0, CC-1) are randomized to or not to receive HIPEC with cisplatin 75 mg/m^2 over 60 min at 41.5°C. A following chemotherapy treatment based on a platinum compound is recommended. This trial, together with similar ones, is necessary to understand definitively the real efficacy of the IP hyperthermic approach in such patients and establish the possible advantage or disadvantage compared with CRS alone.

In patients with platinum-sensitive recurrent OC, a nonrandomized, phase I, single-center trial (Bonn, Germany) is ongoing at this time [40] to determine safety, feasibility, maximum tolerated dose (MTD), pharmacokinetics, and pharmacodynamics of cisplatin use in HIPEC. Three liters of normal saline is used to deliver a single dose of cisplatin IP with a closed-abdomen technique over 90 min at 41–43°C. The liquid is then drained, and irrigation is performed with 2–3 l normal saline solution to wash away any residual chemotherapeutic agent. A phase III multicenter RCT, the Hyperthermic Intra-Peritoneal Chemotherapy (HIPEC) in Relapse Ovarian Cancer Treatment (CHIPOR) study [41], is evaluating the effect of HIPEC on OS in patients treated for unresectable late first relapse of OC after second-line chemotherapy. The main objective is to improve OS at 12 months in patients in the arm with HIPEC versus patients in the arm without HIPEC. In fact, patients undergoing six cycles of second-line platinum-based chemotherapy are once again scheduled for surgery (5–12 weeks following the last cycle of chemotherapy). If CC is achieved, patients are randomized to receive or not receive HIPEC with cisplatin 75 mg/m^2. The advantages seen in this study are the possibility of providing CRS plus HIPEC to a larger number of patients (adding those initially unresectable) and reducing morbility in women who previously received intensive treatment. In patients in whom it is not possible to perform primary tumor debulking surgery, for those whose condition was unfavorable for such surgery, or for those with residual disease > 1 cm following primary debulking surgery, secondary debulking could be performed. A phase III trial from The Netherlands [42] is evaluating the efficacy of HIPEC in such cases. After surgery, patients will be randomized to receive or not receive HIPEC (with platinum 100 mg/m^2). The primary outcome of this trial is to evaluate recurrence-free survival (RFS), and secondary outcomes are toxicity, morbidity, QoL, tumor response, and OS.

A US phase II randomized trial [43] aims to evaluate the outcome of secondary CRS with (arm 1) or without (arm 2) carboplatin-based HIPEC followed by systemic combination chemotherapy for recurrent platinum-sensitive ovarian, fallopian tube, and primary peritoneal cancer. Both arms will receive a standard platinum-based systemic chemotherapy. Primary outcome is to evaluate the proportion of patients without evidence of disease progression at 24 months following treatment: > 40 % is consider acceptable; < 25 % is not. Secondary outcomes are to determine toxicity and postoperative complication rates, completion rate of four cycles, and pharmacokinetics.

Interesting is the use of IP treatment on an outpatient basis. A US phase II, open-label, single-center study [44] is evaluating the effectiveness of this treatment regimen with cisplatin and doxorubicin given on days 1 and 8 over a 3-week cycle. The target is patients with recurrent ovarian, primary peritoneal, or fallopian tube cancer who have already been treated with surgery and HIPEC with cisplatin. Outcomes are toxicity, adverse event rate, time to serum cancer antigen 125 (CA125) nadir and/or chemotherapy response, and OS. Protocol drug regimens are cisplatin 75 mg/m^2 at 40.5–42°C intraoperatively, followed by a courses of IP chemotherapy with cisplatin 75 mg/m^2 on day 1, week 1, followed by doxorubicin 25 mg on day 8, week 2 for four sequential 3-week cycles.

Another clinical trial is evaluating other drug regimens [45]. Cisplatin, carboplatin, paclitaxel, pegylated liposomal doxorubicin, hydrochloride, and gentamicin act via differing mechanisms to stop the growth of the neoplastic cells. Primary outcomes are to determine whether CRS plus HIPEC followed by postoperative normothermic IP chemotherapy is feasible and safe and to evaluate toxicity during treatment and follow-up. Secondary objectives are to determine QoL in comparison with historical regimens, to evaluate PFS and OS, and to perform correlative studies focused on understanding the mechanisms of HIPEC on EOC. During HIPEC, patients receive cisplatin for 60 min; the week after surgery, they receive carboplatin, paclitaxel, pegylated liposomal hydro-chloride, or gentamicin either IP or IV.

A phase III RCT from the National Cancer Institute, the Carboplatin, Paclitaxel and Gemcitabine With or Without Bevacizumab After Surgery in Treating Patients With Recurrent Ovarian Epithelial Cancer, Primary Peritoneal Cavity Cancer, or Fallopian Tube Cancer trial [46], is the only ongoing trial testing a new regimen for HIPEC. In fact, these drugs work in different ways to stop the growth of tumor cells: some block the ability of tumor cells to grow and spread; others help kill tumor cells or carry tumor-killing substances to them.

This study aim is to determine whether combination chemotherapy is more effective when given with or without bevacizumab after surgery.
Table 25.1 summarizes trials for treating primary and recurrent OC.

25.8 New Trials in Gastric Cancer

Regarding the treatment of GC, a recent French protocol is ongoing: Glehen et al. [11] stress the importance of validating HIPEC efficacy in European and Caucasian patients with IP recurrence from GC, as was previously done in Asian patients [11]. The objective of the D2 Resection and HIPEC (Hyperthermic Intraperitoneal Chemoperfusion) in Locally Advanced Gastric Carcinoma (GASTRICHIP) prospective, open, randomized, multicenter, phase III clinical study is to evaluate the effects of HIPEC with oxaliplatin 250 mg/m^2 at 42–43°C for 30 min.

Research is focusing on new drugs with different targets. Recent studies analyzed the importance of vascular endothelial growth factor (VEGF) in malignant ascites to improve peritoneal liquid production and neoangiogenesis [47, 48]. In EOC, bevacizumab IV was tested. The only indication for this treatment is in patients with advanced OC with poor prognostic indicators (stage IV or suboptimal debulking) [49]. Nevertheless, trials with other antiangiogenic drugs are ongoing. Their use has also been studied in HIPEC. The Lyon group, in a recent randomized phase II study [47] of patients with malignant ascites from GC with synchronous PC, obtained a clinical effect after IP infusion of catumaxomab—a nonhumanized chimeric antibody that blocks epithelial-cell adhesion molecule (EpCAM), T lymphocyte, CD3, accessory-cell, and Fcγ receptors. Indeed, in GC, this molecule is expressed in 90 % of cases, and IP infusion of catumaxomab could efficiently treat microscopic residual disease after CRS.

The aim of a US safety/efficacy study [50] is to determine the safety of a laparoscopic approach for HIPEC administration. Primary outcome is OS; secondary outcomes are safety and toxicity. The study arm receives mitomycin-C and cisplatin for 1 h on day 1 through three or four small abdominal incisions. After IP chemotherapy, the liquid is removed and a peritoneal washing and, eventually, biopsies are performed. Patients receive sodium thiosulfate IV to protect the kidneys.

Another ongoing US study [51] is evaluating technical parameters (CRS CC, achievement of hyperthermia, and morbidity and mortality rates) in patients with PC from CRC, GC, appendiceal, pseudomyxoma peritonei (PMP), and malignant peritoneal mesothelioma (MPM) origin undergoing CRS plus HIPEC with mitomycin-C (40 mg for 90 min).

The aim of a Spanish nonrandomized multicentric phase II study [52] is 1C level of evidence in terms of DFS and OS in patients with PC from GC. The strategy is to validate two new treatment schemas in three phases: In phase I, patients undergo IP infusion (through a peritoneal catheter implant) of docetaxel (30 mg/m^2) and cisplatin (30 mg/m^2) and IV administration of 5-FU (200

Table 25.1 Ongoing clinical trial on HIPEC in ovarian cancer. PLDH: pegylated liposomal doxorubicin hydrochloride

Study	Type of study	Phase	Time	Drug	Id number*	Country
Feasibility Study of HIPEC for Patients With Stage III or Only Pleural Stage IV Ovarian Carcinoma in First-Line Therapy	Safety/efficacy	II-III	Primary	Cisplatin	NCT01709487	Belgium
Phase 3 Trial Evaluating Hyperthermic Intra-peritoneal Chemotherapy in Upfront Treatment of Stage IIIC Epithelial Ovarian Cancer (CHORINE)	Randomized	III	Primary	Cisplatin + paclitaxel	NCT01628380	Italy
Quality of Life and Survivorship Care in Patients Undergoing Hyperthermic Intraperitoneal Chemotherapy (HIPEC) (HOPE)	Efficacy	n.p.	Primary recurrence		NCT01126346	USA
Surgery and Chemotherapy With or Without Chemotherapy After Surgery in Treating Patients With Ovarian,	Safety	n.p.	Primary recurrence	Cisplatin, carboplatin, PLDH, Paclitaxel, gentamicin	NCT01970722	USA

(cont.) →

Table 25.1 (*continued*)

Fallopian Tube, Uterine, or Peritoneal Cancer						
Intraoperative Hyperthermic Intraperitoneal Chemotherapy With Ovarian Cancer	Randomized	III	Primary recurrence	Cisplatin	NCT01091636	Korea
Safety and Pharmacokinetics of Intraoperative Hyperthermic Intraperitoneal Chemoperfusion (HIPEC) With Cisplatin to Treat Platinum-sensitive Recurrent Ovarian Cancer	Nonrandomized	I	Recurrence	Cisplatin	NCT01387399	Germany
Hyperthermic Intraperitoneal Chemotherapy (HIPEC) in Ovarian Cancer Recurrence (HORSE)	Randomized	III	Recurrence	Cisplatin	NCT01539785	Italy
Outcomes After Secondary Cytoreductive Surgery With or Without Carboplatin Hyperthermic Intraperitoneal	Randomized	II	Recurrence	Carboplatin	NCT01767675	USA

(*cont.*) →

Table 25.1 (*continued*)

Chemotherapy (HIPEC) Followed by Systemic Combination Chemotherapy for Recurrent Platinum-Sensitive Ovarian, Fallopian Tube, or Primary Peritoneal Cancer						
A Phase II Combined Modality Protocol of Debulking Surgery With HIPEC Followed by Intraperitoneal Chemotherapy for the Treatment of Recurrent Ovarian, Primary Peritoneal and Fallopian Tube Cancers	Safety/efficacy	II	Recurrence	Cisplatin	NCT01659554	USA
Secondary Debulking Surgery ± Hyperthermic Intraperitoneal Chemotherapy in Stage III Ovarian Cancer (OVHIPEC)	Randomized	III	Recurrence	Cisplatin	NCT00426257	Netherlands

(*cont.*) ↓

Table 25.1 (*continued*)

Hyperthermic Intra-Peritoneal Chemotherapy (HIPEC) in Relapse Ovarian Cancer Treatment (CHIPOR)	Randomized	III	Recurrence	Cisplatin	NCT01376752	France
Carboplatin, Paclitaxel and Gemcitabine With or Without Bevacizumab After Surgery in Treating Patients With Recurrent Ovarian Epithelial Cancer, Primary Peritoneal Cavity Cancer, or Fallopian Tube Cancer	Randomized	III	Recurrence	Carboplatin, paclitaxel, gemcitabine, bevacizumab	NCT00565851	USA

*From www.clinicaltrials.gov; n.p., not provided

mg/m^2/day, 7 days/week for 2 weeks) simultaneously with two cycles of IP administration. Phase II involves CRS plus HIPEC (mitomycin-C 15 mg/m^2 plus Adriamycin 15 mg/m^2 at 42–43°C for 60 min) and simultaneous IV administration of 5-FU (400 mg/m^2) plus leucovorin (20 mg/m^2) for 10 min at the beginning of peritoneal perfusion. In the phase III, adjuvant chemotherapy with docetaxel (75 mg/m^2), cisplatin (75mg/m^2), and 5-FU (750mg/m^2 day) is administered 8–12 weeks after surgery.

A German RCT study [53] compared patients with GC with IP free tumor cells (≥ T2, < T4, M0, N±) in two arms: in the experimental arm, HIPEC with mitomycin-C and cisplatin was administered after gastrectomy. In the control group, surgery only was performed. The primary outcome is PC-free survival at 5 years; the seconds is DFS at 5 years. A Chinese trial [54] is comparing different chemotherapy regimens with oxaliplatin and paclitaxel in HIPEC from GC to evaluate OS as primary outcome and safety and adverse events.

Table 25.2 summarizes new trials for treating GC.

25.9 New Trials in Colorectal Cancer

Ongoing is a US randomized phase II trial [55], the first study comparing EPIC vs. HIPEC for CRC and appendiceal cancer after CRS (< 2.5 mm). Drug regimens used during HIPEC and EPIC are mitomycin-C for the first one and floxuridine and leucovorin for the second one. Primary outcome is DFS at 3 years. A French multicenter phase III randomized trial [56] compares follow-up with explorative laparotomy plus HIPEC to simple follow-up in patients with CRC initially treated with surgery and adjuvant chemotherapy and are at high risk of developing PC. After the first tumor resection, patients undergo adjuvant treatment [6 months with 5-fluorouracil, leucovorin, and oxaliplatin (FOLFOX-4) regimen]. If the recurrence risk is low, the patient is not randomized; if it is high, the patient will be randomized to surveillance alone (control group) or exploratory laparotomy plus HIPEC (experimental group).

Regarding follow-up in patients with PC from mucinous CRC, a randomized phase II trial from Italy [57] aims to compare a second-look laparoscopy with standard follow-up in patients with no radiological evidence of disease 6 months after complete resection. The purpose is to evaluate whether a second-look laparoscopy improves OS in patients who undergo CRS, peritonectomy, and HIPEC or systemic chemotherapy.

Table 25.3 summarizes new trials in CRC.

25.10 Future

A further frontier is represented by using a minimally invasive approach to CRS with or without HIPEC for patients with isolated disease. Recent studies report

Table 25.2 Ongoing clinical trial on HIPEC in gastric cancer

Study	Type of study	Phase	Drug	ID number*	Country
D2 Resection and HIPEC (Hyperthermic Intraperitoneal Chemoperfusion) in Locally Advanced Gastric Carcinoma (GASTRICHIP)	Randomized	III	Oxaliplatin	NCT01882933	France
Laparoscopic Hyperthermic Intraperitoneal Chemoperfusion (HIPEC) for Metastatic Gastric Cancer	Safety/efficacy	II	Mitomycin-C, cisplatin	NCT02092298	USA
Single-Arm Study Treating Patients of Peritoneal Surface Malignancy (Colorectal, Appendical, Pseudomyxoma, Gastric) With Cytoreductive Surgery and Hyperthermic Intraperitoneal Mitomycin C	Safety/efficacy	II	Mitomycin-C	NCT02040142	USA
Clinical Trial at Neoadjuvant Peritoneal and Systemic Chemotherapy Plus HIPEC in Gastric Carcinomatosis	Safety/efficacy	II	Docetaxel, cisplatin, mitomycin-C, Adriamycin, leucovorin Mitomycin-C	NCT01342653	Spain
Randomized Controlled Trial to Prevent Peritoneal Seeding in Gastric Cancer (HIPEC Stomach)	Randomized	II-III	Mitomycin-C, cisplatin	NCT01683864	Germany
Sequential HIPEC of Oxaliplatin and Paclitaxel for Gastric Cancer Patients With Peritoneum Metastasis (SHOP-G01)	Safety	II	Oxaliplatin, paclitaxel	NCT01471132	China

*From www.clinicaltrials.gov

Table 25.3 Ongoing clinical trials on HIPEC in colorectal cancer

Study	Type of study	Phase	Drug	ID number*	Country
Trial Comparing Simple Follow-up to Exploratory Laparotomy Plus "in Principle" Hyperthermic Intraperitoneal Chemotherapy (HIPEC) in Colorectal Patients (Prophylo-CHIP)	Randomized	III	-	NCT01226394	France
Second-Look Laparoscopy in Colorectal Cancer (HIPEC)	Randomized	II	Folinic acid, 5-fluorouracil, oxaliplatin	NCT01628211	Italy
ICARuS Post-operative Intraperitoneal Chemotherapy (EPIC) and Hyperthermic Intraperitoneal Chemotherapy (HIPEC) After Optimal Cytoreductive Surgery (CRS) for Neoplasms of the Appendix, Colon or Rectum With Isolated Peritoneal Metastasis	Randomized	II	Mitomycin-C, floxuridine + leucovorin	NCT01815359	USA

*From www.clinicaltrials.gov

encouraging data about the feasibility of laparoscopic treatment in well-selected, platinum-sensitive patients with localized recurrence [58, 59]. In this context, a remarkable role was played by preoperative radiologic examination, and possibly IP laparoscopic evaluation, to better identify the appropriate subset of patients for this treatment regimen. Moreover, HIPEC can be safely administered in combination with minimally invasive surgical procedures, such as laparoscopic peritonectomy, both in animal models and patients with OC and platinum-sensitive recurrent disease [58, 60]. Furthermore, it is plausible that a larger number of patients with recurrent disease will benefit in the future from minimally invasive techniques, greater accuracy in assessing disease extension, wider diffusion of robotic/laparoscopic approaches, and increased surgeon expertise.

References

1. Van der Speeten K, Stuart OA, Sugarbaker PH (2009) Using pharmacologic data to plan clinical treatments for patients with peritoneal surface malignancy. Curr Drug Discover Technol 6:72-81
2. Jacquet P, Sugarbaker PH (1996) Peritoneal-plasma barrier. Cancer Treat Res 82:53–63
3. Montori G, Coccolini F, Ceresoli M et al (2014) The treatment of peritoneal carcinomatosis in advanced gastric cancer: state of the art. Int J Surg Oncol 2014:912418
4. Chua TC, Liauw W, Saxena A et al (2011)Evolution of locoregional treatment for peritoneal carcinomatosis: single-center experience of 308 procedures of cytoreductive surgery and perioperative intraperitoneal chemotherapy. Am J Surg 201:149-156
5. Spratt JS, Adcock RA, Muskovin M et al (1980) Clinical delivery system for intraperitoneal hyperthermic chemotherapy. Cancer Res 40:256–260
6. Dedrick RL (1986) Interspecies scaling of regional drug delivery. J Pharmacol Sci 75:1047–1052
7. Sugarbaker PH (1995) Peritonectomy procedures. Ann Surg 221:29–42
8. Sommariva A, Pilati P, Rossi CR (2012) Cyto-reductive Surgery combined with Hyperthermic Intra-Peritoneal Chemotherapy for Peritoneal Surface Malignancies: Current treatment and results. Cancer Treat Rev 38:258–268
9. Markman M, Bundy BN, Alberts DS et al (2001) Phase III trial of standard-dose intravenous cisplatin plus paclitaxel versus moderately high-dose carboplatin followed by intravenous paclitaxel and intraperitoneal cisplatin in small-volume stage III ovarian carcinoma: an intergroup study of the Gynecologic Oncology Group, Southwestern Oncology Group, and Eastern Cooperative Oncology Group. J Clin Oncol 19:1001–1007
10. Rietbroek RC, van de Vaart PJ, Haveman J et al (1997) Hyperthermia enhances the cytotoxicity and platinum-DNA adduct formation of lobaplatin and oxaliplatin in cultured SW 1573 cells. J Cancer Res Clin Oncol 123:6-12
11. Glehen O, Passot G, Villeneuve L et al (2012) GASTRICHIP: D2 resection and hyperthermic intraperitoneal chemotherapy in locally advanced gastric carcinoma: a randomized and multicenter phase III study. BMC Cancer 14:183
12. Jemal A, Siegel R, Xu J, Ward E (2010) Cancer statistics, 2010. CA Cancer J Clin 60:277–300
13. http://www.aiom.it/area+pubblica/area+medica/prodotti+scientifici/linee+guida/1%2C333%2C1%2C
14. Coccolini F, Gheza F, Lotti M et al (2013) Peritoneal Carcinomatosis. World JGastroenterol 19:6979-6994
15. Heintz APM, Odicino F, Maisonneuve P et al (2006) Carcinoma of the ovary. Int J Gynecol Obstet 95:S161–192

16. Leitao MM Jr, Chi DS (2009) Surgical Management of Recurrent Ovarian Cancer. Semin Oncol 36:106-111
17. Bristow RE, Puri I, Chi DS (2009) Cytoreductive surgery for recurrent ovarian cancer: a meta-analysis. Gynecol Oncol 112:265–274
18. Al Rawahi T, Lopes AD, Bristow RE et al Surgical cytoreduction for recurrent epithelial ovarian cancer. Cochrane Database Syst Rev 2:CD008765. doi: 10.1002/14651858
19. Waddell T, Verheij M, Allum W et al (2013) Gastric cancer : ESMO-ESSO-ESTRO clinical practice guidelines for diagnosis, treatment and follow-up. Ann of Oncol 24:vi57-vi63
20. Armstrong DK, Bundy B, Wenzel L et al (2006) Intraperitoneal cisplatin and paclitaxel in ovarian cancer. N Engl J Med 354:34-43
21. Alberts DS, Liu PY, Hannigan EV et al (1996) Intraperitoneal cisplatinplus intravenous cyclophosphamide versus intravenous cisplatin plus intravenous cyclophosphamide for stage III ovarian cancer. N Engl J Med 335:1950–1955
22. Yonemura Y, Bando E, Kawamura T et al (2007) Cytoreduction and intraperitoneal chemotherapy for carcinomatosis from gastric cancer. Cancer Treat Res 134:357-373
23. Coccolini F, Cotte E, Glehen O et al (2014) Intraperitoneal chemotherapy in advanced gastric cancer: Meta-analysis if randomized trials. Eur J Surg Oncol 40:12-26
24. Yonemura Y, De Aretxabala X, Fujimura T et al (2001) Intraoperative chemohyperthermic peritoneal perfusion as an adjuvant to gastric cancer : final results of a randomized controlled study. Hepatogastroenterology 48:1776-1782
25. Verwaal VJ, van Ruth S, de Bree E et al (2003) Randomized trial of cytoreducion and hyperthermic intraperitoneal chemotherapy versus systemic chemotherapy and palliative surgery in patients with peritoneal carcinomatosis of colorectal cancer. J Clin Oncol 21:3737-3743
26. Elias D, Gilly F, Boutitie F et al (2010) Peritoneal colorectal carcinomatosi treated with surgery and perioperative intraperitoneal chemotherapy: retrospective analysis of 523 patients in a multicentric French study. J Clin Oncol 28:63-68
27. Deraco M, Kusamura S, Virzì S et al (2011) Cytoreductive surgery and hyperthermic intraperitoneal chemotherapy as upfront therapy for advanced epithelial ovarian cancer: multiinstitutional phase-II trial. Gynecol Oncol 122:215–220
28. Sugarbaker PH (1996) Peritoneal Carcinomatosis: Principles of Management. Kluwer Academic, Boston, USA
29. Piso P, Dahlke MH, Loss M, Schlitt HJ (2004) Cytoreductive surgery and hyperthermic intraperitoneal chemotherapy in peritoneal carcinomatosis from ovarian cancer. World J Surg Oncol 2-21
30. http://www.clinicaltrials.gov/ct2/show/ NCT01091636
31. http://www.clinicaltrials.gov/ct2/show/NCT01709487
32. http://www.clinicaltrials.gov/ct2/show/NCT01628380
33. Di Giorgio A, Naticchioni E, Biacchi D et al (2008) Cytoreductive surgery (peritonectomy procedures) combined with hypertermic intraperitoneal chemotherapy (HIPEC) in the treatment of diffuse peritoneal carcinomatosis from ovarian cancer. Cancer 113:315–325
34. Passot G, Bakrin N, Roux AS et al (2014) Quality of life after cytoreductive surgery plus hyperthermic intraperitoneal chemotherapy: A prospective study of 216 patients. EJSO 40:529-535
35. http://www.clinicaltrials.gov/ct2/show/NCT01126346
36. Fagotti A, Paris I, Grimolizzi F et al (2009) Secondary cytoreduction plus oxaliplatin-based HIPEC in platinum-sensitive recurrent ovarian cancer patients: a pilot study. Gynecol Oncol 113:335-340
37. Fagotti A, Costantini B, Vizzielli G et al (2011) HIPEC in recurrent ovarian cancer patients: Morbidity-related treatment and long-term analysis of clinical outcome. Gynecol Oncol 122:221–225
38. Fagotti A, Costantini B, Petrillo M et al (2012) Cytoreductive surgery plus HIPEC in platinum-sensitive recurrent ovarian cancer patients: a case–control study on survival in patients with two year follow-up. Gynecol Oncol 127:502–505
39. http://www.clinicaltrials.gov/ct2/show/NCT01539785

40. http://www.clinicaltrials.gov/ct2/show/NCT01387399
41. http://www.clinicaltrials.gov/ct2/show/NCT01376752
42. http://www.clinicaltrials.gov/ct2/show/NCT00426257
43. http://www.clinicaltrials.gov/ct2/show/NCT01767675
44. http://www.clinicaltrials.gov/ct2/show/NCT01659554
45. http://www.clinicaltrials.gov/ct2/show/NCT01970722
46. http://www.clinicaltrials.gov/ct2/show/NCT00565851
47. Goere D, Gras-Chaput N, Auperin A et al (2014) Treatment of gastric peritoneal carcinomatosis by combining complete surgical resection of lesions and intraperitoneal immunotherapy using catumaxomab. BMC Cancer 14:148
48. Saada E, Follana P, Peyarde F et al (2011) Pathogenesis and management of refractory malignant ascites. Bull Cancer 98:697-687
49. Ledermann JA, Raja FA, Fotopoulou C et al (2013) Newly diagnosed and relapsed epithelial ovarian carcinoma: ESMO Clinical Practice Gluidelines for diagnosis, treatment and followup. Ann Oncol 24:vi24-vi32
50. http://www.clinicaltrials.gov/ct2/show/NCT02092298
51. http://www.clinicaltrials.gov/ct2/show/NCT02040142
52. http://www.clinicaltrials.gov/ct2/show/NCT01342653
53. http://www.clinicaltrials.gov/ct2/show/NCT01683864
54. http://www.clinicaltrials.gov/ct2/show/NCT01471132
55. http://www.clinicaltrials.gov/ct2/show/NCT01815359
56. http://www.clinicaltrials.gov/ct2/show/NCT01226394
57. http://www.clinicaltrials.gov/ct2/show/NCT01628211
58. Fagotti A, Petrillo M, Costantini B et al (2014) Minimally invasive secondary cytoreduction plus HIPEC for recurrent ovarian cancer: A case series. Gynecol Oncol 132:303-306
59. Gallotta V, Fagotti A, Fanfani F et al (2014) Laparoscopic surgical management of localized recurrent ovarian cancer: a single-institution experience. Surg Endosc 28:1808-1815
60. Ferron G, Gesson-Paute A, Classe JM, Querleu D (2005) Feasibility of laparoscopic peritonectomy followed by intra-peritoneal chemohyperthermia: an experimental study. Gynecol Oncol 99:358–361

MIX
Papier aus verantwortungsvollen Quellen
Paper from responsible sources
FSC® C105338

If you have any concerns about our products,
you can contact us on
ProductSafety@springernature.com

In case Publisher is established outside the EU,
the EU authorized representative is:
Springer Nature Customer Service Center GmbH
Europaplatz 3, 69115 Heidelberg, Germany

Printed by Libri Plureos GmbH
in Hamburg, Germany